Hand Injuries In Athletes

Hand Injuries In Athletes

James W. Strickland, M.D.

Clinical Professor, Department of Orthopedics
Indiana University School of Medicine
Indianapolis, Indiana

Arthur C. Rettig, M.D.

Clinical Assistant Professor, Department of Orthopedics
Indiana University School of Medicine
Indianapolis, Indiana

W.B. SAUNDERS COMPANY

Harcourt Brace Jovanovich, Inc.

Philadelphia London Toronto
Montreal Sydney Tokyo

W. B. SAUNDERS COMPANY
Harcourt Brace Jovanovich, Inc.

The Curtis Center
Independence Square West
Philadelphia, PA 19106

Library of Congress Cataloging-in-Publication Data

Hand injuries in athletes / [edited by] James W. Strickland, Arthur C. Rettig.
p. cm.
ISBN 0-7216-2779-X
1. Hand—Wounds and injuries. 2. Sports—Accidents and injuries. I. Strickland, James W. II. Rettig, Arthur C. [DNLM: 1. Athletic Injuries. 2. Hand Injuries. WE 830 H23093]
RD559.H3593 1992 617.5′75044—dc20
DNLM/DLC 90-9124

Developmental Editor: Lawrence J. McGrew
Designer: Bill Donnelly
Production Manager: Bill Preston
Manuscript Editor: Ellen Murray
Illustration Coordinator: Cecilia Roberts
Indexer: Dena Sher
Cover Designer: Dorothy Chattin

Hand Injuries in Athletes ISBN 0-7216-2779-X

Printed in the United States of America

Last digit is the print number: 9 8 7 6 5 4 3 2 1

CONTRIBUTORS

Thomas R. Dennis, M.D. Fellow, Hand Surgery, Joseph H. Boyes Fellow, Los Angeles, California

Jorge M. Gabrera, M.D. Clinical Assistant Professor, University of Miami, Miami, Florida; Team Physician, Florida International University and Miami Dade College, Miami, Florida; Team Physician, ASL Miami Freedom; Consultant, U.S. Olympic Soccer Federation, Miami, Florida

Jeffrey P. Groner, M.D. Assistant Professor of Surgery (Plastic and Reconstructive), Washington University School of Medicine, St. Louis, Missouri; Plastic Surgeon, Barnes Hospital, St. Louis Children's Hospital, Jewish Hospital, and St. Louis Regional Medical Center, St. Louis, Missouri

Hill Hastings, II, M.D. Chief of Hand Surgery, Department of Orthopedic Surgery, Wishard General Hospital, Indianapolis, Indiana; Clinical Assistant Professor, Department of Orthopedics, Indiana University Medical Center, Indianapolis, Indiana; Assistant Clinical Professor, Department of Surgery, College of Medicine, University of Kentucky, Lexington, Kentucky; Attending Staff, St. Vincent Hospital and Health Care Center, Indiana University Medical Center, and Wishard Memorial Hospital, Indianapolis, Indiana

Jan M. Koepfer, O.T.R. The Hand Rehabilitation Center of Indiana, Indianapolis, Indiana

Joseph P. Leddy, M.D. Clinical Professor of Surgery—Orthopedic, Robert Wood Johnson Medical School, University of Medicine and Dentistry of New Jersey, New Brunswick, New Jersey; Senior Attending Staff and Chief Hand Surgery Service, Robert Wood Johnson University Hospital, New Brunswick, New Jersey; Senior Attending Staff, Chief of Orthopedic and Hand Surgery, St. Peter's Medical Center; Courtesy Staff, Princeton Medical Center and Consultant, McCosh Infirmary, Princeton University, Princeton, New Jersey; Consultant, Rutgers University Athletic Teams and Hurtado Health Center, New Brunswick, New Jersey

Frank C. McCue, III, M.D. Alfred R. Shands Professor of Orthopaedic Surgery and Plastic Surgery of the Hand; Director, Division of Sports Medicine and Hand Surgery; and Team Physician, University of Virginia, Department of Athletics, Charlottesville, Virginia; Courtesy Staff, University of Virginia Page Memorial Hospital, Luray, Virginia; Courtesy/Surgical Staff, Community Memorial Hospital, South Hill, Virginia; Courtesy/Surgical Staff, Johnston Memorial Hospital, Abingdon, Virginia; Courtesy/Surgical Staff, Byerley Hospital, Hartsville, South Carolina

Robert J. Neviaser, M.D. Professor and Chairman, Department of Orthopaedic Surgery, George Washington University School of Medicine, Washington, D.C.; Director, Hand and Upper Extremity Service, George Washington University Medical Center, Washington, D.C.

Arthur C. Rettig, M.D. Clinical Assistant Professor, Department of Orthopedics, Indiana School of Medicine, Indianapolis, Indiana; Attending Staff, Methodist Hospital, St. Vincent Hospital, Indianapolis, Indiana

George A. Richardson, M.D. Attending Staff, Humana Brazos County Hospital, Bryan, Texas

Ramon O. Ryan, M.S., M.D. Attending Staff, St. Vincent's Hospital and Health Care Centers, Indianapolis, Indiana

Jill A. Sadler, O.T.R. Guest Lecturer, University of Indianapolis Occupational Therapy Program, Indianapolis, Indiana; Clinical Supervisor, The Hand Rehabilitation Center of Indiana, Indianapolis, Indiana

Jennifer A. Stone, M.S., A.T.C. Head Athletic Trainer, Olympic Training Center, Colorado Springs, Colorado

James W. Strickland, M.D. Clinical Professor, Department of Orthopedics, Indiana University School of Medicine, Indianapolis, Indiana; Hand Surgery Associates of Indiana, Inc., Indianapolis, Indiana

Julio Taleisnik, M.D. Clinical Professor, Orthopaedic Surgery, University of California, Irvine, California

Paul M. Weeks, M.D. Professor of Surgery (Plastic and Reconstructive), Washington University School of Medicine, St. Louis, Missouri; Plastic Surgeon in Chief, Barnes Hospital, St. Louis Children's Hospital, Jewish Hospital, and St. Louis Regional Medical Center, St. Louis, Missouri

James H. Whitaker, M.D. Assistant Clinical Professor, Department of Surgery, Kansas Medical School and University of Missouri Medical School, Kansas City, Missouri; Chairman of Orthopedic Surgery, Research Medical Center, Kansas City, Missouri

E. F. Shaw Wilgis, M.D. Associate Professor of Orthopedics and Plastic Surgery, Johns Hopkins University, Baltimore, Maryland; Chief, Division of Hand Surgery, Union Memorial Hospital, Baltimore, Maryland

Norman P. Zemel, M.D. Associate Clinical Professor, Department of Orthopaedic Surgery, University of Southern California School of Medicine, Los Angeles, California; Active Staff, Centinela Medical Center, Los Angeles, California; Associate, Kerlan-Jobe Orthopaedic Clinic, Los Angeles, California

PREFACE

Injuries to the wrist and hand are an all-too-frequent consequence of athletic participation. Competitive and recreational athletes sustain a wide variety of soft tissue, bone, ligament, tendon, vessel, and nerve damage to their upper extremities. With the maturation of sports medicine as a distinct discipline, it is important that team physicians and orthopedic surgeons be well versed in the diagnosis and treatment of these disorders.

In this volume, we have asked a number of surgeons who are recognized for their astuteness in the management of various types of hand disorders to provide a succinct and up-to-date account of the best methods of diagnosis and treatment. Emphasis has been given to those methods that assure the athlete the best possible result with as rapid a return to competition as is reasonably possible.

The book begins with a dissertation on philosophical and practical approaches to the management of hand injuries in sports participants and proceeds to a discussion of the healing processes in the soft tissues and bones of the hand. An overview of the epidemiology of athletic hand injuries and their pathomechanics is provided, followed by sections discussing common digital joint injuries and disruption of the collateral ligaments of the thumb. The current thinking regarding the management of ligamentous injuries, cartilage tears, and instability of the wrist is then presented, followed by chapters dealing with the management of metacarpal and phalangeal fractures, carpal fractures, and tendon injuries in athletes. The volume concludes with discussions of compression neuropathies and vascular injuries and an in-depth analysis of splinting and rehabilitation of the injured hand.

We believe that this book provides those involved in the diagnosis and treatment of athletic hand injuries with practical and current information to meet the challenge of providing the best possible care of the injured part while returning the participant to his or her athletic endeavor in an expeditious manner.

James W. Strickland, M.D.
Arthur C. Rettig, M.D.

CONTENTS

CHAPTER 1
A Philosophy for the Management of Athletic Injuries of the Hand and Wrist **1**
James W. Strickland, M.D.

CHAPTER 2
Healing of Hard and Soft Tissues in the Hand **7**
Jeffrey P. Groner, M.D.
Paul M. Weeks, M.D.

CHAPTER 3
Epidemiology of Hand Injuries in Sports **37**
Arthur C. Rettig, M.D.
Ramon O. Ryan, M.S., M.D.
Jennifer A. Stone, A.T.C.

CHAPTER 4
Common Athletic Digital Joint Injuries of the Hand **49**
Frank C. McCue, III, M.D.
Jorge M. Cabrera, M.D.

CHAPTER 5
Collateral Ligament Injuries of the Thumb Metacarpophalangeal Joint **95**
Robert J. Neviaser, M.D.

CHAPTER 6
Soft Tissue Injuries of the Wrist **107**
Julio Taleisnik, M.D.

CHAPTER 7
Management of Extra-articular Fractures of the Phalanges and Metacarpals **129**
Hill Hastings, II, M.D.

CHAPTER 8
Carpal Fractures **155**
Norman P. Zemel, M.D.

CHAPTER 9
Tendon Injuries **175**
Joseph P. Leddy, M.D.
Thomas R. Dennis, M.D.

CHAPTER 10
Compressive Neuropathies **209**
James H. Whitaker, M.D.
George A. Richardson, M.D.

CHAPTER 11
Vascular Injuries to the Athletic Hand **229**
E. F. Shaw Wilgis, M.D.

CHAPTER 12
Rehabilitation and Splinting of the Injured Hand **235**
Jill A. Sadler, O.T.R.
Jan M. Koepfer, O.T.R.

Index **277**

Hand Injuries In Athletes

CHAPTER

1

A Philosophy for the Management of Athletic Injuries of the Hand and Wrist

James W. Strickland, M.D.

There is a great tendency to downplay the importance of upper extremity injuries to athletic competitors. Because the obvious disability resulting from contusions, strains, sprains, ligament or cartilage tears, or fractures of the legs is absent, great pressure is frequently placed on the athlete to continue to play after similar insults to the wrist or hand. It is a curious phenomenon that coaches, spectators, and even some trainers and physicians regard an injured toe as a greater impediment to sports participation than an injured finger. This attitude, unfortunately, may lead to a compromise in the quality of medical care for many athletes, who are allowed to return to competition without adequate diagnosis or treatment of their upper extremity condition and often to worsening of their injury and long-term complications.

Given the increasing number of physicians who supplement their residency training with fellowships in hand and upper extremity surgery, it is surprising how often athletes with wrist and hand problems are managed by orthopedic surgeons or team physicians with little or no training in this area. It is by no means axiomatic that a superb sports medicine physician, highly skilled in the diagnosis and treatment of knee injuries, can provide the same expert care for an injured wrist, with its tremendous number of subtle instability patterns requiring complex diagnostic studies. In fact, a cavalier attitude toward hand injuries often prevails, and the affected athlete is allowed to return to competition with little or no protection of the injured part. The result of this attitude may be chronic pain or instability that will be much more difficult to effectively manage.

Good sports medicine begins with recognition of the full magnitude of the specific injury. Fractures are obvious and their impact on athletic participation is reasonably well appreciated. If displaced, they must be reduced, and when reduced, they must be carefully immobilized and protected. Time to healing is well documented and most physicians discourage athletic participation that may in any way jeopardize the healing sequence. Still, there is a disturbing tendency to find ways to return the athlete to competition, often in violation of the time-honored tenets of fracture management. There is no question that the development of fixation devices that provide strong stability to fractures of the carpal bones, metacarpals, or phalanges has given rise to the temptation to return the athlete to competition often well in advance of bone healing. Before embarking on this type of aggressive management, the team physician has the obligation to pose a number of pertinent questions and to answer those questions with absolute honesty, unbiased by zeal to get the player back to the game or by the pressures to do so from the athlete, other players. coaches, fans, faculty, and alumni. Those questions include

1. If this fracture had occurred in a nonathlete or in the off-season, would I manage it in the same manner?
2. Is the method of treatment that I have selected the most appropriate for this injury and can it be expected to provide the best long-term result?
3. Are the potential complications of the treatment method significantly greater than might be expected from a more conservative approach?
4. Will the treatment allow the athlete to return to competition with little or no risk of re-injury or the possibility of decreased long-term function?

If the physician concludes from this self-interrogation that the method of treatment selected is the best for a particular fracture, that it carries a low risk of complications, and that it should allow the best long-term performance for the affected wrist or hand, he is justified in proceeding.

After carrying out fracture fixation, the decision as to when to return the athlete to competition is often a difficult one. The physician must be quite confident that there is little or no likelihood that the fracture and its fixation device can be in any way disrupted by the vigorous stresses that will occur during a hard-fought game. The designers of fracture fixation devices have not intended or recommended that these materials be subjected to the tremendous forces that are incurred in many individual and team sports. While they have created screws, plates, and wiring techniques that can be shown to impart considerably greater resistance to deformity than no fixation or the simple use of one or more Kirschner wires, the main advantage of these devices has been to provide accurate reduction and stability sufficient to allow early joint motion in an effort to minimize the stiffness that so often results from wrist and hand fractures. To apply these methods with the expectation that the extremity can perform as though there was no fracture at all is wishful thinking, totally unsupported by any scientific investigation. Even the provision of additional external support to the part following open reduction and internal fixation is of little value when one or more strong insults occur during competition.

The treating physician must have an understanding of the stresses to which the wrist and hand of the patient-athlete will be subjected during the course of a game. The specific performance demands at the particular level of competition, the forces that will be generated by the competitive activities of a certain position, and the peculiarities of the individual player's method of participation are important considerations, as are the number and magnitude of the insults to the part that might be expected in a given game or practice. A "worst case" scenario must be developed, taking into account the consequences of a violent fall or strong physical contact with another player, the field, the floor, or athletic equipment. The questions must be: What is the worst thing that could happen and how will it affect the injury and its treatment? What are the long-term sequelae of such an event? Could the athlete actually lose more playing time because of re-injury than if competition were avoided for a period of time commensurate with safe healing of the fracture? Will malunion or nonunion be more likely and could any long-term or permanent disability result from the decision to allow participation? Only after considerable soul-searching and honest dialogue with the athlete and family (not with coaches, fans, or even highly involved fellow physicians) can a logical decision be made regarding the return to competition following osseous injury of the wrist or hand.

Two years ago, I placed a Herbert screw in an acute scaphoid fracture in a 6′6″, 230 lb, power forward on a Division I college basketball team. He was midway through a tremendous season and had already used his "red shirt" year. The team relied heavily on his performance and the coach was a very good friend of mine. I had found that the Herbert screw provided extremely strong fixation for displaced midscaphoid fractures and considered it to be an appropriate (actually conservative) treatment for this notoriously poorly healing bone. It therefore seemed reasonable to internally fix the fracture and return the player to action after several weeks rather than resorting to prolonged casting with the obligatory loss of competition for the remainder of the season and, potentially, all or part of the next season should the bone go on to nonunion. Secure fixation was achieved, the wound healed uneventfully, and at 3 weeks, the boy returned to basketball. With minimal discomfort, he scored 30 points in the second game following his return, averaged 24.5 points for the remainder of the season, and was a First Team, All Conference selection. When he returned for a postseason checkup, I was dismayed to find that not only had the fracture not healed, it had collapsed into a "hump back" deformity with obvious absorption around the threads at both ends of the screw. Fortunately, iliac wedge grafting with the insertion of a new Herbert screw and 3 months of immobilization resulted in complete union without deformity. In the following season, this player averaged 26 points and was runner-up for Player of the Year in his league. While the boy and his family have no regrets and would pursue the same course of treatment again, I must question my decision to internally fix this particular fracture and allow the rapid return to competition when I knew that there would be tremendous stress on the wrist during the course of each practice and game when he would frequently dive on the floor after loose balls and bang his hand against the backboard or other players. In retrospect, the likelihood that scaphoid union would occur even with the strong fixation provided by the screw was not great. While my colleagues and I have had success with this technique in acute scaphoid fractures in other athletes (even basketball players), it would appear that they played a less violent game than the boy in question. This experience would temper my decision to allow other athletes to resume competition following this method of treatment. Again, consideration of the particular stresses placed on the wrist and hand during the course of practices and games is extremely important.

Similarly, educated judgments must be tempered regarding the return to competition following soft tissue injuries of the wrist and hand. The treating physician must be absolutely sure that the risk of significant re-injury is not great and that, were it to occur, it would not compromise the final healing and long-term performance of the injured part. Dislocations of the digital joints, in particular, stand out as athletic injuries for which there is often too little appreciation of the magnitude of the damage to the periarticular support structures. It should be recognized that any dislocation causes disruption of restraining tissues opposite the deviated or displaced bone. For example, a dorsal dislocation of the proximal interphalangeal joint must have a concomitant rupture of the palmar plate, while lateral dislocations always tear the collateral ligaments on the opposite side of the joint. Failure to protect these structures fully until complete healing has occurred can result in chronic instability of the joint with considerable functional disability and significant technical difficulty attendant to secondary reconstructive procedures. While small splints or buddy taping may suffice following the anatomic reduction of proximal interphalangeal dislocations, it is again important to carefully consider the impending stresses of competition and worst case possibilities before permitting athletic participation.

The terms "sprains" and "strains" are employed with considerably less frequency now than in days gone by. A plethora of literature has evolved regarding ligamentous injury in the upper extremity, and the wrist in particular has been the subject of intense investigation. We are now confronted with a tremendous array of intracarpal instability patterns that weaken hand function and produce considerable pain. Rotatory subluxation of the scaphoid, scapholunate instability, lunotriquetral instability, midcarpal instability, and similar conditions can result from athletic injuries and are often so subtle in their presentation that they go unrecognized, particularly by the physician not accustomed to diagnosing wrist pathology. Injuries to the triangular fibrocartilage complex, occult ganglion cysts, and overuse or repetitive trauma syndromes are also acknowledged sequelae of athletic competition. The diagnosis of many of these conditions requires the use of provocative physical examination maneuvers or special radiographic techniques (cineradiography, bone scintigraphy, arthrography, tomography, computed tomography, and magnetic resonance imaging) to establish the diagnosis. Prompt recognition and treatment of these conditions may be necessary to prevent chronicity and the need for late reconstructive surgery, which almost always involves some permanent loss of function. The physician managing these injuries must understand the anatomy and kinesiology of the wrist and the many potential conditions that can arise from athletic injury. A high degree of awareness is necessary to ensure that these conditions are not dismissed as contusions, sprains, or tendinitis with the inevitable compromise of immediate and long-term performance.

The athlete's age and level of performance are factors that must be considered in any decision concerning a return to competitive participation following athletic injuries to the upper extremity. The delicate status of the musculoskeletal system of the preadolescent makes the athlete quite vulnerable to injury, and there is absolutely no reason to cut any corners in the management of these conditions. Epiphyseal fractures, in particular, should be appropriately reduced, casted, and allowed to heal, and ligament and tendon injuries in these skeletally immature individuals should be treated with great respect, with no effort made to prematurely return the child to sports activities. Unfortunately, the pressures of parents and coaches are often considerable following injury to young athletes, and it is the obligation of the treating physician to temper these inappropriate passions by a rational and conservative course of treatment designed to ensure the best long-term performance. Obviously, older athletes may have somewhat different competitive obligations and desires, and in most instances, they can be provided with a rational explanation of the nature of their injury and the consequences of returning to competition and, at least to some extent, may participate in the decision as to whether or not to do so. The professional athlete may often choose to "play hurt" even with some risk of re-injury or worsening of the condition. Again, considerable input by the physician as to the potential long-term consequences of such a decision must be provided and, in some cases, documented in writing before the athlete can be allowed to return to the fray.

I am reminded of a particular day in my office when I saw two football players with identical acute ruptures of the flexor digitorum profundus tendon from the distal phalangeal insertion of the dominant ring finger. The first, a high school senior, was without any consideration to the contrary taken to surgery for tendon repair. Although he missed the remainder of the season, he recovered excellent digital function that would serve him for the rest of his life. The second, a professional lineman, aware that he might never recover distal interphalangeal joint flexion, elected to forego surgery and to immediately resume his competitive activity to avoid risking the loss of his job. These radically different approaches to the same injury exemplify the need to consider each injury individually, not only from the point of view of the most efficacious medical management, but also with regard to the unique circumstances of the particular athlete.

In some instances the informed willingness of the athlete to take a reasonable risk of jeopardizing treatment and the future function of the part may have to be honored, although the "worst possibility" must be thoroughly reviewed. One cannot overemphasize the obligation on the part of the physician to offer information and advice that will allow the athlete and his coaches to fully appreciate the potential consequences of returning to competition after a given injury. In the last analysis, the decision to return to athletic competition following wrist or hand injury will depend on the nature of the injury and the unique requirements of the injured competitor. Our obligation is to fully inform the athlete of the nature of the injury, the proposed treatment, the anticipated time to heal, the methods that can be employed to protect the part during practice or game situations, the likelihood of re-injury, and the effect on healing, treatment, and the long-term function that re-injury might have. It is the athlete who must decide what best suits not only the immediate situation but also long-term needs and goals.

The use of local anesthetic agents to alleviate the discomfort emanating from an injured part is a subject of considerable debate. Again, one must weigh the potential damage that could occur during an athletic event if the athlete fails to recognize pain at the affected area. It would seem that little harm could arise from a single injection into an area of bruising, strain, or inflammation if there is little or no likelihood that additional damage could occur during the practice or game. In particular, trigger areas of capsular inflammation or tendinitis without any alteration of structural integrity are candidates for local anesthetic instillation prior to competition, provided the procedure does not compromise proper management, the injections are not carried out on a repetitive basis, and the patient is fully aware of what is being done. On the other hand, to arrest pain in an area of recent fracture or dislocation or around partial or complete ligamentous disruptions where reinjury would increase the severity of the condition is an absolutely unacceptable part of the precompetition regimen. In these instances, the benefits of playing without pain are strongly outweighed by the protective benefits of discomfort at the site of injury. In truth, the indications for the pregame use of a local anesthetic in the upper extremity are extremely limited.

As physicians dealing with athletic injuries to the wrist and digits, we have consummate responsibility to fully appreciate the magnitude and severity of the condition and we must make treatment decisions that are consistent with the time-honored principles of managing musculoskeletal pathology. Decisions cannot be tempered by the considerable pressures that will be generated by all concerned to get the athlete back into competition as soon as possible. Unfortunately, one of those mitigating pressures often emanates from the physician himself as he strives to contrive a treatment alternative that will publicly demonstrate his abilities to rapidly deal with sports injuries and to contribute to the success of a team with which he may have close personal loyalties. It is better for the physician to detach himself from such pressures and consider only the best treatment for the particular injury of the individual athlete. Treatment in all cases must be that which will provide the most predictable healing of the injured tissues with the fewest complications and the best long-term functional prognosis. While athletic participation is sometimes not inconsistent with those treatment principles, the risks must be recognized and fully appreciated by all concerned.

CHAPTER

2

Healing of Hard and Soft Tissues in the Hand

Jeffrey P. Groner, M.D.
Paul M. Weeks, M.D.

Tissue repair and regeneration determine the initial management and subsequent follow-up care of hand injuries. A solid understanding of the principles and events of tissue healing is the foundation of optimal care. This chapter summarizes the biologic phenomena of repair and regeneration to provide a better appreciation of why the particular techniques of management described in subsequent chapters are utilized.

Soft Tissue Injury

Skin and soft tissues are subject to contusion, abrasion, laceration, and avulsion either alone or in association with other tissue injuries. Because it is representative of healing processes in other soft tissues, the stages of healing of a skin laceration will be described in detail.

Injury elicits a programmed succession of cellular activities beginning with vessel disruption and clot formation. The clot develops an internal fibrin and fibronectin lattice, and within 12 hours an inflammatory cell reaction occurs. Macrophages remove debris and initiate cellular events including fibroblast recruitment, wound vascularization, and collagen production and degradation. Within 48 hours, fibroblasts have developed from undifferentiated mesenchymal cells and migrate along the fibrin/fibronectin network of the clot.[6] Capillary buds appear and follow the advancing front of fibroblasts. Between the second and fourth days, fibroblasts begin synthesis of collagen precursors. Type III collagen first appears in the wound between the fourth and sixth days, and by the seventh day a fine collagen framework is established. Fibroplasia and collagen production increase rapidly and reach a plateau lasting for 2 to 4 weeks. Thereafter, the fibroblast population and collagen synthesis gradually decrease, although net accumulation of collagen may continue for several months. After the fourth week, tissue remodeling is the major activity in the wound. Collagen synthesis and degradation continue: type III collagen is gradually replaced by type I collagen, and progressive orientation and stabilization by crosslinking occurs. This may continue for up to 2 years following the original injury.[7]

The events of the first 4 to 6 days, including inflammation, clot organization, fibroblast recruitment, and cellular enzyme induction constitute the *lag* or substrate phase. Fibroplasia and collagen production appear at the fifth or sixth day, then plateau before activity gradually decreases 3 to 4 weeks postwounding. The phase of remodeling follows and may continue for 2 years after injury.

Wound tensile strength gain bears a direct relationship to the ongoing cellular events and processes. Wound strength is very limited during the lag phase. Initially, tensile strength (strength per unit of scar tissue) is derived from the fibrin in the clot and, by the second or third day, by the spanning of the wound by epithelial cells and capillaries. With fibroplasia and collagen synthesis there is a significant gain in tensile strength that rises rapidly owing to the accretion of collagen. By the midpoint of the lag phase the wound has gained sufficient strength to resist mild shear. In a rat skin wound, 15 percent of preinjury burst strength (strength of the entire wound) is regained by 3 weeks and over 70 percent by 9 weeks.[4] After suture repair of skin lacerations in rats, wound strength diminishes initially, reaching a low point at 5 days, before it begins to increase. This may be due to the initial peak of inflammatory changes, which weaken the tissues about the sutures. Wound tensile strength develops at a slow but sustained rate throughout the period of wound remodeling but never equals the strength of nonwounded skin. The accumulation of breaking strength follows a sigmoidal curve. Various factors such as sex, nutritional status, and patient age can affect the healing process.[2]

Epithelial regeneration occurs by multiplication and migration of the basal cells of the epidermis. Intracellular activity is noted within 12 hours after injury, and the cells become detached from the basement membrane within 24 hours. Mitosis increases and the cells migrate onto vascularized denuded tissue surfaces. After the defect is covered with epithelium, the cells continue to divide, differentiate, and keratinize, increasing epithelial thickness and durability. In a sutured wound or minor abrasion, coverage with epithelium can occur within 48 hours.[5]

Wound healing and epithelialization may be enhanced through the application of growth factors—substances that promote cell migration or synthesis of reparative substances. A mixture of platelet-derived growth factors obtained from the patient's own blood has been used to promote healing of chronic cutaneous wounds.[3] Epidermal growth factor has been used successfully to enhance epithelialization of split-thickness skin graft donor sites.[1]

Bone

To fulfill its primarily structural function, bone must resist deformation without being brittle and allow for the effective transmission of voluntary movement while helping to absorb and dissipate potentially dangerous loading stress. The bones of the hand do this through a highly complicated linked series of joints and musculotendinous units. The bones are tubular (phalanges and metacarpals) or cuboidal (the carpal bones). Each is composed of an outer cortex and inner cancellous matrix. The cortex is thicker in the center of tubular bones where the maximal stresses occur. Cuboidal bones have greater cartilaginous surfaces than tubular bone. Except for the articular surfaces and musculotendinous and ligamentous attachments, the bones are covered by periosteum, a thin, tough, fibrous membrane that is relatively loosely attached in children and becomes more firmly adherent as the bone matures. Bone is supplied with blood vessels, nerves, and lymphatics.

Cancellous bone is morphologically analogous to a calcified sponge but has a definite structure: its bony plates are disposed perpendicular to the long axis of a bone to resist stresses. Cancellous bone serves to modulate compressive forces across joints. Cortical and cancellous bones are composed of mineralized plates that in cancellous bone form trabeculae and in cortical bone are arranged in concentric circles about a central artery and vein to form an osteon.

Bone is composed of cells and matrix. The matrix contains organic components and minerals, primarily calcium hydroxyapatite. Type I collagen accounts for about 95 percent of the organic components, with proteoglycans making up the remainder. Collagen is organized in overlapping layers within the mineralized matrix. Each layer has a singular orientation of fibers, and the functional concept is similar to that of plywood. It has been hypothesized that the mineral phase provides resistance to compressive forces (providing stiffness) and the collagen to tensile strain (providing strength); however, experimental models indicate that the mineral component also plays the dominant role in tensile resistance.[4]

There are three types of cells within the matrix: (1) osteoblasts, found in areas of bone formation, where they produce organic matrix components and promote mineralization; (2) osteoclasts, which degrade mineral and organic matrix through an array of enzymes; and (3) osteocytes, the resident cells in mature bone that maintain extracellular calcium and phosphorus ion concentrations.[8]

Cortical and cancellous bones are constantly undergoing remodeling. In cancellous bone, trabeculae are simultaneously resorbed by osteoclasts and replaced by osteoblasts, a process termed creeping substitution. In cortical bone, remodeling occurs along the structured lines of the osteon. An array of osteoclasts tunnel through the cortex followed by vascular buds and osteoblasts, which produce new bone and create a new osteon. A steady state between destruction and formation is reached that can be altered to increase bone strength or to conserve tissue efficiency and economy. Bone remodeling occurs in response to functional strains within the bone (Wolfe's law). Elements of these remodeling processes accompany the healing of fractures.

Fracture healing entails three overlapping phases: inflammation, repair, and remodeling.[11] Cortical and cancellous bones proceed through these steps somewhat differently. The initial inflammatory stage is characterized by hematoma formation and local cellular response. Damaged cells release vasoactive substances. Marked vasodilatation and hyperemia of the soft tissues about the bony injury occur within hours. A nonspecific inflammatory response occurs, mediated by histamine, kinins, prostaglandins, and the complement system. The area becomes swollen. During the initial 24 hours, damaged vessels thrombose. These events reduce blood flow to the ends of the fractured bone, and this, combined with the force of the original injury, results in cell death within 2 to 4 days after injury. Monocytes and multinucleated cells phagocytize debris, a process that may require several days to weeks depending on the severity of the injury. Local vessels send endothelial buds into the hematoma, and a network of capillaries begins to form within 2 to 3 days and becomes marked by 1 week. Fibroblasts migrate along the fibrin network of the clot. The hematoma is rapidly replaced by granulation tissue, leading to the formation of soft callus. The events of hematoma formation, vascularization, and fibroblast colonization are common to both cortical and cancellous bone repair. The different mechanisms of fracture healing include formation of an external callus, a medullary callus, and primary bone union.[11]

The external callus is a product of the periosteum, which consists of an outer fibrous layer and an inner cellular layer termed the cambium. Within 12 to 16 hours after injury, mitosis increases in the cambial layer across the entire extent of the bone and reaches a peak within the first 24 to 48 hours after injury.[17, 18] After this initial peak, mitotic activity is confined to the fracture site. These proliferating cells form a collar about the opposite ends of the fracture, which coalesce to form a bridge that unites and stabilizes the fracture. These cells differentiate into osteoblasts, which produce primitive bone lacking organization of organic matrix. In areas of low oxygen tension, chondroblasts rather than osteoblasts are formed. The resulting callus is fibrocartilaginous and can be converted to bone by endochondral ossification if it becomes adequately vascularized.

The internal or medullary callus arises from cancellous bone. The initial vascular response lags behind that of the periosteum, although proliferation of osteoprogenitor cells is noted within the medullary cavity within a few days.[2] These cells migrate into the hematoma at the fracture gap and differentiate into osteoblasts and chondroblasts before producing fibrocartilage and depositing trabeculae of primitive bone. Creeping substitution of dead cancellous bone by adjacent living cancellous bone occurs, a process similar to that of bone remodeling.

Primary union occurs when cortical abutment and firm stabilization are provided. Theoretically, this would involve the growth of an osteon across the fracture gap in a manner similar to that in cortical bone remodeling.[16] On a cellular level, however, stabilization necessary for this type of union would be difficult to achieve and likely would require the initial step of medullary callus formation on a microscopic scale.[1]

Because the cellular processes involved in these types of union are different, there are corresponding differences in the speed of union and the ability to bridge gaps. Formation of external callus with its rich periosteal blood supply and rapidly proliferating cambial osteoprogenitor cells is the fastest of these processes but fades after an initial burst of activity. Medullary union is somewhat slower but endures longer and is able to bridge a greater gap between fracture fragments. Primary union, with its characteristics of cortical bone remodeling, is very slow and, by definition, unable to bridge any gap.

The relative stability of the fracture fragments has an important impact on the mechanism and outcome of the attempt at healing.[1, 5, 10, 14] Periosteal callus formation is tolerant of motion at the fracture site and may even be stimulated by it. Medullary callus formation is less tolerant of motion, and healing by primary union cannot occur when even the slightest amount of instability is present. Rigid stability between fracture fragments has an inhibitory effect on periosteal callus formation and may completely ablate the process. Medullary callus formation tolerates interfragmentary stability well. Absolute rigidity is fundamental to the concept of primary cortical repair.

Fractures of a given type within a similar population tend to heal within a few weeks of each other. A *delayed* union occurs when the healing time is considered to be much longer than that required for routine healing of the fracture type. A *nonunion* is present when the fracture remains unhealed beyond the ordinary period and demonstrates no progress toward further healing. Factors that may retard or impair healing in the hand include the stability, reduction, or distraction of the fracture fragments; the blood supply of the healing bones; and the nature of the surrounding soft tissue bed.[13]

The lack of adequate fracture stabilization may lead to a proliferation of unstable callus and the development of a fibrous union. Subsequent immobilization of the fragments may lead to the formation of a bony union.[5] If the distance between fracture fragments is large, then the initial periosteal callus reaction will not be able to bridge the gap and union will have to be carried out by the much slower process of medullary callus formation. Movement at the fracture site may further impede medullary callus formation. Complicating matters more, there may be soft tissue ingrowth from surrounding tissues that may present as a mechanical barrier to fracture bridging.[6] The loss of direct blood supply to a bone fragment requires either the recruitment of a new blood supply by vascular ingrowth from surrounding tissues or the much slower replacement of necrotic bone through the unilateral endeavors of the vascularized fracture fragment.[13]

The interplay of these factors is demonstrated in the healing of a scaphoid fracture. This cuboidal carpal bone is covered on many of its surfaces by articular cartilage and so lacks a periosteal sheath with its inherent rapid callus formation. Healing will take place through the slower, less motion-tolerant route of medullary callus formation. In addition, the proximal pole of the scaphoid may be devascularized by this injury, requiring its eventual replacement through the process of creeping substitution.

Many other local and systemic factors can contribute to delayed healing or nonunion, and in some instances these cannot be discerned. The rationale of reliable treatment for these problems must rest upon the recognition of the cause. In the treatment of delayed union, additional immobilization of the fracture fragments by closed or open means is often attempted. Stimulation of union with electrical fields has met with success in many instances. Established nonunions most often require some type of operative intervention, commonly debridement and fixation of the bone ends and often bone grafting.

The placement of bone graft in a fracture gap has several positive effects. It provides a population of cells in a normal matrix that may be amenable to revascularization.[12] The matrix may also induce bone formation through the induction of undifferentiated mesenchymal cells to switch from a fibrogenic to an osteogenic pattern of development.[15] These cells may be obtained from the surrounding soft tissues or possibly the circulation. Once induced they establish cell lines whose progeny function as chondroblasts or osteoblasts. This inductive substance, termed bone morphogenic protein (BMP),[7, 15] is obtained from the bone matrix and is found in greater quantities in cortical than in cancellous bone.[9] In animal experiments, the amount of new bone formed through the action of BMP is directly proportional to the amount used.

Healing fractures slowly acquire strength, proceeding through a continuum of increased mechanical durability. Determination of the time at which a fracture has healed sufficiently to allow a return to activity depends on several factors. Distorting forces in the hand are limited, and motion of the joints and tendons is important in the prevention of soft tissue changes. Immobilized bone undergoes a net decrease in calcium content.[8] For these reasons mobilization of soft tissues and bone should probably be initiated as soon as this activity will not prove detrimental to fracture healing.[3]

In the event of rigid internal stabilization of tubular bones, motion can often be initiated after the immediate postoperative period. Otherwise, the callus of tubular bones in the hand will have usually acquired sufficient rigidity by the third or fourth week to begin nonloaded mobilization.[3] This will, of course, depend on the nature of the injury and condition of the soft tissues. Suitability for mobilization can be clinically ascertained through palpation of the callus and the determination of a rubbery or firm consistency and the absence of pain at the site. Healing of carpal bones, with their large cancellous component, requires a correspondingly longer period of immobilization, often in the range of several months. Healing is by medullary callus, and even the small amount of motion experienced after internal fixation of these bones may impede healing. Assessment of healing of these bones relies upon the diminution of site tenderness and on radiographic (including tomography) and magnetic resonance imaging findings.

Cartilage

A prerequisite for smooth, painless joint function is an undamaged articular cartilage surface. The primary function of articular (hyaline) cartilage is to provide a low friction interface between opposable joint surfaces that can resist and readily recover from compressive deformation. The efficacy and durability of this tissue is attested to by the fact that the thinnest articular surfaces in the body are located in the interphalangeal joints of the fingers.

Articular cartilage is composed of a small number (usually less than 5 percent by volume) of cells dispersed within an extracellular matrix.[10] This matrix consists of collagen fibers in a hydrated glycoprotein gel. The collagen fibers (primarily type II) impart tensile strength, and proteoglycans provide stiffness and compressive strength.[18] Proteoglycans compose 40 percent of the dry weight of the matrix.[2] Hydrophilic proteoglycan aggregates attract water molecules, which account for 75 percent of the wet weight of cartilage. Matrix water contributes to the ability of cartilage to resist compression and to regain its normal shape after deformation. Water content is highest just below the articular surface and aids in joint lubrication. The temporary swelling that may develop after exercise is attributed to absorption of water from the joint surface.[22] Drying of cartilage is rapid and deleterious. In a rabbit knee model, necrotic changes extended to the middle layers after 30 minutes and to the entire thickness after 60 minutes of drying in room air.[17]

Articular cartilage contains no nerve, vascular, or lymphatic tissue.[2] Its metabolic activity requires oxygen and nutrients obtained by diffusion from the synovial fluid.[11] In the adult human hand there is no significant nutritional contribution from underlying bone.

In normal cartilage, the cells do not replicate and serve only in the maintenance of matrix through enzymatic degradation and collagen and glycosaminoglycan production.[19] Fifty percent of the glycosaminoglycan is replaced annually, and 50 percent of the cartilage is replaced every 10 years. All matrix degradative enzymes are produced by chondrocytes, with the exception of hyaluronidase, which is produced by the synovial membrane.

The articular surface can be divided into four zones of varying matrix composition, collagen fiber orientation, and cellularity.

Zone 1. The superficial or tangential zone (termed the lamina splendens by Hunter) is a fine, transparent layer that can be peeled from the cartilage surface as a thin sheet. It is firmly attached at the articular margins, where it blends with the periosteum. The collagen fibers are oriented tangentially to the surface. The fibril pattern exhibits a specific pore size that allows passage of nutrients and some synovial fluid molecules but excludes larger molecules such as proteins and hyaluronic acid. This layer is relatively metabolically inactive.

Zone 2. The collagen is oriented obliquely to the surface. The chondrocytes are more numerous and metabolically active than those in zone 1.

Zone 3. This is the thickest portion of the articular cartilage. Chondrocytes are numerous and oriented in columns. The collagen fibers are vertically oriented, and some of these fibers pass through the tidemark (the basophilic boundary of zones 3 and 4) to enter the zone of calcified cartilage and subchondral bone. It is not present in the developing animal but becomes apparent after endochondral ossification has ceased. The collagen above and below the tidemark is continuous and serves to anchor the articular cartilage to the underlying calcified structures.

Zone 4. In adults the zone of calcified cartilage separates the hyaline cartilage from subchondral bone. Before maturity it appears to be a site of endochondral ossification with degenerating chondrocytes. By maturity the matrix has become calcified, with the level of calcification advancing with age.

Injury can result in cell death and collagen fibril disruption, depending on the rate and magnitude of loading. A single blunt impact exceeding a critical threshold or multiple insults of sufficient magnitude can produce irreversible damage.

Damage of hyaline cartilage is followed by increased metabolic activity, including (1) an increase in DNA synthesis; (2) an increase in synthesis of acid polysaccharides; (3) an increase in synthesis of protein for protein polysaccharides and perhaps for collagen; and (4) an increase in size and number of nucleoli, the sites of ribosomal RNA precursors concerned with protein synthesis.

Articular surface injuries can be roughly grouped into two categories, partial and full thickness. Partial-thickness injuries involve the articular cartilage surface down to any level but not involving the subchondral bone; in full-thickness tears there is subchondral involvement. The routes of repair for these two different lesions diverge, perhaps owing to the unusual nature of hyaline cartilage itself.

Because cartilage is an avascular tissue, injuries that are confined to the articular cartilage do not elicit a vascular proliferative, inflammatory, or fibroblastic response.[11, 13] There is no increase in substrate or oxygen supply for repair, no organized hematoma to serve as a scaffold or connective tissue matrix or as an attractant for fibroblasts, and no source of undifferentiated pluripotential cells that can become chondroblasts and so create new cartilage. The entire process must rely upon the generative reserve of the chondrocytes themselves. In adults, the chondrocytes are well-differentiated, functionally distinct cells and although it has not been conclusively demonstrated in mature animals that these cells have retained the ability to undergo mitosis in vivo, several studies indicate that this may occur.[5, 9] In partial-thickness injuries, the initial increased metabolic activity soon fades, and new cartilage tissue formation is not demonstrated to any appreciable extent.[6, 8, 11, 14] There have been contradictory studies regarding partial-thickness defect healing in immature animals, with some reports noting healing of partial-thickness defects in a minority of immature test animals.[13]

There does appear to be some healing of defects in injuries that involve the subchondral bone.[3, 4, 6] In this instance, fracture of the subchondral bone leads to hematoma formation, a nonspecific inflammatory response, and fibroblast and vascular proliferation and ingrowth. The area of damaged subchondral bone heals but does not extend into the cartilage. Granulation tissue fills the cartilage defect, organizes, and becomes fibrocartilage.[15] With proper physiologic loading some remodeling of the fibrocartilage may occur, allowing it to take on properties of articular cartilage. Displaced articular fractures are likely to remain fibrocartilage, and the articular surface to remain discontinuous. The fibrocartilage lacks the resiliency of a hyaline surface, and the development of post-traumatic arthritis is promoted.[1, 12]

Fractures of the articular surface involving subchondral bone that are stabilized by compression screws appear to heal without an intermediate stage of fibrocartilage.[16] There is some evidence that, in this instance, there may be proliferation of chondrocytes from a source within the articular surface itself. The remodeled cartilage appears to have a collagen and proteoglycan orientation similar to that found in normal hyaline cartilage.

Immobilization is deleterious to cartilage, causing irreversible joint surface changes in some animal models in as little as 30 days. This may be due to a decrease in the physiologic circulation of the tissue, which is dependent on joint motion. Continuous passive motion (CPM) after full-thickness injury appears to lead to a more rapid and complete transformation from fibro- to hyaline-appearing cartilage.[20, 21] In one experiment involving rabbit knees, CPM had a significant effect when used in the first week postinjury but was of no added benefit after this time in another rabbit knee model. Sensory denervation elicited degenerative changes in addition to those seen with immobilization.[7]

Ligaments

These sturdy, flexible bands of fibrous connective tissue link the bones of the skeleton. They allow full function while maintaining joint integrity and stability, thereby preventing dislocation. They create a discrete joint space and help to generate a physiologic pressure on the articular surface, which is important in articular cartilage maintenance and joint lubrication. Intrinsic and extrinsic innervation provides proprioceptive and kinesthetic feedback.

Ligaments of the hand may be intracapsular or capsular. Intracapsular ligaments, such as the collateral ligament of the interphalangeal joints, exist as easily identifiable structures within a synovial membrane. Capsular ligaments, such as the accessory collateral ligaments of the interphalangeal joints, may be so closely bound to the capsule that grossly they may not be easily identified as separate structures.

On a microscopic level, ligaments appear as organized tissue composed of cells within an organic matrix. The matrix consists primarily of fibers with a smaller amount of amorphic ground substance. These fibers are primarily collagen, although small amounts of reticular and elastic fibers are also present. Ninety percent of the collagen is of the type I variety with the majority of the remainder being of the type III variety.[3] The fibers are arranged in a wavy pattern called the "crimp" of a given ligament.[9] The amorphic ground substance consists primarily of two mucopolysaccharides, hyaluronic acid and chondroitin sulfate. Glycosaminoglycans account for an additional 0.5 percent of the dry ligament weight. Though collagen makes up 75 percent of the dry weight of a ligament, a physiologically hydrated ligament is two thirds water.[9] Glycosaminoglycans help to maintain hydration and arrangement of ligament components.[11]

The predominant cell type of the ligament is the fibroblast. These are oriented along the axis of the ligament collagen fibers and are usually found singly or in widely dispersed groups within the substance of the ligament where they produce the acellular components. In order to carry out their function, ligaments must be tightly bound to bone. There is a continuation of the body of the ligament into the bone, which on a microscopic level appears as a gradual transmission of collagen fibers through layers of fibrocartilage and mineralized fibrocartilage into the subchondral bone.[10]

Ligaments are anisotropic, oriented to resist tension along their long axis.[11] They possess time- and history-dependent viscoelastic properties.[14] Tested in vitro with longitudinal tensile loading, they exhibit nonlinear mechanical behavior. The initial portion of the stress-strain curve displays a shallow slope demonstrating an intraligamentous compensation of loading, which is attributed to a straightening of the fiber crimp with a progressive recruitment of fibers.[25] As more fibers come into tension, levels of stress increase until all fibers are loaded, and as the percentage of unloaded fibers diminishes the slope of the curve increases. If tensile strain continues to increase, fibers will begin failing microscopically, leading ultimately to ligament rupture.[13] In practical terms, this curve means that the ligaments will allow for some joint displacement with relatively little effort but will increase resistance as deformation becomes greater.

Ligaments possess an ability, within a given range, to adapt to physiologic demands. They display memory: that is, they respond differently to each stretch in a series.[25] This phenomenon is thought to involve interaction of collagen and other matrix components. If a ligament is loaded in tension and held at physiologic length, stress relaxation will occur, with the stress decreasing at a predictable rate over time. If a ligament is loaded cyclically to this length, peak stresses will also decline. The beneficial effects of stretching before exercise may be a reflection of these observations. Some softening of ligaments also occurs with increased temperature, and this may account for the benefits of local heat in the mobilization of joints. As ligaments are loaded to the point of rupture, there is a progressive microscopic disruption of collagen fibers, leading up to the ultimate failure of the ligament.

Ligament repair entails an ordered sequence of events.[11, 12] A ligament laceration or rupture kills cells, disrupts matrix, and damages blood vessels.[2, 4] Cell death causes the release of the chemical mediators histamine, kinins, and prostaglandins. A nonspecific inflammatory response ensues. The vessel injury and disruption result in a hemorrhagic exudate, which leads to the formation of a clot composed of fibrin, platelets, erythrocytes, and cell and matrix debris. Fibrin provides a framework for fibroblast attachment, migration, and possibly proliferation. Within hours after injury, undamaged local fibroblasts demonstrate an increased amount of endoplasmic reticulum, indicating at least that a signal for protein synthesis has been received.[9]

Within 2 to 3 days, fibroblasts at the injury site are multiplying and have begun collagen synthesis. The entire ligament becomes edematous secondary to vascular dilatation and a heightened inflammatory reaction. Vascular buds begin to enter the clot, and vascular connections across the defect may be seen at 3 to 4 days postinjury.

At 7 to 10 days, the entire ligament has become more swollen, a reflection of increased cellularity and vascularity. Granulation tissue fills the injury gap, establishing vascular continuity. The number of fibroblasts continues to increase, and there is a steady production of collagen. A ligament bearing only a partial cross-sectional lesion would be in particular jeopardy of complete rupture at this time owing to weakening resulting from both the edema and the well-established inflammatory reaction.

At 3 weeks, local edema has diminished somewhat, but the entire ligament remains swollen. The fibroblastic response now involves the entire ligament, and it is at this point in the repair process that the maximum fibroblast density is reached. The matrix and cells at the repair site remain poorly oriented, but the healing area has gained some tensile strength. By 6 weeks, the edema, hypercellularity, and hypervascularity have begun to diminish. Organization of the collagen fibrils and fibroblasts occurs, and tensile strength continues to increase.[13] The fibroblast population and vascularity are significantly diminished from peak levels at 6 months. The collagen fibrils and fibroblasts continue to gain orientation, and the fibroblasts still produce collagen, albeit at a much reduced rate. One year postinjury the scar is still undergoing active remodeling, with a decrease in fibroblast population and vascularity to normal levels. There is increasing orientation of the fibroblasts and matrix. The remodeling process is active during at least the first two years after injury.

Ligamentous strain or tension-induced partial rupture arises when the magnitude of a load exceeds the peak tensile strength of a ligament without exceeding its breaking strength. Injuries of this type occur toward the end of the stress/strain curve. An experimental model utilizing the medial collateral ligament of sheep demonstrated an initial decrease in strength to 13 percent of control levels with a complete recovery at 6 weeks.[16] These injuries appeared to heal through a predominantly fibroblastic reaction lacking a significant inflammatory component. There was complete recovery of strength and a somewhat hypercellular but otherwise essentially normal histologic appearance of the ligament at 6 weeks postinjury.

Repair of ligaments affects final healing strength. Ruptured ligaments allowed to heal by scar formation are consistently weaker at all stages of healing than ligaments repaired by suture.[11, 12] Although the final strength values vary with the particular animal study, sutured ligaments consistently reached a significantly higher healing endpoint strength. Histologic examination reveals a near recapitulation of normal ligamentous structure with suture repair.

Both reinserted ligament and tendon grafts are gradually incorporated into the bony attachment sites. This process occurs over a period of months to years as the bone remodels and requires the participation of bone cells and fibroblasts.[4, 6, 23] Vascularity of the injury site may be important.[5, 18, 24] In patellar tendon reconstruction of anterior cruciate ligaments, the tendon functions as an avascular free graft until it is revascularized by surrounding soft tissues.[4, 7, 8]

Age, conditioning, and immobility may have an important impact on the occurrence of ligament injury or failure. It has been demonstrated that ligaments from younger individuals are stronger than those obtained from older individuals. Also, the bone insertion sites of older individuals appear to be less well mineralized. Failure of these ligaments commonly involves disruption or avulsion of the osseous insertion.[19] A gain in tensile strength and collagen content has been noted in ligaments obtained from individuals subjected to conditioning or training regimens. For example, knee ligaments of exercised dogs contained more collagen and had higher weight-to-length ratios than those of a control group.[2, 21] Immobilization effects may be related to changes both within the ligament and at its bony insertion.[15] Immobilization appears to disrupt the balance between bone breakdown and synthesis, with a relative predominance of osteoclastic (resorptive) activity at the ligament insertion. The weakening of the bony insertion site may lead to a lower load requirement for rupture. In younger individuals, rupture commonly occurs within the body of the ligament. After immobilization, a similar loading stress in the same individual may entail rupture at the insertion site with avulsion of bone.

The initial ligamentous effect of immobilization is a decrease in glycosaminoglycan and water content.[1] Some experimental models demonstrate a hypermetabolic response with both increased synthesis and degradation of matrix components, whereas others show only an increase in degradation.[17] In the hypermetabolic model, the increased metabolic turnover of collagen increases the proportion of new to old collagen. The new collagen may lack orientation and this may translate into a loss of strength. In the medial cruciate ligament of rabbits, there was a 2 percent loss of total collagen mass after 9 weeks of immobilization, indicating at least an initial balance between synthesis and degradation. By 12 weeks, however, there was a 28 percent loss of total collagen mass, indicating a predominance of degradation.[3]

Most animal models of ligament instability support the contention that immobility precipitates a decrease in collagen and mucopolysaccharide content and strength. There is also wide agreement that a relatively short period of immobilization may generate mechanical changes that require a prolonged period of recovery.[18, 20]

Animal studies demonstrate an increase in ligament strength accompanying training. Increased ligament size, higher collagen content, and larger fiber size are noted in trained animals.[22] After ligament repair, exercise may serve to increase collagen deposition and realignment of fibers.[13] If trends demonstrated in animal studies can be applied to human ligament healing, then even a small amount of excessive immobilization may be detrimental, whereas appropriately applied rehabilitation exercises may actually speed healing.

Tendons

Tendons serve as the physical link between muscle and bone. They transmit the force of muscle contraction and, along with retinacula and fibrous pulleys, may help to provide a degree of mechanical advantage. They eliminate the need for muscle to span the entire length between origin and insertion and enable the muscle belly to be located at some distance from the joint on which it acts. Toward fulfillment of this role, they must be tough and inelastic so as not to fail under repetitive loading and to efficiently transmit the full strength of muscular contraction.

Tendons consist of three regions: the origin at the musculotendinous junction, the tendon proper, and the insertion into bone. (Tendons may also insert into other tendons; however, this does not change the structure or function of the tendon in transmitting force.) At the musculotendinous junction, there is an interdigitation of muscle cell and tendon, with collagen fibrils of the tendon lying adjacent to the basement membrane of the muscle cell. Here dense intercellular connections serve to transmit the contractile force of the myofibrils to the collagen fibers marking the true microscopic origin of the tendon. At the tendon's insertion into bone, there is a transmission of collagen fibers across zones of increasing stiffness. The continuous collagen fibers pass through progressive zones of fibrocartilage, calcified fibrocartilage, and bone.[1]

As tendons proceed from origin to insertion, they may pass through specialized connective tissue sheaths. The histologic and healing characteristics of these intrasynovial tendons differ somewhat from those of extrasynovial tendons. Tendons in the upper extremity are composed predominantly of type I collagen fibers in a linear array oriented parallel to the longitudinal axis of the tendon. Tenocytes, the fibroblast-like cells located within the tendon, are fusiform and sparsely dispersed throughout the substance of the tendon either singly or in small groups. Longitudinally oriented connective tissue septa that pass inward from the outer surface of the tendon constitute the endotenon and serve to divide the tendon into groups of collagen fibers or fascicles. A thin layer of cells and connective tissue, the epitenon, is continuous with the endotenon and sheathes the outer surface of the tendon. At the origin of the tendon, the epitenon is continuous with the epimysium of the attached muscle. In extrasynovial tendons the epitenon is surrounded by a loose connective tissue layer called the peritenon. It is elastic and yielding and is composed of collagen and elastic fibers. It provides a smooth low-resistance bed for the tendon and carries blood vessels that contribute to the nutritional support of the tendon. Histologically, the epitenon is more clearly defined when the course of the tendon becomes intrasynovial. Intrasynovial tendons have a connective tissue mesentery, the mesotenon, that assumes the function of the peritenon in the transmission of blood vessels to the tendon.

The vascular supply of the tendon travels within the endotenal septa. The vessels gain entry through the peritenon or, in the case of intrasynovial tendons, through the mesotenon. In the digital flexor sheaths, the mesotenon, here called the vincular system, is discontinuous. It enters the tendon at discrete points, and tissue far removed from these areas has a less extensive vascular supply. The volar, mechanical surface of these tendons is largely devoid of vessels. It has been demonstrated that within the digital flexor sheaths and within the sheaths of the extensor retinaculum, the tendons obtain the bulk of their metabolic needs through diffusion from the synovial fluid.

Injury to the tendon may occur as a rupture at the origin, insertion, or body of the tendon, or there may be a physically inflicted transection of the tendon substance. A rupture at the origin of the tendon may heal spontaneously or may require surgical repair if a significant portion has become detached. A separation at the insertion often entails avulsion of a bone fragment to which the tendon is attached. If this fragment does not disrupt the joint surface and remains in close apposition to the avulsion site, then bony healing will occur and continuity of the tendon-bone unit will be re-established. However, when the tendon has become completely separated from bone, it must be surgically reattached. As the bone remodels, the substance of the tendon is incorporated into the site and a new physiologic insertion will form.

Ruptures within the body of the tendon are preceded by some abnormality or deterioration of the tendon, usually inflammation or mechanical abrasion. After complete transection or rupture, the functional re-establishment of tendon continuity must rely upon the physical apposition of the two tendon ends in order for healing to take place. After the repair of a lacerated extrasynovial tendon, healing likely takes place through the efforts of all tissues involved in the area—the one wound/one scar theory. A blood clot forms, and a nonspecific inflammatory reaction occurs. A fibrin network is established and the clot is populated by fibroblasts and advancing capillary buds. Collagen and ground substance are produced, and the wound gradually gains in tensile strength. The collagen and scar tissue slowly become remodeled along the lines of functional stress, and histologically the repair site resembles the uninjured tendon. Adhesions of the extrasynovial tendon may occur, but the tissue bed through which it passes is often elastic and yielding. The extrasynovial tendon heals in a well-vascularized, nonrigid environment from which it can obtain a convenient population of undifferentiated mesenchymal and collagen-producing cells.

Synovial tendons exist as discrete structures surrounded by fluid within a connective tissue tunnel sealed at both ends. There has been a long and extensive debate over whether the cells responsible for the repair of intrasynovial tendons are obtained from the tendon itself or from the sheath or surrounding tissues. Strong experimental evidence points to the possibility of contributions from either tissue site.[6, 8] It is conceivable that intrasynovial tendon healing is not an exclusive process, but that as in other tissues, a physical insult will generate contributions from all adjacent repair-capable tissues.

As the suture-repaired intrasynovial tendon heals, it passes through stages characterized by different cellular processes.[5, 9] By the third day strands of fibrinous material bridge the repair site at the tendon surface. Small blood clots may be present at gaps between the opposing tendon ends. There is a proliferation of epitenon cells at the laceration and around suture sites. This collar of cells is thicker when there is a larger gap between tendon ends. The fibrin strands may act as a framework for the migration of the epitenon cells, and by the seventh day these cells have migrated into the repair site and begun producing collagen.[2] Capillary buds then begin to enter the repair site, and by the tenth day collagen strands bridge the repair site, and the new intratendinous vascular supply has become more prominent. At some point during the following week, evidence of collagen production will be seen within the endotenon. It is unclear whether this collagen is produced by the resident cellular population or by the migrating epitenon cells. Collagen production continues, and there is some evidence that it peaks at the third or fourth week after repair.

The strength of the repaired tendon diminishes over the first 3 to 5 days postoperatively and then gradually increases. In animal models, a more rapid increase in the breaking strength of tendons is noted, with early postoperative active loading of the tendon to some degree. Animal models also demonstrate that immobilization of healthy tendons for even relatively short periods of time (3 weeks) may lead to significant diminution of strength. Continuous passive motion of the tendons in the immobilized extremity markedly diminished these changes.[4] In another model utilizing partially lacerated, nonrepaired chicken flexor tendons, a more rapid gain in tensile strength was noted among the mobilized group of animals.[10, 11]

The repair of partial tendon lacerations was evaluated in a chicken flexor tendon model. Tendons were transected across 25 to 75 percent of their cross-sectional area and then repaired or allowed to heal spontaneously. At all stages in the repair process, the nonsutured tendons appeared to have significantly greater rupture strength as compared with the repaired tendons.[7] A prospective human study demonstrated excellent function in 16 of 17 human partial flexor tendon lacerations treated with early mobilization.[10] In a primate model utilizing partial cross-sectional excision of tendon substance and early unrestricted motion, ruptures occurred only in tendons rendered ischemic by ligature.[8]

The healing of the intrasynovial tendon is accompanied by the cellular repair processes of the interrupted synovial sheath and adjacent tissues. The hematoma, fibrin strands, and nonspecific inflammatory response engendered by this process may play a role in the development of adhesions from the sheath and surrounding tissues to the tendon. It has also been postulated that epitenon cells may migrate toward the sheath, creating adhesions. The inner surface of the synovial sheath, unless very badly damaged, generally regains its former appearance and function.

Repair or excision of the sheath does not affect the net matrix formation of the healing tendon.[3] Passive flexion and active extension of digits with lacerated tendons have been used as a strategy to overcome adhesion formation. This regimen, however, does not provide a great deal of tendon excursion within the sheath, and it may be that reflex contraction of the muscle bellies improves excursion, increasing the length and flexibility of the adhesions.

Although increased rate of tensile strength gain is seen in mobilized tendon repair models, this must be weighed against the possibility of stress-induced tendon repair rupture. Similarly, although the strength of unrepaired partial lacerations may be greater than that in repaired tears, this must be balanced against the possibility of adhesion formation and late tendon triggering. The type of injury and condition of the adjacent tissues must be factored into the repair and rehabilitation of the injured tendon.

Muscles

Motor function of the hand is provided through the action of voluntary striated muscle fibers. The extrinsic muscles are located within the forearm and supply their motor force through the action of tendons; the intrinsic musculature is located in the hand. Muscle is well vascularized and has a high functional metabolic demand for oxygen and substrate. An undamaged nerve supply is essential for the function and maintenance of muscle tissue.[6, 11, 18] Muscle is composed of muscle cells, connective tissue, and a well-defined nerve and vascular supply. The basic unit of muscle is the fiber. The muscle cell, or myofiber, is a single multinucleated cell that contains an assembly of contractile material, called myofibrils, that extends throughout its length. The myofiber cell wall contains three layers. The innermost layer, the sarcolemma, is an excitable electrically polarized membrane. The middle layer of the cell wall, the basement membrane, consists of proteins and polysaccharides. The endomysium, the external layer, is composed of collagen fibers. The endomysium and the basement membrane together make up the basal lamina; their longitudinal construct (in which the individual fiber resides) is called the myotube. The nuclei of the myofiber are located peripherally in the sarcoplasm (cytoplasm) just beneath the sarcolemma. Between the sarcolemma and the basement membrane are located small collections of tightly crowded satellite cells.[6, 14] These cells vary in number throughout life, accounting for as much as one half of all muscle cell nuclei in the newborn but less than 5 percent in the mature adult.[1]

There are three levels of macroscopic connective tissue organization in fully formed skeletal muscle.[6] The external surface of the muscle is covered by a sheath of connective tissue termed the epimysium. The interconnected septa extending through the muscle that sheathes the fascicles (or bundles) of myofibers are termed the perimysium. The individual myofibers are bound by the endomysium. Blood vessels and nerves travel through these connective tissue planes to invest the muscle cells. Capillaries and fine nerve elements are found in the endomysium investing each nerve fiber.

A specialized extension of the intracellular filaments is transmitted across the sarcolemma and basal lamina in continuity with extracellular collagen fibers. At a microscopic level this represents the muscle-tendon interface. Laminin and type IV collagen are found in this area. On a macroscopic level there is an interdigitation, or folding, of the tendon-muscle interface that serves to increase the surface area and reduce tensile stress. Still, the most common location of acute stretch-induced failure is at the musculotendinous junction.[15]

An increase in contractile activity short of macroscopic damage may lead to an adaptive increase in the strength or endurance of a muscle.[9, 10] The number of mitochondria and amount of energy-producing enzymes may increase,[7, 8] and substrate metabolism may become more efficient, boosting potential work output.[3] Motor-unit fiber recruitment is improved. The tissue mass may increase as evidenced by a greater cross-sectional area of the muscle, which may be due either to an increase in the content of myofibrils within the individual muscle cells or to an absolute increase in the number of muscle fibers. The increase in the number of myofibers may be accounted for by either one of two processes. There is a large body of evidence that indicates that the satellite cells may serve as a reservoir for muscle regeneration or stress-induced hyperplasia. There is also some evidence indicating that under certain conditions, muscle cells may split or branch to form new fibers. Increased muscle capacity then may be a result of larger or more efficient fibers or an increase in the number of fibers, or both.[12, 17]

After injury to a muscle, repair processes attempt to regenerate structure and re-establish function. The degree of injury determines the mechanism of repair. A mild tear will leave a large population of myofibers and satellite cells (to regenerate the damaged cellular population) as well as an intact connective tissue envelope to provide a framework for the repair.

The connective tissue framework of the muscle may serve as a guide for the regenerating muscle cells. When injury has not disrupted the myotube, the multiplication of satellite cells and formation of new muscle fibers take place within this structure. When the myotube is ruptured, the satellite cells may migrate into the external matrix or blood clot and form new muscle fibers there. The connective tissue orientation here is important and provides orientation for the regenerating fibers; minced explants of muscle tissue placed in a collagenous framework will grow along the axis of that framework.

A major tear or laceration will involve some degree of scarring with a postrepair increase in muscle connective tissue content.[20] The reparative process, to some degree, involves a competition between fibroblasts of the connective tissue component and regenerating muscle cells. If the fibroblasts form a scar, then continuity of the regenerating muscle mass will be interrupted. After transection of a muscle, all devascularized tissue will necrose. If both sides of the muscle are vascularized but are not in close apposition, fibrous tissue may grow into the gap, preventing reinnervation and/or the re-establishment of muscle fiber continuity across the transection site. As a general rule, the more severe the damage, the greater the resultant increase in the proportion of intramuscular connective tissue. The most severe forms of injury involve either crushing or ischemia.[20] The resultant widespread cell death with a concomitant loss of regenerative cell population means that these injuries are repaired predominantly by connective tissue scarring. Innervation may be significantly disrupted as well, further complicating functional recovery.[11]

In a minor muscle injury, such as a strain or tourniquet ischemia of limited duration (less than 3 hours), repair of damaged muscle fibers takes place rapidly and completely.[19] With somewhat greater disruption of tissue, regeneration may still occur within existing myotubes with excellent functional recovery. With greater degrees of injury, there is a progressive increase in the amount of connective tissue scarring and a proportionate decrease in the degree of functional return.

The cellular processes and time scale of muscle repair have been demonstrated in animal models.[6] Closed trauma was inflicted to a degree sufficient to cause necrosis of individual muscle fibers without devascularizing or grossly destroying large areas of the muscle, creating lesions similar to a contusion or severe muscle strain. By the end of the first day degenerating myofibers and an inflammatory and a nonspecific inflammatory cell infiltrate were noted. The nuclei of the satellite cells increased in size. By the second day tissue macrophages had migrated beneath the basement membrane and were engaged in the phagocytosis of myofibrillar debris. Mitosis of the satellite cells begins at this time and occurs synchronously for the first few divisions. The progeny of the satellite cells, the myoblasts, remain attached to the inner aspect of the basement lamina and expand along the length of the myotube. The cell membranes gradually merge and form a syncytium, which becomes a new muscle fiber.[15] The division of satellite cells and phagocytosis of debris occur simultaneously in the regeneration process. A certain proportion of the satellite cells do not differentiate along myoblast lines, maintaining the population of these regenerative cells.

By the fourth day there may be several new myofibers within the lumina of the original myotube. These adjacent fibers may fuse laterally or remain detached and become separated by the development of their own basal lamina. By 3 months the mature myotubes have detached and clusters of new muscles fibers are no longer apparent. It may take up to 6 months or more to regain normal muscle morphology.

With more severe injury and disruption of the myotubes, the satellite cell progeny grow along the outer aspect of the basal lamina in a spiral or parallel configuration. Fusion of the myoblasts occurs, and the process continues as described. It should be noted that regeneration is facilitated following injuries that leave the myotubes intact. This serves to maintain the satellite cell progeny in one population, prevents dilution of this population by nonmuscle cells, and leads to a higher collision and fusion frequency between the myoblasts. With an even greater degree of injury a blood clot forms, with the subsequent development of a collagenous framework and an attempt by myoblasts to re-establish fiber continuity across the hematoma gap before a scar barrier is formed.

Immobilization causes widespread biochemical and morphologic changes within muscle. Strength declines and fatigability increases rapidly after limb immobilization. A significant decrease in the rate of protein synthesis is observable by the sixth hour of limb immobility. Lower levels of enzymes responsible for the oxidation of substrate and the production of energy are apparent. After 4 weeks, the muscle tissue of experimental animals demonstrates a wasting of mass and a lower total content and tissue concentration of myofibrillar proteins. This development of disuse atrophy occurs rapidly in the immobilized muscle and may require a long recovery.[5] Conversely, there is some evidence that the speed and completeness of soft tissue recovery may be enhanced by the physiologic use of the injured limb. Muscles immobilized in stretched, neutral positions appear to atrophy less rapidly than those in shortened positions.[13] Healing of muscle injuries varies with age and is slower in older animals. A reduction in muscle fiber size is seen in older humans (>65 years of age), which may be attributable in part to low physical activity.[4] Resolution of inflammation takes longer, and a delayed recovery of strength is seen.

After injury there is a gradual decrease in muscle tensile strength over a period of 4 to 5 days. This is likely attributable to the initial inflammatory response. This loss of tensile strength may be alleviated somewhat by the administration of anti-inflammatory drugs though at the cost of somewhat delayed muscle regeneration.[2]

Nerves

Nerves may contain either motor and sensory fibers or only motor or sensory fibers. Nerve fibers in the hand and forearm have three levels of organization. The basic unit is the neuron and its supporting elements. The efferent cytoplasmic process of a neuron is an axon. Each axon is accompanied by satellite cells (for nutrition) and Schwann cells and connective tissue. Motor and larger sensory nerve fibers have a myelinated sheath associated with a single Schwann cell. Conversely, groups of unmyelinated fibers are sheathed by a single non–myelin sheath-producing Schwann cell. The nerve/Schwann cell array is enveloped by a connective tissue tube (the endoneurium) composed primarily of collagen and an occasional fibroblast. The discontinuity of the myelin sheath that occurs between successive Schwann cells is termed a node of Ranvier.

Nerve fibers are grouped into a fascicle that is bounded by a connective tissue sheath (perineurium). Peripheral nerves may contain one or more fascicles. A heavier, although loosely applied, connective tissue cover, the epineurium, encases each peripheral nerve and sends extensions centrally in a multifascicular nerve framework to bind together and maintain the positions of the fascicles. The fascicular pattern is more or less consistently located when comparing nerves from different individuals.

When a nerve fiber is disrupted, the distal axon is devitalized and undergoes wallerian degeneration. There is disintegration of myelin and a proliferation of Schwann cells. The Schwann cells phagocytize cellular debris, and with time the endoneurial tubes collapse, presenting a potential, rather than an actual, conduit for nerve regrowth.

The proximal portion of the axon usually degenerates proximal to the first node of Ranvier. Within a few days, axonal sprouting occurs. A single axon will produce multiple sprouts that extend toward the distal segment in an attempt to grow down the distal endoneurial tubes. A molecular gradient of neuronotrophic factors may help to direct sprouts toward target cells.[6] Growth occurs at the rate of approximately 1 to 1½ mm per day. This progression distally can be demonstrated by an advancing Tinel's sign. Reinnervation of the motor end plates is possible up to 2 years after injury. Reinnervation of sensory organs can occur later, and protective sensation can be re-established after nerve repair several years after injury. The inconsistent and often disappointing results after nerve repair can be understood by recognizing the fascicular complexity (and interfascicular branching) and the many obstacles that the axonal sprouts must encounter in their attempt to re-establish neural continuity.

The severity of nerve injury depends on the degree of physical disruption of the functional unit. The least severe injury, neuropraxia, produces an electrochemical conduction block within the axon that prevents transmission of nerve impulses. All elements of the nerve are intact, and complete recovery may occur in a few hours or may require months. The longer recovery period reflects a more severe injury.

Axonotmesis occurs only when the axon has been interrupted; all other elements, including the endoneurial sheaths, remain intact. Wallerian degeneration is followed by axonal sprouting. Since the endoneurial tubes are intact, regeneration to normal or near normal levels occurs within several months. A more severe injury occurs with endoneurial sheath disruption. Axonal sprouting will not be as well directed, and scarring of the endoneurium will further impede recovery. When all axons are not disrupted at one level, a neuroma in continuity will form. If all axons are disrupted, the nerve may remain in continuity, yet no axon sprouts will enter the endoneurial sheaths distally. Tinel's sign will not advance distally.

Neurotmesis is associated with transection of the nerve, including the epineurium and fascicles. Surgical repair is required. Early and accurate diagnosis is important in obtaining optimal outcome. When motor nerves are injured, splinting and passive range of motion exercises are necessary to prevent contracture and soft tissue resorption.

Following neuropraxia and axonotmesis injuries, damaged nerves exhibit changes in mechanical properties. There is an initial decrease in strength and rigidity and an increase in elasticity followed by a subsequent increase in strength and stiffness and a decrease in elasticity. In animal experiments, stiffness and strength reach control levels by the sixth day after injury. All changes appeared to be most prominent at or just distal to the injured nerve segment.[1] Early immobilization of the segment may possibly prevent further damage during this initial response to injury.

Following surgical repair, bursting strength gradually increases. In rats, bursting strength is 25 and 42 percent of control values at 2 and 3 weeks, respectively. There is little gain in strength between 3 and 9 weeks after repair, but a significant increase occurs by the twelfth week. In monkeys, the bursting strength of sutured nerves is 77 percent of control values by the fourth week after repair.[4]

Nerve elasticity is derived primarily from the perineurium. The greater the percentage of fascicular area in cross-sectional diameter, the greater will be the tensile strength of the nerve.[11, 12] With increasing levels of tension, histologic changes vary from hyperemia to intraneural hematoma, axonal disruption, and, finally, nerve rupture.

Tension has important effects on intraneural microvascular flow. In a rabbit model, tension producing a 5 to 10 percent elongation of nerve is sufficient to affect venous flow. Intraneural circulation was completely arrested with 11 to 18 percent elongation.[5, 7–9] Great amounts of tension will produce gapping or tearing of sutures at the repair site, whereas lesser amounts will interfere with intraneural venous or arterial flow, leading to a hypoxic, ultimately fibrotic, nerve end.

Recovery of sensation after peripheral nerve repair is a function of the characteristics of specific nerve fiber types supplying sensory end organs.[3, 13] The return of pain sensibility is seen first, followed by perception of 30 cps vibratory stimuli, followed closely by moving touch and, several months later, by perception of constant touch.[2] It is generally agreed that the best functional results after nerve repair are obtained in children.[10]

Electrical Stimulation

Wolff's law (adaptive structural change occurs in response to mechanical stress) hints at the relationship between biologic and physical processes in bone. The search for a putative means of translating mechanical forces into biologic signals led investigators to consider the possibility that electrical fields might have some effect on bone remodeling.[5, 15]

Bone generates electric potentials in three ways.[23, 27] Strain-related or piezoelectric potentials are associated with mechanically stressed bone, with areas of compression being electronegative and areas of tension electropositive. These potentials arise from the organic matrix, are proportional to the rate and amount of strain, and are independent of cell viability. Bioelectric potentials are dependent on the viability of cells and rely upon chemical gradients generated by metabolic effort. Electrokinetic or streaming potentials may be the major component of mechanically generated potentials. They are created by the stress-induced flow of an ion-containing fluid (tissue fluid) through a solid matrix bearing an electric countercharge (bone).

In rabbit tibias, the metaphysis was shown to be electronegative relative to the epiphysis; a fracture of the diaphysis was noted to greatly increase the degree of electronegativity. In vitro experiments demonstrated that low-level electrical currents could affect cell activation and bone growth, and these and similar observations led to the therapeutic use of electrical stimulation in the treatment of delayed healing of fractures.

Electrical signals are supplied in one of three ways.[6, 8] In the faradic system, electrodes are placed within the tissue and a potential is applied, generating an ionic current flow.[22] In a capacitive system of delivery, electrodes are placed externally on the opposite sides of the limb at the level of the delayed union. An oscillating external potential is applied and a time-varying electrical field is generated within the tissues.[17] In the inductive system of signal delivery, a coil or pair of coils is placed externally so that an imaginary extension of the coil's axis will pass through the limb near the fracture site.[3, 4] Time-varying voltages are passed through these coils, generating a time-varying magnetic field. The magnetic field induces the production of a secondary time-varying electrical field within the tissues themselves.

All types of electrical delivery appear to improve healing of delayed unions and nonunions. The increase in rate or quality of healing appears to be unrelated to the type of stimulation employed.[9, 10, 27] In comparing human bones in similar therapeutic trials, the percentage of successful union varies between approximately 70 and 85 percent.[2] In the hand, a similar range is encountered with different stimulation systems used in the treatment of scaphoid fractures.[21] It is theorized that the biologic action of electromagnetic fields may occur through the increased ossification of callus, improved rate of revascularization, or increased osteogenesis.[4, 6, 18] The rate of success in treatment of scaphoid fractures is about 85 percent and approaches that of bone grafting.[7] The electrical field is commonly applied for 3 to 5 months in scaphoid fracture treatment.[2, 7, 12, 15, 21] There may be a synergistic effect when bone grafts and electrical stimulation are used concurrently.[2, 3] Failure of electrical stimulation has been attributed to senile and disuse osteoporosis, pseudarthrosis, obesity, and osteomyelitis.[8, 10, 15]

When electrical stimulation was applied in a normal rabbit fracture healing model, a more rapid gain in tensile strength was noted during the midphase of fracture healing.[14] Final union strength was identical in the experimental and the control groups, which seems to indicate that there is a specific cellular scenario during which the application of current is most effective. In stimulation of human nonunions, the greatest success and most rapid response are seen in treatment of the proliferative type of fibrous nonunion, where rapid calcification of the fibrous callus is induced with an attendant gain in fracture stability.[21]

The anecdotal reports of improvement of sensory return or cutaneous wound healing at bone electrical stimulation sites led to investigations of soft tissue electrical stimulation.[13, 26] Electrical stimulation has been used in human subjects in the successful treatment of recalcitrant cutaneous burns and in the rescue of ischemic skin flaps.[11, 16] Animal studies demonstrate improved growth and physiologic parameters of Schwann cells grown in culture; improved regeneration in a rat nerve transection model; increased incorporation of labeled proline and hydroxyproline in an in vitro tendon culture assay; improved ligament healing with shift toward mature wound collagen types in a rabbit model; and diminution of elevated bone resorption rates and stimulation of bone formation in a rat osteoporosis model.[1, 9, 19, 20, 24, 25] Various strategies for the delivery of electrical stimulation were used in these models, but the common implication is that, at least under certain situations, cellular activity can be modified toward healing or tissue maturation by application of an exogenous electric field.

Steroid Effects

Joint and tendon inflammations are painful conditions that can weaken these structures, increasing their susceptibility to damage or rupture. Injection of corticosteroids into tendon sheaths and joint capsules is an accepted, widely used therapeutic measure for tenovitis and synovitis. However, there are many anecdotal reports citing spontaneous rupture of tendons or ligaments and accelerated erosion or necrosis of joint surfaces after corticosteroid administration.[1, 4, 7–9]

Systemic corticosteroids were administered to rats in a wound healing, bursting strength model. The steroid-affected wounds gained

immobilization: A correlative biomechanical and histological study in primates. Clin. Orthop. 123:210, 1977.
18. Noyes, F.R., Butler, D.L., Paulos, L.E., et al.: Intra-articular cruciate reconstruction: Perspectives on graft strength, vascularization and immediate motion after replacement. Clin. Orthop. 172:71, 1983.
19. Noyes, F.R., Grood, E.S.: The strength of the anterior cruciate ligament in humans and rhesus monkeys: Age-related and species-related changes. J. Bone Joint Surg. 58A(8):1074, 1976.
20. Noyes, F.R., Torvik, P.J., Hyde, W.B., et al. Biomechanics of ligament failure: An analysis of immobilization, exercise, and reconditioning effects in primates. J. Bone Joint Surg. 56A(7):1406, 1974.
21. Tipton, C.M., James, S.L., Mergner, W., et al.: Influence of exercise on strength of medial collateral knee ligaments of dogs. Am. J. Physiol. 218(3):894, 1970.
22. Vidik, A.: Elasticity and tensile strength of the anterior cruciate ligament in rabbits as influenced by training. Acta Physiol. Scand. 74:372, 1968.
23. Whiston, T.B., Walmsley, R.: Some observations on the reaction of bone and tendon after tunnelling bone and insertion of tendon. J. Bone Joint Surg. 42B(2):377, 1960.
24. Whiteside, L.A., Sweeney, R.E.: Nutrient pathways of the cruciate ligaments: An experimental study using the hydrogen wash-out technique. J. Bone Joint Surg. 62A:1176, 1980.
25. Woo, S.L.-Y., Gomez, M.A., Woo, Y.K., Akeson, W.H.: Mechanical properties of tendons and ligaments. Biorheology 19:385, 1982.

TENDONS

1. Elliott, D.H.: Structure and function of mammalian tendon. Biol. Rev. 40:392, 1965.
2. Garner, W.L., McDonald, J.A., Koo, M., et al.: Identification of the collagen-producing cells in healing flexor tendons. Plast. Reconstr. Surg. 83:875, 1989.
3. Kain, C.C., Russell, J. E., Rouse, A.M., et al.: Regional differences in matrix formation in the healing flexor tendon. Clin. Orthop. 229:308, 1988.
4. Loitz, B.J. Zernicke, R.F., Vailas, A.C., et al.: Effects of short-term immobilization versus continuous passive motion on the biomechanical and biochemical properties of the rabbit tendon. Clin. Orthop. 244:265, 1989.
5. Manske, P.R.: Review article: Flexor tendon healing. J. Hand Surg. 13:237, 1988.
6. Mass, D.P., Tuel, R.: Human flexor tendon participation in the in vitro repair process. J. Hand Surg. 14:64, 1989.
7. Ollinger, H., Wray, R.C., Weeks, P.M.: Effects of suture on tensile strength gain of partially and completely severed tendons. Surg. Forum 26:63, 1974.
8. Seyfer, A.E., Bolger, W.F.: Effects of unrestricted motion on healing: A study of posttraumatic adhesions in primate tendons. Plast. Reconstr. Surg. 83:122, 1989.
9. Strickland, J.W.: Flexor tendon injuries. Part 1. Anatomy, physiology, biomechanics, healing, and adhesion formation around a repaired tendon. Orthop. Rev. 25(10):632, 1986.
10. Wray, R.C., Holtmann, B., Weeks, P.M.: Clinical treatment of partial tendon lacerations without suturing and with early motion. Plast. Reconstr. Surg. 59:231, 1977.
11. Wray, R.C., Ollinger, H., Weeks, P.M.: Effects of mobilization on tensile strength of partial tendon lacerations. Surg. Forum 26:557, 1975.

Background Reading

Hunter, J., Schneider, L., Mackin, E.: Tendon Surgery in the Hand. St. Louis, C.V. Mosby, 1987.

MUSCLES

1. Allbrook, D.B., Han, M.F., Hellmuth, A.E.: Population of muscle satellite cells in relation to age and mitotic activity. Pathology 3:233, 1973.
2. Almekinders, L.C., Gilbert, J.A.: Healing of experimental muscle strains and the effects of nonsteroidal, antiinflammatory medication. Am. J. Sports Med. 14(4):303, 1986.

3. Anderson, P., Henriksson, J.: Training induced changes in the subgroups of human type II skeletal muscle fibres. Acta Physiol. Scand. 99:123, 1977.
4. Aniansson, A., Zetterberg, C., Hedberg, M., et al.: Impaired muscle function with aging. Clin. Orthop. 191:193, 1984.
5. Booth, F.W.: Physiologic and biochemical effects of immobilization on muscle. Clin. Orthop. 219:15, 1987.
6. Carlson, B.M.: The regeneration of skeletal muscle: A review. Am. J. Anat. 137:119, 1973.
7. Costill, D.L., Daniels, J., Evans, W., et al.: Skeletal muscle enzymes and fiber composition in male and female track athletes. J. Appl. Physiol. 40:149, 1976.
8. Friden, J., Seger, J., Sjostrom, M., et al.: Adaptive response in human skeletal muscle subjected to prolonged eccentric training. Int. J. Sport Med. 4:177, 1983.
9. Friden, J., Sjostrom, M., Ekblom, B.: A morphological study of delayed muscle soreness. Experientia 37:506, 1981.
10. Friden, J., Sjostrom, M., Ekblom, B.: Myofibrillar damage following intense eccentric exercise in man. Int. J. Sports Med. 4:170, 1983.
11. Guth, L., Albuquerque, E.: The neurotrophic regulation of resting membrane potential and extrajunctional acetylcholine sensitivity in mammalian skeletal muscle. In Bischoff, R., Carlson, B., Shafiq, S., et al. (eds.): Muscle Regeneration. New York, Raven Press, 1979.
12. Hay, E.D.: Skeletal-muscle regeneration. N. Engl. J. Med. 284:1033, 1971.
13. Jokl, P., Konstandt, S.: The effect of limb immobilization on muscle function and protein composition. Clin. Orthop. 174:222, 1983.
14. Lipton, B.H., Schultz, E.: Developmental fate of skeletal muscle satellite cells. Science 205:1292, 1979.
15. Miller, W.A.: Rupture of the musculotendinous juncture of the medial head of the gastrocnemius muscle. Am. J. Sports Med. 5:191, 1977.
16. Nichols, J., Shafiq, S.: Morphological changes in satellite cells in regenerating pectoralis muscle of the chicken. In Bischoff, R., Carlson, B., Shafiq, S., et al. (eds.): Muscle Regeneration. New York, Raven Press, 1979.
17. Schiaffino, S., Bormioli, S., Aloisi, M.: Fiber branching and formation of new fibers during compensatory muscle hypertrophy. In Bischoff, R., Carlson, B., Shafiq, S., et al. (eds.): Muscle Regeneration. New York, Raven Press, 1979.
18. Thompson, N.: Autogenous free grafts of skeletal muscle. Plast. Reconstr. Surg. 48:11, 1971.
19. Tountas, C.P., Bergman, R.A.: Tourniquet ischemia: Ultrastructural and histochemical observations of ischemic human muscle and of monkey muscle and nerve. J. Hand Surg. 2:31, 1977.
20. Walton, M., Rothwell, A.G.: Reactions of thigh tissues of sheep to blunt trauma. Clin. Orthop. 176:273, 1983.

Background Reading

Walton, J.: Disorders of Voluntary Muscle. New York, Churchill Livingstone, New York, 1988.

NERVES

1. Beel, J.A., Groswald, D.E., Luttges, M.W.: Alterations in the mechanical properties of peripheral nerve following crush injury. J. Biomech. 17(3):185, 1984.
2. Dellon, A.L., Curtis, R.M., Edgerton, M.T.: Evaluating recovery of sensation in the hand following nerve injury. Johns Hopkins Med. J. 130:235, 1972.
3. Dellon, A.L., Munger, B.L.: Correlation of histology and sensibility after nerve repair. J. Hand Surg. 8(6):871, 1983.
4. Higgs, P.E., Weeks, P.M.: The rate of bursting strength gain in repaired nerves. Ann. Plast. Surg. 3(4):338, 1979.
5. Lundborg G.: Structure and function of the intraneural microvessels as related to trauma, edema formation, and nerve function. J. Bone Joint Surg. 57A(7):938, 1975.
6. Lundborg, G., Dahlin, L., Danielsen, N., et al.: Nerve regeneration across an ex-

tended gap: A neurobiological view of nerve repair and the possible involvement of neuronotrophic factors. J. Hand Surg. 7(6):580, 1982.
7. Lundborg, G., Rydevik, B.: Effects of stretching the tibial nerve of the rabbit: A preliminary study of the intraneural circulation and the barrier function of the perineurium. J. Bone Joint Surg. 55B(2):390, 1973.
8. Miyamoto, Y., Watari, S., Tsuge, K.: Experimental studies on the effects of tension on intraneural microcirculation in sutured peripheral nerves. Plast. Reconstr. Surg. 63(3):398, 1979.
9. Ogata, K., Naito, M.: Blood flow of peripheral nerve effects of dissection, stretching and compression, J. Hand Surg. 11B(1):10, 1986.
10. Poppen, N.K., McCarroll, H.R., Jr., Doyle, J.R., et al. Recovery of sensibility after suture of digital nerves. J. Hand Surg. 4(3):212, 1979.
11. Sunderland, S., Bradley, K.C.: Stress-strain phenomena in human peripheral nerve trunks. Brain 84:102, 1961.
12. Sunderland, S., Bradley, K.C.: Stress-strain phenomena in denervated peripheral nerve trunks. Brain 84:125, 1961.
13. Yamauchi, S., Nomura, S. Yoshimura, M., et al.: A clinical study of the order and speed of sensory recovery after digital replantation. J. Hand Surg. 8(5, Part 1):545, 1983.

Background Reading

Lundborg, G.: Nerve Injury and Repair. New York, Churchill Livingstone, 1988.

ELECTRICAL STIMULATION

1. Akai, M., Oda, H., Shirasaki, Y., et al.: Electrical stimulation of ligament healing. Clin. Orthop. 235:296, 1988.
2. Bassett, C.A.L., Mitchell, S.N., Gaston, S.R.: Pulsing electromagnetic field treatment in ununited fractures and failed arthrodeses. JAMA 247:623, 1982.
3. Bassett, C.A.L., Mitchell, S.N., Schink, M.M.: Treatment of therapeutically resistant non-unions with bone grafts and pulsing electromagnetic fields. J. Bone Joint Sur. 64(A):1214, 1982.
4. Bassett, C.A.L., Valdes, M.G., Hernandez, E.: Modification of fracture repair with selected pulsing electromagnetic fields. J. Bone Joint Surg. 64(A):888, 1982.
5. Bassett, C.A.L., Pawluk, R.J.: Effects of electric currents on bone in vivo. Nature 204:652, 1964.
6. Black, J.: Electrical stimulation of hard and soft tissues in animal models. Clin. Plast. Surg. 12:243, 1985.
7. Bora, F.W., Osterman, A.L., Woodbury, D.F., et al.: Treatment of nonunion of the scaphoid by direct current. Orthop. Clin. North Am. 15:107, 1984.
8. Brighton, C.T.: The treatment of non-unions with electricity. J. Bone Joint Surg. 63(A):847, 1981.
9. Cruess, R.L., Kan, K., Bassett, C.A.L.: The effect of pulsing electromagnetic fields on bone metabolism in experimental disuse osteoporosis. Clin. Orthop. 173:245, 1983.
10. Esterhai, J.L., Brighton, C.T., Heppenstall, R.B., et al.: Nonunion of the humerus. Clin. Orthop. 211:228, 1986.
11. Fakhri, O., Amin, M.A.: The effect of low-voltage electric therapy on the healing of resistant skin burns. J. Burn Care Rehab. 8:15, 1987.
12. Frykman, G.K., Taleisnik, J., Peters, G., et al.: Treatment of nonunited scaphoid fractures by pulsed electromagnetic field and cast. J. Hand Surg. 11A(3):344, 1986.
13. Glassman, L.S., McGrath, M.H., Bassett, C.A.L.: Effect of external pulsing electromagnetic fields on the healing of soft tissue. Ann. Plast. Surg. 16:287, 1986.
14. Goh, J.C.H., Bose, K., Orth, M.C. et al.: Effects of electrical stimulation on the biomechanical properties of fracture healing in rabbits. Clin. Orthop. 233:268, 1988.
15. Lavine, L.S., Grodzinsky, A.J.: Current concepts review: Electrical stimulation of repair of bone. J. Bone Joint Surg. 69(A):626, 1987.
16. Lundeberg, T., Kjartansson, J., Samuelsson, U.: Effect of electrical nerve stimulation on healing of ischaemic skin flaps. Lancet 2:712, 1988.

17. May, H.U., Nippel, F.J., Hansjurgens, A., et al.: Acceleration of ossification by means of interferential current. In Dixon, A.D. (ed.): Normal and Abnormal Bone Growth: Basic and Clinical Research. Alan R. Liss, New York, 1985.
18. Nannmark, U., Albrektsson, T.: Influence of direct currents on bone vascular supply. Scand. J. Plast. Reconstr. Surg. Hand Surg. 22:113, 1988.
19. Nessler, J.P., Mass, D.P.: Direct-current electrical stimulation of tendon healing in vitro. Clin. Orthop. 217:303, 1987.
20. Norton, L.A.: Pulsed electromagnetic field effects on chondroblast culture. Reconstr. Surg. Traumatol. 19:70, 1985.
21. Osterman, A.L., Bora, F.W.: Electrical stimulation applied to bone and nerve injuries in the upper extremity. Orthop. Clin. North Am. 17:353, 1986.
22. Paterson, D.C., Lewis, G.N., Cass, C.A.: Treatment of delayed union and nonunion with an implanted direct current stimulator. Clin. Orthop. 148:117, 1980.
23. Pollack, S.R.: Bioelectrical properties of bone. Orthop. Clin. North Am. 15:3, 1984.
24. Raji, A.M.: An experimental study of the effects of pulsed electromagnetic field (diapulse) on nerve repair. J. Hand Surg. 9B: 105, 1984.
25. Raji, A.R.M., Bowden, R.E.M.: Effects of high-peak pulsed electromagnetic field on the degeneration and regeneration of the common peroneal nerve in rats. J. Bone Joint Surg. 65B:478, 1983.
26. Stromberg, B.B.: Effects of electrical currents on wound contraction. Ann. Plast. Surg. 21:121, 1988.
27. Zoltan, J.D.: Electrical stimulation of bone: An overview. Semin. Orthop. 1:242, 1986.

STEROID EFFECTS

1. Anderton, J.M., Orth, M. CH., Helm, R.: Multiple joint osteonecrosis following short-term steroid therapy. J. Bone Joint Surg. 64A(1):139, 1982.
2. Baxter, J.D., Forsham, P.H.: Tissue effects of glucocorticoids. Am. J. Med. 53:573, 1972.
3. Behrens, F., Shepard, N., Mitchell, N.: Alteration of rabbit articular cartilage by intra-articular injections of glucocorticoids. J. Bone Joint Surg. 57A(1):70, 1975.
4. Bell, M.J., McMurtry, R.Y.: Volar intercalated segment instability as a result of spontaneous rupture of the supporting ligaments of the wrist due to longterm systemic steroid medication. J. Hand Surg. 10B(3):395, 1985.
5. Avioli, L.V., Peck, W., Ciennari, C., et al: Round table discussion: corticosteroids. Calcif. Tissue Int. 36:4, 1984.
6. Ehrlich, H.P., Hunt, T.K.: Effects of cortisone and vitamin A on wound healing. Ann. Surg. 167(3):324, 1968.
7. Fisher, D.E., Bickel, W.H.: Corticosteroid-induced avascular necrosis: A clinical study of seventy-seven patients. J. Bone Joint Surg. 53A(5):859, 1971.
8. Ismail, A.M., Balakrishnan, R., Rajakumar, M.K.: Rupture of patellar ligament after steroid infiltration. J. Bone Joint Surg. 51B(3):503, 1969.
9. Kleinman, M., Gross, A.E.: Achilles tendon rupture following steroid injection. J. Bone Joint Surg. 65A(9):1345, 1983.
10. Mankin, H.J., Conger, K.A.: The acute effects of intra-articular hydrocortisone on articular cartilage in rabbit. J. Bone Joint Surg. 48A(7):1383, 1966.
11. Noyes, F.R., Grood, E.S., Nussbaum, N.S., et al: Effect of intra-articular corticosteroids on ligament properties: A biomechanical and histological study in rhesus knees. Clin. Orthop. 123:197, 1977.
12. Noyes, F., Nussbaum, N.S., Torvik, P.J., et al.: Biomechanical and ultrastructural changes in ligaments and tendons after local corticosteroid injections. J. Bone Joint Surg. 57A(6):876, 1975.
13. Vogel, H.G.: Correlation between tensile strength and collagen content in rat skin. Effect of age and cortisol treatment. Connect. Tissue Res. 2:177, 1974.

CHAPTER

3

Epidemiology of Hand Injuries in Sports

Arthur C. Rettig, M.D.
Ramon O. Ryan, M.D.
Jennifer A. Stone, A.T., C.

This chapter addresses itself to the prevalence of various hand injuries in a number of different sports. A literature review, data from the Olympic Training Center in Colorado Springs, and the experience over a 1-year period from the Methodist Sports Medicine Center in Indianapolis have been utilized to draw a perception of the types of injuries and the sports with which they are most commonly associated. It is hoped that this chapter will give practitioners a greater understanding of the types of hand injuries they may expect to encounter when dealing with a variety of sports. The diagnosis and treatments of these injuries are discussed in subsequent chapters.

Literature Review

In a study at the Cleveland Clinic by Bergfeld and colleagues, a series of 113 hand and wrist injuries were examined.[1] There were 13 sprains, 4 dislocations, and 96 fractures. Ninety-seven of the injuries occurred in football, 6 in soccer, 3 in wrestling, 3 in baseball, 2 in basketball, 1 in ice hockey, and 1 in rugby. Metacarpal fractures were the most common (38) of the 96 fractures. Also noted were 27 injuries to the thumb, 32 to the wrist, and 14 to the fingers. Fractures of the distal radius (12) and the scaphoid (11) were the most common wrist injuries. Ulnar collateral ligament tears (12) and proximal phalangeal fractures (10) were the most common thumb disorders.

In an article evaluating athletic injuries, DeHaven and Lintner described several hand injuries based on data obtained from a population of 3,431 cases treated at the University of Rochester's sports medicine department.[3] Hand injuries represented 5 percent (171) of all cases treated. Injuries occurred more often in men (151) than in women (20). The most common injury was fracture (102), representing 60 percent of all hand injuries. Sixty-three of the fractures occurred in football. There were 72 phalangeal fractures, 27 metacarpal fractures, 2 carpal fractures, and 7 fracture/dislocations. Sprains and strains of the hand made up 2.1 percent (58) and wrist sprains/strains 0.6 percent (17) of all injuries in males. Sprain/strain injuries accounted for a significant amount of the hand injuries—43.36 percent. The incidence in females of both hand and wrist sprain/strain injuries was approximately 1.5 percent of total injuries.

In an article by Dawson and Pullos, softball and baseball injuries to the hand, excluding the wrist, were reported from a 150-bed general hospital in a surburban area over a 3½-month period.[2] Of the 153 patients in the study, the greatest number were injured in June at the beginning of baseball season. The majority of injuries were caused by direct hits with the ball; only a small percentage occurred secondary to striking another player or objects. Sprains accounted for 33½ percent of the injuries (53) and fractures represented 46.2 percent (73). Other injuries noted were fracture/dislocations (6), dislocations (10), tendon ruptures (7), lacerations (3), and contusions (6). It was also observed that a greater percentage of injuries occurred when a larger softball (16 inch) was used, probably due to failure to use a glove with the larger ball. The 153 baseball/softball injuries represented 2.2 percent of the total number of cases treated in this hospital's emergency room over the 3½-month period.

Ellsasser and Stein reported on significant hand injuries that occurred over a 15-year period in a professional football team.[4] There were 46 major hand injuries involving 21 offensive and 25 defensive players. Fingers were injured most frequently (12), with three fractures, seven dislocations, one profundus tendon avulsion, and a fracture/dislocation. There were nine wrist injuries, five fractures, two fracture/dislocations, one dislocation, and one sprain. Hand injuries consisted of eight metacarpal fractures and one laceration. There were five ulnar collateral ligament sprains, two metacarpophalangeal dislocations, and two Bennett fractures of the carpometacarpal joint of the thumb. The authors stated that the majority of phalangeal injuries involved attempts to handle the football. Injuries involving the metacarpal and wrist regions were nearly all sustained in tackling activities. In this group, 12 of the 14 injuries occurred in defensive players, 7 of whom were linebackers.

Sixteen case reports of hand injuries in sports were presented by Kalenak and co-workers.[6] Eleven of these injuries were fractures, eight of which involved phalanges, and four were fracture/dislocations. They also noted two boutonnière deformities, two mallet fingers, a ruptured profundus tendon, and a ruptured radial collateral ligament of the thumb. Eight of the 16 injuries occurred in football.

Nutton and Guy reported eight rugby injuries involving the hand.[9] There were seven dislocations of proximal interphalangeal joints, all occurring during tackling, and one fracture of a metacarpal secondary to a hyperextension injury. Four of the seven dislocations developed boutonnière deformities. The major mechanism of injury was the catching of the fingers in the opponent's clothing.

A note in the *Journal of the American Medical Association* by Kirk noted two lacerations occurring to the side of the hand in a basketball tournament secondary to hitting a sharp edge on the rim of a basketball hoop.[7]

Ho and associates described aneurysms of the hand following sports injuries in two athletes.[5] One occurred in a 31-year-old male lacrosse player after he was struck in the left hand with a lacrosse ball and the other in a 35-year-old female volleyball player who bruised her palm while playing.

The National Athletic Trainers' Association compiled statistics for injuries occurring in high school football during the 1986 season.[8] Of the 636,279 injuries, 92,655 involved the forearm, wrist, and hand (14.6 percent). In general, strains/sprains, contusions, and lacerations made up 88.3 percent and fractures 6.6 percent of all injuries.

Methodist Sports Medicine Center Survey

In a 1-year survey of all hand injuries presenting to the Methodist Sports Medicine Center in Indianapolis, 213 injuries were seen in 207 people. This represented approximately 3 percent of the total number of new patients seen at the center during this period. There were 125 fractures, 13 dislocations, 45 sprains, and 27 other injuries. Twenty-eight different types of injuries were seen and 29 different sports were represented (Tables 3–1 and 3–2). Forty-one of the injuries were suffered by females (19.25%), and 172 injuries occurred in males (80.75%).

Eight sports were selected from the 29 sports represented in the survey to be evaluated more closely (softball and baseball were combined). These sports represented 84.04% (179) of the total hand injuries (213) seen. All of these sports had five or more hand injuries represented in the surveyed year. The pattern in the subgroup with regard to quantity and type of injury was the same as in the overall group, i.e., fractures were the most common, with 55.31 percent (99); followed by sprains, 21.11 percent (36); others, 11.7 percent (20); and finally, dislocations, 7.26 percent (13). Table 3–3 gives the incidence of fractures, dislocations, sprains, and other injuries in each of eight sports expressed as both a number and a percentage. The total number of injuries per sport and the percentage of injuries in each sport, as compared with the total number of hand injuries recorded (213), is also presented. A large range in days lost from competition/practice due to injury can be seen for each of the sports, as would be anticipated with a variety of injuries in each sport. Overall, for all sports in this study, the average number of days lost was 16.74, with a range from 0 to 84. In the eight sport subgroup, the average number of days lost was somewhat higher (17.98), but the range was the same.

Table 3–4 lists each of the eight sports in reference to site of injury and the percentage that each site represents in comparison with the other

Table 3–1 HAND INJURIES SEEN OVER A ONE-YEAR PERIOD—METHODIST SPORTS MEDICINE CENTER

Injury	Number
Carpal tunnel syndrome	2
DeQuervain's disease	6
Tenosynovitis—wrist	10
Ganglion	3
Mallet finger	4
Boutonnière deformity	2
Fracture—distal radius	13
Fracture—ulnar styloid	2
Fracture—lunate	4
Fracture—triquetrum	2
Fracture—hamate	3
Fracture—metacarpals	39
Fracture—Bennett's	1
Fracture—phalanges	41
Fracture dislocation—PIP*	1
Dislocation—thumb	2
Dislocation—MP†	1
Dislocation—thumb MP	1
Dislocation—PIP	8
Dislocation—thumb PIP	1
Sprain—wrist	9
Sprain—hand	1
Sprain—finger	10
Sprain—collateral ligament thumb	12
Sprain—gamekeeper's thumb	3
Sprain—MP	8
Sprain—PIP	3

* PIP = proximal interphalangeal
† MP = metacarpophalangeal

injury locations in the same sport. Football caused both the greatest number of injuries and the highest percentage of fractures (52.52%), dislocations (61.54%), and sprains (38.89%) of the eight sports. Basketball was the next highest in those three areas, with fractures representing 32.32 percent; dislocations, 15.38 percent; and sprains, 25 percent. Baseball/softball accounted for 13.13 percent of fractures and 16.66 percent of sprains but caused no dislocations. Wrestling caused a relatively high percentage of dislocations (15.38%). Fractures made up two thirds of the hand injuries in baseball/softball, football, and basketball. Football caused a relatively high percentage of dislocations, with 10 percent of its injuries falling into that category. Only 4.17 percent of basketball injuries were dislocations. Sprains were common in all three sports, constituting approximately 20% of injuries in football and in basketball and 30 percent in baseball/softball.

Another parameter that was evaluated was the locale in which the injuries occurred, i.e., practice, competition, recreational competition, and others. Table 3–5 shows the number and percentage of injuries that occurred in each situation.

Table 3–2 NUMBER OF HAND INJURIES PER SPORT—METHODIST SPORTS MEDICINE CENTER

Sport	Number
Aerobics	1
Baseball*	10
Basketball†	48
Cycling	1
Bowling	4
Cheerleading	2
Dodgeball	1
Football†	78
Golf†	5
Gymnastics†	6
Hockey	2
Horseback riding	1
Ice skating	2
Jogging	1
Kickball	1
Physical education class	1
Racquetball	2
Rodeo	1
Roller skating	3
Rugby	1
Skate boarding	1
Skiing	1
Soccer	3
Softball*	10
Swimming	1
Tennis†	7
Volleyball†	7
Wrestling†	8
Weight lifting	1

* Combined into one sport—baseball/softball.
† Included in eight-sport group.

Table 3–3 EIGHT SPORT SUBGROUP, METHODIST SPORTS MEDICINE CENTER SURVEY—TYPES OF INJURY

Sport	Fractures	Dislocations	Sprains	Other	Days Lost	Total No. of Injuries*	Percentage of Total Injuries (213†)
Baseball/Softball	13/65‡	0/0	6/30.00	1/5.00	18.62/0–63§	20	9.39
Basketball	32/66.67	2/4.17	9/18.75	5/10.42	17.31/0–63	48	22.54
Football	52/66.67	8/10.26	14/17.95	4/5.13	13.56/0–84	78	36.62
Golf	2/40.00	0/0	2/40.00	1/20.00	7.00/0–28	5	2.32
Gymnastics	3/50.00	0/0	2/33.33	1/16.67	28.00/0–84	6	2.82
Tennis	3/42.86	0/0	0/0	4/57.14	27.29/14–56	7	3.29
Volleyball	1/14.29	1/14.29	3/42.86	2/28.57	18.67/0–77	7	3.29
Wrestling	3/37.50	2/25.00	1/12.50	2/25.00	13.42/0–42	8	3.76
Total	99/55.31	13/7.26	36/20.11	20/11.17	17.98/0–84	179	84.04

* In eight sport subgroup.
† In all sports.
‡ Number/percent.
§ Average/range.

Table 3–4 EIGHT-SPORT SUBGROUP, METHODIST SPORTS MEDICINE CENTER SURVEY—SITE OF INJURY

Sport	Total No. of Injuries	Wrist	Thumb	Hand	Finger
Baseball/Softball	20	7/35.00*	5/25.00	2/10.00	6/30.00
Basketball	48	15/31.25	2/4.17	13/27.08	18/37.50
Football	78	15/18.99	8/10.13	20/25.32	35/44.30
Golf	5	4/80.00	0	0	1/20.00
Gymnastics	6	5/83.33	0	0	1/16.67
Tennis	7	5/71.43	1/14.29	1/14.29	0
Volleyball	7	2/28.57	2/28.57	0	3/42.86
Wrestling	8	1/11.11	1/11.11	2/22.22	5/55.55
Total	179	54/30.17	19/10.61	38/21.23	69/38.55

* Number/percent.

It is interesting to compare the location of fractures in various sports. Football had a high percentage of metacarpal fractures (19/48.72%) compared with all 29 sports, and basketball had 30.77 percent (12) of all the metacarpal fractures. Basketball had eight scaphoid fractures (38.10%) while football had six (28.57%). Phalangeal fractures were high in football (22/50%), basketball had eight (19.51%), and baseball, four (9.09%). Hamate fractures were seen in two sports—golf (2) and baseball/softball (1). Four lunate fractures were noted: two in baseball/softball and two in basketball. A triquetrum fracture was also reported in these two sports.

Certain trends as to the site of injury were observed. A low total number of injuries occurred in golf, gymnastics, and tennis, but a predominance of wrist injuries occurred: 80 percent, 83.33 percent and 71.43 percent, respectively. Wrestling had a high percentage of finger injuries (55.55%); football had 44.30 percent; volleyball, 42.86 percent, and basketball, 37.50 percent. In all of these sports, fingers were the most frequent site of injury. Football, basketball, and baseball/softball all had a fairly

Table 3–5 EIGHT SPORT SUBGROUP, METHODIST SPORTS MEDICINE CENTER SURVEY—SITUATION IN WHICH INJURY OCCURRED

	Number	Percent
Practice	57	28.2
Competition	83	41.1
Recreational competition	32	15.8
Other	30	14.9

well-distributed site-of-injury profile, with finger injuries more prevalent than wrist, hand, or thumb injuries in football and basketball. Baseball/softball had the highest percentage (25%) of thumb injuries.

Olympic Training Center Survey

The Olympic Training Center in Colorado Springs, Colorado, recorded 8311 injuries from January 1, 1977, to October 31, 1986. Seven hundred twenty-nine of the injuries reported were hand/wrist injuries, representing 8.77 percent of all injuries recorded. Thirty-six sports were represented in their records in 731,004 athletic days accrued over this time period.

The highest percentage of hand injuries occurred in roller hockey with 30 percent (6 of 20 injuries). The highest number of injuries occurred in judo with 1691 total injuries and 101 hand injuries (5.97%). Boxing had 81 hand injuries and wrestling, 82 hand injuries, which represented 17.42 percent and 7.19 percent of total injuries, respectively. Other sports with a high percentage of hand injuries were basketball (16.95%/20 of 118), ice hockey (12.16%/53 of 463), softball (24.49%/12 of 49), baseball (25%/1 of 4), volleyball (13.17%/64 of 486), and weight lifting (12.93%/30 of 232).

Table 3–6 lists the number of total injuries, hand/wrist injuries, percentage of injuries that were to hand/wrist, and the sport they occurred in over the 10-year period at the Olympic Training Center.

Tables 3–7 and 3–8 show the sports with the highest percentage of hand injuries and the sports with the greatest number of total injuries. Fifteen sports are listed, and they account for more than 85 percent of all hand injuries noted over the 10-year period at the Olympic Training Center. Injuries to the fingers were the most prevalent, occurring in 214 of the 667 hand injuries within the 15 sport group. There were 204 wrist, 143 thumb, and 106 hand injuries. Sprains were the most common injuries, representing 325 of the 667 (48.73%) hand injuries in this group. The next most frequent injuries were contusions (14.69%/98) and fractures (10.19%/68).

Tables 3–7 and 3–8 focus on the 15 sports that had the highest percentage of hand injuries and compare these sports as to site and type of injury. Fingers suffered the most dislocations and about the same number of lacerations as did hands. The fingers also had the highest number of overall injuries. The fingers had the highest number of fractures, but hands also had a high number of fractures (metacarpal). Hands suffered the most contusions. Wrists, thumbs, and fingers all suffered approximately the same number of sprains.

Judo, with the greatest number of hand injuries (101), demonstrated a high percentage for all four sites of injury. Judo had the highest percentage of wrist and thumb injuries, 20.10% and 18.88%, respectively. It had the third highest number of finger injuries and the fourth highest number of hand injuries. (It should be remembered that the highest number of injuries in general was also reported in judo.) Team handball had a high percentage of injuries to the fingers, representing 18.23 percent of all hand injuries. Boxing had the highest percentage of hand injuries—31.13 percent. Vol-

Table 3–6 THIRTY-SIX SPORT GROUP, OLYMPIC TRAINING CENTER SURVEY—TOTAL HAND INJURIES

Sport	Total No. of Injuries	No. of Hand Injuries	Percent Hand Injuries
Archery	29	3	10.34
Athletics (track and field)	117	5	4.27
Baseball*	4	1	25.00
Basketball†	118	20	16.95
Biathleton	2	0	0
Boxing*	465	81	17.42
Canoeing/kayak	5	0	0
Cycling†	535	47	8.79
Fencing†	23	2	8.70
Artistic gymnastics†	236	28	11.86
Rhythmic gymnastics	65	4	6.25
Field hockey†	470	24	5.11
Ice hockey†	436	53	12.16
Roller hockey	20	6	30.00
Luge	13	0	0
Modern pentathalon	11	0	0
Racquetball	45	2	4.44
Rowing	0	0	0
Shooting†	206	24	11.63
Figure skating	14	0	0
Roller speed skating	295	7	2.37
Ice speed skating	92	3	3.26
Alpine skiing	12	1	8.33
Freestyle skiing	3	0	0
Nordic skiing	20	2	10.00
Soccer†	354	19	5.37
Softball*	49	12	24.49
Swimming	80	7	8.75
Synchronized swimming	21	1	4.76
Tae kwon do	166	9	5.42
Team handball†	689	75	10.89
Volleyball†	486	64	13.17
Water polo	170	15	8.82
Weight lifting†	232	30	12.93
Wrestling†	1141	82	7.19
Judo†	1691	101	5.97

* Baseball and softball were combined in the 15 sport subgroup.
† Included in the 15 sport subgroup with most frequent hand injuries.

leyball, wrestling, and team handball each recorded an 11.18 percent incidence of thumb injuries when compared with the other 15 sports, and volleyball represented 15.42 percent of all finger injuries in this group.

Team handball, boxing, and ice hockey had the greatest percentage of fractures, 14.8 percent, 13.8 percent, and 13.28 percent, respectively. Dislocations were seen most frequently in volleyball (27.27%), team handball (18.18%), and basketball (18.18%). Judo led the field again with sprains (17.53%), but wrestling (15.38%), volleyball (14.46%), and team handball (14.46%) also had high percentages. Boxing recorded the highest percentage of contusions (28.57%), almost double that of the next highest—ice hockey, with 16.33%.

CHAPTER

4

Common Athletic Digital Joint Injuries of the Hand

Frank C. McCue, III, M.D.
Jorge M. Cabrera, M.D.

Injuries to the hand are the most common type of athletic trauma. The hand is used in various ways in a majority of sports and is characteristically held in front of the athlete to absorb initial contact.[35, 36, 38] The joints are extremely well designed to provide stability, mobility, and sensibility but remain vulnerable to extremes of external force and internal stress that can damage the supporting soft-tissue structures. There is a tendency to minimize the severity and importance of these injuries, since the functional loss does not usually completely disable the athlete. This is particularly true of the young, poorly supervised athlete who tends to return to vigorous activity and unprotected use before adequate healing has occurred.

The key to proper care of hand injury is early diagnosis and accurate precise treatment followed by an appropriate rehabilitation program and adequate protection on return to activity.[19] Management of these injuries may have a significant impact not only on competitive activities but also on the athlete's selection of an occupation in later life. It is also psychologically important that athletes be allowed to return to their particular sport as quickly as possible.

Conservative treatment is preferable for the majority of injuries to the hand. Most patients can rapidly return to their normal activities with adequate protection. However, even seemingly minor injuries must be carefully evaluated and treated by a physician. Primary surgical repair is indicated in a small percentage of patients, and secondary reconstructive surgery may be necessary in an even smaller number. When surgical repair is indicated, it is important for the surgeon to be well trained and familiar with hand and wrist surgical techniques.

Metacarpophalangeal Joint of the Finger

ANATOMY

The metacarpophalangeal (MCP) joint is a condyloid joint in which the metacarpal head is narrow dorsally with a widened volar flare, thus increasing its distal surface, which increases the intra-articular contact with the base of the proximal phalanx as flexion increases. This creates a cam type effect due to the head contour, with the collateral ligaments being loose in extension. With increasing flexion, the collateral ligaments become more taut, which allows abduction and adduction in extension and stability in full flexion in the lateral direction. Because of this, the joint should be splinted in at least 45° of flexion to maintain ligamentous length. Shortening of a collateral ligament will cause limitation of flexion, which creates an appreciable functional deficit that is difficult or impossible to overcome. This optimal position may be altered in certain injuries due to the necessity of positioning, requiring a greater degree of extension; early motion should be carried out if at all possible.

The capsule is a reeler in the normal joint dorsally, but a loose insertion of the extensor digitorum communis to the base of the proximal phalanx is present. This capsule may thicken significantly when reactive conditions are present. The volar plate has a thick fibrocartilaginous distal portion attached to the base of the proximal phalanx with a membranous proximal portion that allows adequate room for the proximal phalanx in flexion. This volar plate is securely attached to the proximal phalanx with the deep transverse metacarpal ligaments supporting the proximal phalanges. There are no sturdy proximal check rein ligaments present as are found in the proximal interphalangeal (PIP) joint. The lateral bands of the intrinsic muscles provide secondary reinforcement and primarily give dynamic abduction and adduction when the joint is in extension.

The MCP joints of the fingers are well protected due to this natural ligamentous support and their protective position at the base of the fingers.

DISLOCATIONS

The most common injury of the MCP joint is dorsal dislocation of the proximal phalanx, which is actually a volar displacement of the metacarpal head through a buttonhole rent in the volar plate between the lumbricals, long flexors, and other soft tissue structures in the palm of the hand. The mechanism of this injury is usually forced hyperextension of the digits, as occurs in striking the heel of an opponent in a diving attempt to tackle or in falling on the outstretched hand. The complete dorsal dislocation has been designated the "complex" or "irreducible dislocation" with the anatomic pattern making reduction extremely difficult, and in most cases, impossible by closed means.[21, 24, 46] The differential diagnosis of subluxation and dislocation is important, as an incomplete subluxation may be converted into a complete dislocation on attempted closed manipulation as described by McLaughlin.[43] The volar plate remains attached with the proximal phalanx in subluxation, and if the deformity is significantly increased by hyperextension or traction, the entire volar plate may slip dorsally and interpose between the base of the proximal phalanx and the metacarpal head, producing the "complete complex" or "irreducible dislocation." Reduction of the subluxation and occasionally the complete dislocation can be done by relaxing the flexor tendons with the wrist in volar flexion and creating a controlled increase of the deformity. A volar directed pressure to the dorsal base of the proximal phalanx by the physician's thumb forces it into the flexed position and through the rent in the capsule.

MCP dislocations are most commonly seen in the outer digits of the hand. Individually, the little finger and especially the index finger are most frequently affected, although all digits, and occasionally more than one, can be involved.[21, 24] The finger is angulated toward the more central digit in the index finger, ulnarly overlapping the adjacent long finger with volar dimpling of the skin in the area of the midpalmar crease. The MCP joint is held in slight extension with the distal joint in flexion, and a prominence is felt in the palm over the metacarpal head.

The volar plate ruptures in the membranous portion with the metacarpal head in the index finger displacing between the flexor tendons ulnarly and the lumbrical on the radial side (Fig. 4–1). The volar plate is impinged between the articular surfaces with the tightly displaced flexor tendons maintaining tension on the volar plate and the tight constriction about the neck of the metacarpal proximal to the bulbous articular surface. Longitudinal traction following this injury actually prevents reduction because of the nooselike constriction about the metacarpal neck in much the same fashion as a Chinese finger traction apparatus.

Radiographs may show widening of the joint space caused by interposition of the volar plate and occasionally a sesamoid may be visible within the joints. Occasional osteochondral fractures or injury to the articular surface may be visible, especially in the metacarpal head.

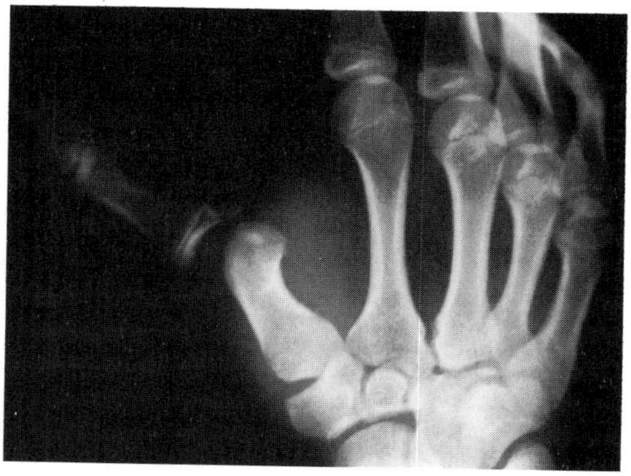

Figure 4–1 Complex dorsal dislocation of the index MCP joint. Note the radial lumbrical and neurovascular bundle and the nooselike effect of the flexor tendons ulnarly. (From Poznanski, A.K.: The Hand in Radiologic Diagnosis. Philadelphia, W.B. Saunders, 1984, p. 686.)

Treatment

The older the dislocation, the greater the likelihood of stiffness, pain, and degenerative arthritis.[46] However, satisfactory results have been reported as long as 6 months after the date of injury, although both dorsal and volar surgical approaches are usually necessary to correct the cases.[46]

While many surgeons still advocate dorsal incision, the complex volar structures that prevent reduction are dealt with more easily through the volar or volar midline incision.[21, 43, 46] The volar approach in the index finger is through an oblique palmar incision between the midpalmar and distal palmar creases extending radially to the midlateral line (Fig.4–2). Great care must be taken to prevent damage to the prominent palmar structures, especially the radial neurovascular bundle, which is stretched as it diagonally proceeds across the prominent metacarpal head.[21] This structure may be damaged at the time of injury and should be repaired under magnification.

The approach to the little finger is similar in the reversed position with the ulnar neurovascular bundle being more prominent. Tension is maintained by the dorsal displacement of the flexor tendons in the sheath with the volar plate being the main deterrent to reduction. Release of this sheath and the A-1 pulley relaxes this tension, and the volar plate is returned to the normal position as reduction occurs. After reduction, the joint is surprisingly stable, and early motion is desirable.[21] We maintain the MCP joint in approximately 30° of flexion until the reaction has abated, usually within 7 to 10 days. Then active flexion in this position is begun, with dorsal protective splinting for approximately 5 weeks to prevent extension or hyperextension. However, earlier active flexion may be possible as soft tissue reaction allows. If the finger is maintained in flexion for too long, full extension may never be regained. The patient should obtain complete flexion by the time the splint is removed.

COLLATERAL LIGAMENT INJURIES

Collateral ligament injuries of the MCP joint are not nearly as common or as disabling as those involving the PIP joints and are most often seen in the radial collateral ligament, usually in the ulnar three digits. The

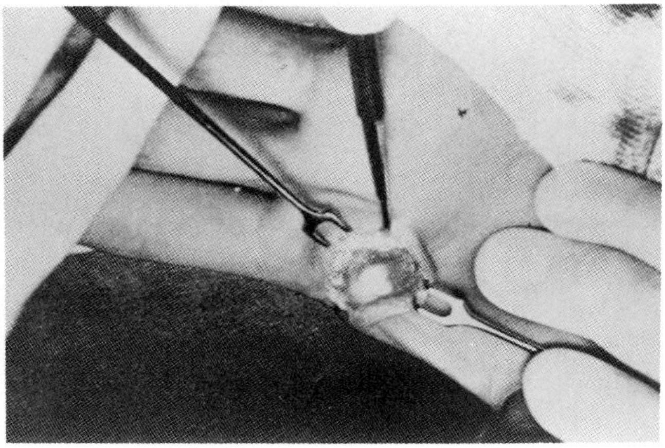

Figure 4–2 This operative picture demonstrates the volar incision most commonly advocated for reduction. If necessary, extension along the radial border of the palm provides greater exposure. (From McCue, F.C., Garroway, R.Y.: Sports Injuries to the Hand and Wrist. In: Schneider, R.C., Kennedy, J.C., Plant, M.L. (eds): Sports Injuries: Mechanisms, Prevention and Treatment. Baltimore, Williams & Wilkins, 1985, p. 750.)

mechanism of injury is deviation away from the injured collateral ligament, generally in some degree of flexion. Radial or ulnar control of the joint is maintained by the intrinsic muscles; consequently, lateral instability is not a usual functional problem. A history of trauma, direct point tenderness, and pain on lateral deviation are the most common diagnostic findings in the acute injury. Initial treatment should consist of immobilization in slight flexion for 3 weeks followed by buddy taping to the adjacent digits for an additional 3 weeks until the pain has abated, particularly during the athletic season. If symptoms persist, surgical reconstruction of the ligament may be necessary to obtain functional return.

This diagnosis should be entertained in cases of persistent discomfort in the area of the MCP joint with point tenderness, soft-tissue reaction, and thickening of the collateral ligament on clinical examination. If the symptoms are disabling and persist, surgery may be necessary for either repair or reconstruction of the ligament. Occasionally, an avulsion fracture, particularly of the distal attachment of the collateral ligament, may be seen interposed in the joint on the x-ray film.

RUPTURE OF THE EXTENSOR HOOD OF THE EXTENSOR DIGITORUM COMMUNIS

As the extensor digitorum communis and its associated extensor indicis proprius and extensor digiti quinti tendons pass over the metacarpal head, they are stabilized by the extensor hood or sagittal fibers. These structures arise from the extensor tendons and insert into the volar plate. The fibers move in a sagittal plane as the central tendons move in a distal proximal motion in MCP joint flexion and extension. This extensor hood has several functions, the most essential of which is centralization of the extensor tendons over the dorsal apex of the metacarpal head during MCP flexion and extension. This is of prime importance in the active motion of the MCP joint.

Rupture of the extensor hood is most common on the radial side, allowing ulnar deviation of the extensor tendon into the valley between the metacarpal heads. Subluxation or dislocation may occur following forceful flexion or extension of the fingers or blunt trauma to the metacarpal head. The patient will have good MCP joint flexion but incomplete active MCP extension and ulnar deviation of the involved digits. If the joint is passively extended to neutral, the tendon reduces, and the patient is able to hold the MCP joint in extension, even against resistance. This test will aid in differentiation between subluxation and division of the central extensor tendon. The middle finger is most commonly involved. A functionally disabling snapping of the tendon in certain individuals may be present as well.

Treatment

If diagnosed early, prior to contraction of the hood fibers, nonoperative treatment may be successful. The proximal phalanges of the involved digit, and most optimally, its radial associated digit, should be splinted in neutral position. PIP motion should be restricted. Exercise may be begun out of the splint at 3 weeks, but a protective splint should be continued except for these exercise periods for 6 to 8 weeks.

Acute tears are satisfactorily treated by a primary suture of the defect. This is usually accomplished under regional anesthesia through a longitudinal skin incision. Exact coaptation of the ruptured hood with interrupted sutures of nonabsorptive material will give consistently good results in cases in which the hood is sufficiently substantial. Postoperative immobilization is similar to that described for nonoperative treatment.

In delayed or subacute injuries, primary repair is generally possible but may be technically difficult due to thinning and retraction of the hood fibers. If repair is impossible owing to contracture or friability of the hood fibers and the considerable tension on joint flexion causing separation of the repair, other reconstructive procedures are available.

The central tendon must be accurately centered over the MCP joint and adequately stabilized to resist recurrence of the subluxation during MCP flexion. Release of the ulnar side of the hood may be necessary in chronic cases. A portion of the juncturae tendinum may be used in which the junctura of the ulnar side is lapped over the extensor tendon and sutured to the joint capsule on the radial side. Use of a slip of the extensor tendon on the radial side of the finger passed around the lumbrical and sutured back on itself is another operative possibility.

In one case, swelling continued to limit the ability of a quarterback to grip the football, and a large mass of granulation tissue had formed by the hypertrophic synovium in the tear. When this was removed and repair of the extensor hood was carried out, full return of function was obtained.

INTRA-ARTICULAR METACARPOPHALANGEAL JOINT FRACTURE

Metacarpal head fractures usually result from direct impact. Owing to the cancellous nature of the bone, extensive comminution is often present. If an appreciable portion of the articular surface is involved, open exploration and anatomic reduction and fixation with multiple small Kirschner wires (K-wires) may be necessary. The collateral ligaments and the volar plate figure prominently, both in the deformity and in attempts at closed reduction. These fractures are best exposed through a dorsal longitudinal incision. The articular impaction defects are generally left to fill in with fibrous tissue. Occasionally, if they are significant in size, the defects should be elevated and filled in with bone grafts from the distal radius. In some comminuted fractures, particularly those distal to the collateral ligament origin, an attempt at closed reduction with molding followed by early protected motion may be the treatment of choice unless joint stability is compromised.

Reconstructive surgery involving arthroplasty with or without a Silastic prosthesis is often necessary in the grossly disrupted joints following the intra-articular injury or after secondary degenerative arthritic changes have occurred. Epiphyseal arrest can occur following metacarpal head fractures in children. In these situations, the cosmetic impairment is generally greater than the functional loss.

Proximal Interphalangeal Joint of the Fingers

ANATOMY

The proximal interphalangeal (PIP) and distal interphalangeal (DIP) joints are quite similar anatomically. Both are hinged condylar joints having essentially one plane of motion—flexion and extension. The proximal and midphalangeal heads are bicondylar in contour, reciprocally fitting with the corresponding biconcave articular surfaces of the proximal middle phalanx and the proximal distal phalanx, respectively. They are supported radially and ulnarly by the corresponding collateral ligaments, which originate from a concave fossa on the respective radial and ulnar sides of the proximal and middle phalangeal heads. They insert across their respective joints into tubercle-like elevations, as well as to the most distal portion of the volar plate. The accessory collateral ligaments are more attenuated and essentially form a contiguous connection between the inferior portions of the collateral ligaments and the volar plate. Dorsally, the PIP joint is covered by the central slip of the extensor apparatus attaching on the dorsal tubercle of the middle phalanx (Fig. 4–3*B*,Q). The radial and ulnar lateral bands pass on either side of the central slip and all three structures are maintained together by the triangular ligament (Fig. 4–3*B*). The oblique retinacular ligament arises from the side of the proximal phalanx and passes lateral to the PIP joint capsule to join the lateral margin of the extensor lateral bands on the dorsal lateral aspect of the middle phalanx[29] (Fig. 4–3*A*,N). The transverse retinacular ligament is superficial to the oblique retinacular ligament arising from the volar aspect of the capsule and the flexor tendon sheath and passes dorsally to be attached to the lateral margins of the lateral bands of the extensor mechanism (Fig. 4–3*A*,O). Milford showed that Cleland's ligament arises from the joint capsule and adjacent bone deep to the transverse retinacular ligament and radiates proximally and distally dorsal to the neurovascular bundle.[11, 44] Grayson's ligament is a transversely directed sheet of fascia arising from the flexor tendon sheath that passes volarly to the neurovascular bundle.[11] The dorsal extensor apparatus of the DIP joint is composed of the confluence of both lateral bands and their oblique retinacular ligaments. They join to insert into the dorsal distal phalanx.

Volarly, the interphalangeal (IP) joints are very similar. The floor of the joints is composed of a thick fibrocartilaginous volar plate that is contiguous with the accessory collateral ligament and the collateral ligament proper. The distal attachment into the proximal volar base of the middle phalanx is quite firm. Proximally, the volar plate becomes attenuated centrally as it thickens laterally where it attaches to the loose areolar tissue of the proximal phalanx, forming the two check-rein ligaments. In the DIP joint, the volar plate is more firmly attached proximally.

The PIP joint is the most commonly injured joint of the hand. This is because of the significant long proximal and distal lever arms that place lateral and torque stresses on a hinge-type joint that has minimal lateral mobility.[37] The PIP joint is particularly important functionally, and any injury resulting in a fixed deformity, either in flexion or extension, can

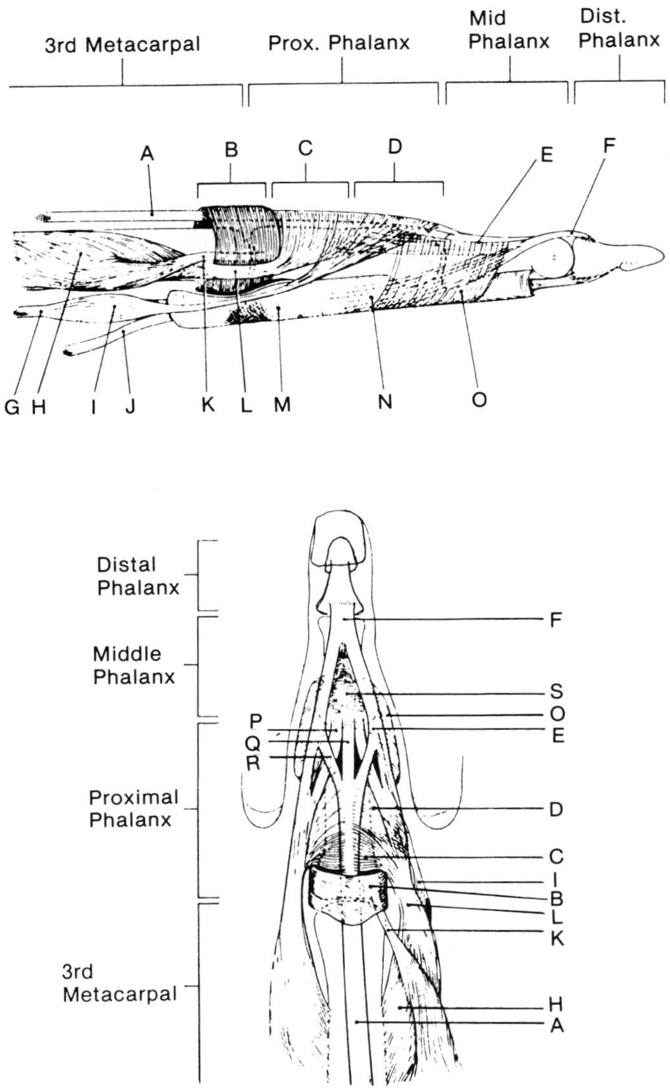

Figure 4–3 Diagrammatic representation (radial view, left middle finger) of the muscles, tendons, and fascia that directly influence the motion of the finger. *A,* Common extensor tendon; *B,* sagittal bands; *C,* transverse fibers of the interossei; *D,* oblique fibers of the interossei; *E,* lateral conjoined tendon; *F,* terminal tendon; *G,* flexor digitorum profundus tendon; *H,* interosseous muscle (second dorsal) deep head; *I,* lumbrical muscle; *J,* tendon of flexor digitorum superficialis; *K,* medial tendon, superficial head of second dorsal interosseous; *L,* lateral tendon of deep head of second dorsal interosseous muscle; *M,* fibrous flexor pulley; *N,* oblique retinacular ligament; *O,* transverse retinacular ligament; *P,* medial interosseous band; *Q,* central slip of the common extensor; *R,* lateral slip of the common extensor; *S,* triangular ligament. (From Smith, R.J.: Balance and kinetics of the fingers under normal and pathological conditions. Clin. Orthop. 104:92, 1974.)

cause significant disability as well as predispose the athlete to re-injury. It is easy to ignore or minimize the severity of these injuries, and athletes often return to competition prematurely without appropriate protection.

Injuries to the PIP joint can be classified as articular fractures, fracture-dislocations, dislocations, collateral ligament injuries, boutonnière deformities, volar plate injuries, and pseudo-boutonnière deformities. Each of these diagnoses will be discusssed individually.

ARTICULAR FRACTURES

Intra-articular fractures of the PIP joint are quite common and may involve either the proximal phalangeal head or the middle phalangeal base. The most common isolated fracture of the PIP joint is the condylar fracture, which can be classified as single, bicondylar, or osteocondylar. The single condylar fracture (Fig. 4–4) may have a long or short oblique fracture component. Other fracture patterns seen are T-bicondylar fractures, middle phalanx intra-articular fractures, and comminuted fractures.

General principles of hand fracture management dictate that one first attempt conservative management as long as this will not compromise the ultimate result. Therefore, as a general rule, intra-articular fractures that are nondisplaced or minimally displaced (less than 1 mm), osteochondral fractures with less than 2 mm displacement, nondisplaced dorsal or volar chip avulsion fractures of the middle phalanx, and small undisplaced osteochondral fractures of the proximal phalangeal head may be treated by splinting or casting. The finger may be placed in an aluminum gutter splint with the PIP joint flexed 30° for 3 weeks, at which time protected active flexion exercises can be started. Splinting should continue during athletic participation for an additional 4 to 6 weeks or until full range of motion is obtained without any tenderness over the site of injury. It is important to follow these fractures with weekly roentgenograms for the first 2 weeks to insure maintenance of reduction. If there is any question as to loss of reduction, closed reduction with percutaneous K-wire pinning or open reduction with pinning of the substantial fracture patterns may be performed. Athletic participation may be allowed in certain stable fractures. In unstable fractures, it is best to wait until significant healing has occurred at 3 to 4 weeks before allowing the athlete to return to competition. It

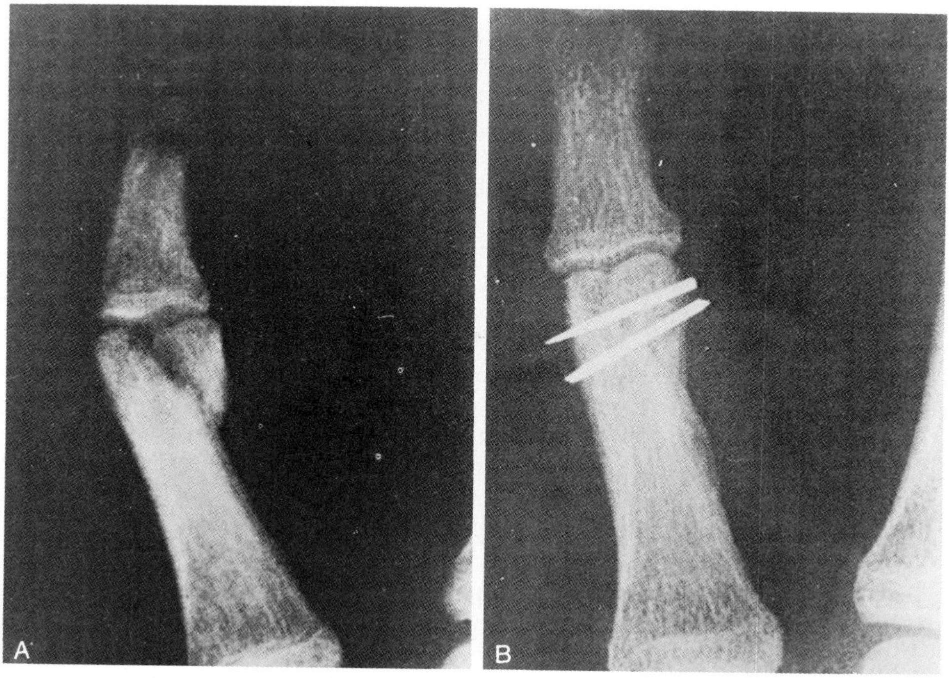

Figure 4–4 *A*, On this preoperative roentgenogram note the displaced single condylar fracture. *B*, Postoperative reduction with internal fixation. (From McCue, F.C., Garroway, R.Y.: Sports injuries to the hand and wrist. In Schneider, R.C., Kennedy, J.C., Plant, M.L. (eds.): Sports Injuries: Mechanisms, Prevention and Treatment. Baltimore, Williams & Wilkins, 1985, pp. 752 and 753.)

would be difficult to justify loss of reduction in an intra-articular fracture because of premature athletic participation.

Indications for surgical treatment of intra-articular fractures include displaced single condylar fractures, displaced T-bicondylar fractures, dorsal or volar middle phalangeal base fractures involving greater than 35 to 40 percent of the articular surface with 3 mm or more of displacement, and comminuted fractures with large fragments. Treatment must be individualized: one cannot percutaneously pin after closed reduction in all cases, and one should not always attempt open reduction and internal fixation. Closed reduction followed by percutaneous K-wire pinning can usually be achieved in a single condylar fracture if it is not significantly displaced. Sometimes, a K-wire can be inserted into the displaced fragment to lever it into a reduced position for internal fixation. If there is any difficulty with this method, one should not hesitate to open the fracture from a dorsal approach to gain adequate reduction.

Open reduction can generally be performed on the PIP through either a dorsal or a midaxial approach, depending on the location of the pathology. Dorsal exposures through a straight longitudinal or semilunar skin incision can be utilized for dorsal middle phalanx fractures, single or T-condylar fractures, and avulsion fractures of the extensor apparatus. After exposure of the dorsal aspect of the joint, one can either split the central extensor slip longitudinally or expose the area through a dorsal radial or dorsal ulnar approach between the oblique retinacular ligament and the inferior border of the lateral band. This will allow adequate reduction of the fragments, and internal fixation can be effected in single condylar fractures with parallel 0.035 K-wires (see Fig. 4–5). In T-condylar fractures, one can attempt diagonal cross-pinning or parallel pinning of the bicondylar fragments, thereby converting the fractures into two fragments, and then adding a third wire in a diagonal fashion. The middle phalanx dorsal fractures are usually attached to a central slip of the extensor apparatus. It is thus crucial to re-attach the fragment using either one or two 0.028 or 0.035 Kirschner wires or a Bunnell suture with 4.0 pull-out wires, which can be tied over a button volarly.

Comminuted fractures are often difficult to manage and usually have a poor prognosis, no matter what treatment is provided. In many cases, the severity of comminution precludes any attempt at open reduction. Generally, if large fragments are noted, an attempt at open reduction is warranted with cross-pinning with K-wires. At the very least, it will provide restoration of bone length and alignment, allowing easier secondary reconstruction if arthrosis becomes incapacitating. If the fracture is severely comminuted, one should attempt molding or closed reduction to improve alignment and splinting or casting for short-term immobilization of 1½ to 2 weeks, at which time early motion can be started.

It is important to emphasize that in open reductions of finger fractures, the dissection must be performed with great care, particularly in condylar fractures that are singly attached by the collateral ligament. Injury to this area of the collateral ligament can jeopardize the blood supply to that condylar fragment and result in avascular necrosis. Postoperative management generally involves either casting or splinting of the finger with the PIP joint in approximately 25 to 30° of flexion for 3 weeks.

Sufficient fracture stability and healing can be assumed when the site is no longer tender to palpation and when roentgenographic evidence of callus deposition or fracture line consolidation is noted, usually within 2 to 4 weeks. At this time, protective flexion exercises are instituted. Again, athletic participation may be allowed with appropriate splinting and protective padding after discontinuation of initial immobilization and removal of internal fixation.

FRACTURE-DISLOCATIONS

Fracture-dislocations are common in athletes. They can take the form of dorsal or volar dislocation with or without collateral ligament tears. The mechanism of injury is an axially directed force coupled with either dorsal or volar forces. In combination injuries, an additional angular force allows injury to the collateral ligament. This mechanism of injury is quite common in football, basketball, and baseball.

The dorsal dislocation of the middle phalanx with a volar lip fracture is the most common fracture-dislocation of the PIP joint.[35, 42, 50] The patient usually presents either with a fusiform swelling of the PIP joint after reduction on the field by the trainer or a teammate or with obvious dorsal deformity. Closed reduction should be performed after digital block or Bier block anesthesia.

Dorsal fracture-dislocations can be classified as stable or unstable. Stable dorsal fracture-dislocations usually have a small volar fragment representing less than 35 to 40 percent of the articular surface. The main portion of the collateral ligaments remains attached to the middle phalanx. Unstable dorsal fracture-dislocations, on the other hand, have a significant volar lip fragment of greater than 35 to 40 percent of the articular surface. Thus, the collateral ligaments remain attached to the volar fragment. In this instance, instability is due both to the lack of volar articular surface and to the lack of collateral ligament support.

Treatment depends on the stability assessment and on the degree of fracture displacement. Those fractures that have concentric reduction of the articular surfaces with less than 2 to 3 mm of displacement or fracture separation can be treated with dorsal splinting of the PIP joint in 30° of flexion for 3 weeks. This is followed by buddy taping as additional protection for another 2 to 3 weeks. One should follow these patients with weekly roentgenograms over the first 2 weeks to insure that displacement has not progressed. If there is any question of progression of displacement, a more aggressive surgical approach should be undertaken. Athletes with significant dorsal fragment size should not be allowed to engage in competitive activities until sufficient healing has occurred (approximately 2 to 3 weeks). One can usually determine healing by the degree to which tenderness has subsided after a period of immobilization. If significant tenderness is still present after 2 to 3 weeks, the athlete should not be allowed to return to vigorous activity. The patient should also be informed that it may take several months for significant swelling and stiffness to subside.

For unstable or significantly displaced fractures of greater than 2 to 3 mm, several management philosophies exist. Some physicians use dynamic skeletal traction devices, a method that requires skill in Kirschner wire placement as well as thorough follow-up.[2, 12, 51] The authors do not feel that this method can be satisfactorily utilized by most surgeons. MacElfrish, Dobyns, and O'Brien have shown very good results with their dynamic extension block splinting technique in fractures involving 30 percent or less of the articular surface.[33]

Open reduction and internal fixation are ideally done through volar or lateral approaches for large volar lip fragments of greater than 35 to 40 percent of the articular surface allowing accurate reduction for fixation. Fixation can be achieved with 0.028 or 0.035 Kirschner wires or Bunnell's sutures with a 4-0 pull-out wire tied over a dorsal button. Postoperative immobilization with a gutter aluminum splint over the volar aspect of the finger can be maintained with the PIP joint held in 20 to 30° of flexion for a total of 3 weeks, at which time protective gentle active exercise is begun in flexion, avoiding extension beyond 30°. If pull-out wires were utilized, they can be removed after 3 to 4 weeks and more active flexion and extension exercises can be instituted. If the fragment is quite comminuted and the volar fragment is of significant size, a volar plate arthroplasty is advocated by Eaton.[16] The volar plate is advanced into the defect in the middle phalanx base created by debridement of the comminuted fragments. A 4-0 Bunnell wire suture is utilized with a pull-out wire for fixation with a dorsal button tied over the finger. A 0.035 transarticular K-wire may be utilized for added immobilization to prevent dorsal subluxation. Postoperatively, the patient is started on protective flexion exercises 2 to 3 weeks after removal of the transarticular K-wire. Full extension beyond 30° is avoided until 4 weeks postoperatively, at which time the pull-out wires are removed and active flexion and extension exercises are instituted. The patient should regain full extension by the fifth week after surgery. If an extension deficit persists, dynamic splinting and more aggressive extension exercises are instituted.

If a collateral ligament injury is associated with either dorsal or volar fracture-dislocations, it should be repaired with direct sutures or a 4-0 pull-out wire technique. The volar plate should be checked for tears and repaired if necessary.

Volar-fracture dislocations with the middle phalanx palmarly dislocated associated with a dorsal lip fracture of the middle phalanx base are extremely uncommon. Management is similar to that for the dorsal fracture-dislocation counterpart. An exception is volar fracture-dislocations, as they are unstable in flexion and should be splinted in extension. A K-wire transarticular excision can also be used for added immobilization.

DISLOCATIONS

Dislocations of the PIP joint may be dorsal, volar, or lateral. These injuries are most commonly seen in ball-handling sports, such as football, basketball, and baseball, but they also occur in a multitude of other sports and are commonly referred to as a "jammed" finger. The untrained coach or overzealous athlete has a tendency to minimize the injury, which can result in serious disability. The mechanism of injury for the more common dorsal dislocation is hyperextension with some degree of axial loading to the PIP joint while it is held in extension. Fracture-dislocations can also result when the primary deforming force is axial loading with an associated dorsal or volar force. In dorsal dislocations, the volar plate ruptures from its distal attachment with or without an avulsion fracture of the base of the middle phalanx.

Closed reduction is usually easily obtainable with a local digital nerve block. At times, athletes present after having had on-field reduction by a teammate or an athletic trainer. If no associated collateral ligament injury or major fracture is noted, these injuries are quite amenable to volar splinting in 20 to 30° of flexion for 2 to 3 weeks. Mobilization time is dependent upon the degree of soft-tissue injury and swelling. Athletes can usually be allowed to participate in athletic endeavors if the finger is appropriately splinted. Additional buddy taping is carried out until the finger can undergo pain-free complete range of motion and no tenderness is present at the PIP joint.

It must be stressed that a thorough examination for dynamic and static stability is required in evaluating all dislocations of the PIP joint. Dynamic assessment is performed by having the patient go through a complete active range of motion of the joint after reduction. Static assessment involves putting the joint under stress, both volar or dorsal and radially or ulnarly, to check for associated collateral ligament injuries as well as to evaluate the instability of the original dislocation.

Volar dislocations (Fig. 4–5), with their associated ligamentous damage, are extremely rare. In 1970, Spinner presented a classic paper

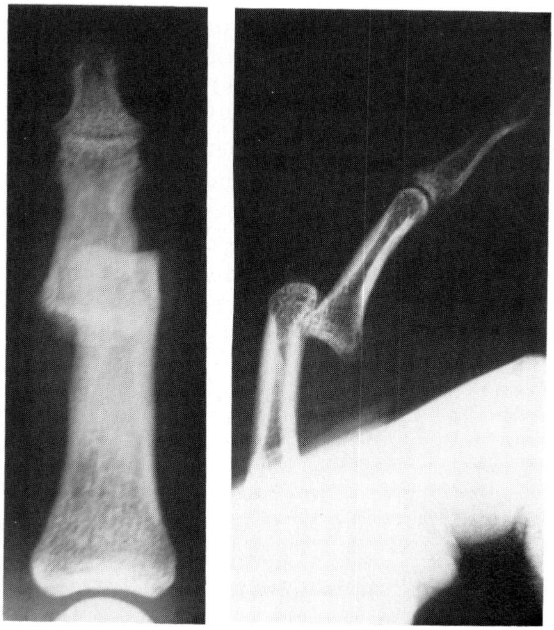

Figure 4–5 Radiographs of a volar PIP dislocation. (From Reider, B.: Sports Medicine: The School Age Athlete. Philadelphia, W.B. Saunders, 1991, p. 224.)

that biomechanically documented the mechanism of injury through cadaveric studies.[57] He also followed a significant number of patients with volar dislocations of the PIP joint and was able to corroborate substantial surgical findings suggested by the biomechanical study. He concluded that a varus or valgus force significant enough to tear one of the collateral ligaments, coupled with a volar thrust of the middle phalanx, would result in volar dislocation. His studies imply that these injuries are associated with central slip avulsions, collateral ligament tears, partial tears of the transverse retinacular ligament, and partial tears of the volar plate. The torn collateral ligament herniates through the transverse retinacular ligament tear on the ipsilateral side of the disruption and is maintained in an unreduced posture. Left untreated, this injury results in a chronic boutonnière deformity as well as collateral ligament instability with its associated disabling consequences.

The associated significant soft-tissue injury makes conservative management of acute cases difficult, if not impossible. It is recommended that all patients with reducible or unreducible acute volar dislocations of the PIP joint and chronic boutonnière deformities with positive varus or valgus stress films undergo open exploration to repair all damaged structures. For chronic cases, the volar plate must usually be excised, as it often is contracted and significantly scarred. Spinner recommends central slip reconstruction via the Pulvertaft technique and release of the contracted retinacular ligaments.[48, 57] A transarticular 0.035 Kirschner wire insures immobilization in extension. Splinting is carried out for 3 weeks, allowing active and passive flexion of the DIP joint. The wire is removed at 3 weeks, and gradual mobilization of the PIP joint is instituted. Athletic competition should be restricted in severe injuries until the K-wire has been removed and significant healing has occurred, usually at least 3 weeks postoperatively.

Lateral PIP dislocations are also quite uncommon. They result in tears of one collateral ligament with an associated partial avulsion of the volar plate from the middle phalanx on the ipsilateral side. As in all dislocations, once closed reduction is obtained, stability assessment in both static and dynamic situations is required. For lateral dislocations with complete tears of the collateral ligament and adequate dynamic stability, some authors recommend closed treatment with splinting followed by mobilization after 2 to 3 weeks. McCue and co-workers recommend primary repair of collateral ligament tears as well as of the volar plate avulsion.[42, 49, 52] In the athlete, it is imperative to insure adequate end-to-end healing and reduce the length of disability. We have seen several athletes with persistent locking, pain, and swelling on the ipsilateral side of the tear, even with adequate immobilization as conservative treatment. Open reduction and repair resolved their symptomatology. Acute repair provided excellent results in the great majority of athletes with collateral ligament–associated tears in McCue's series.[42]

In irreducible volar dislocations, a significant rotatory component may be noted, allowing significant buttonholing of the proximal phalangeal condyle, displacing the lateral band volarly (Fig. 4–6). In this situation, open reduction is recommended.

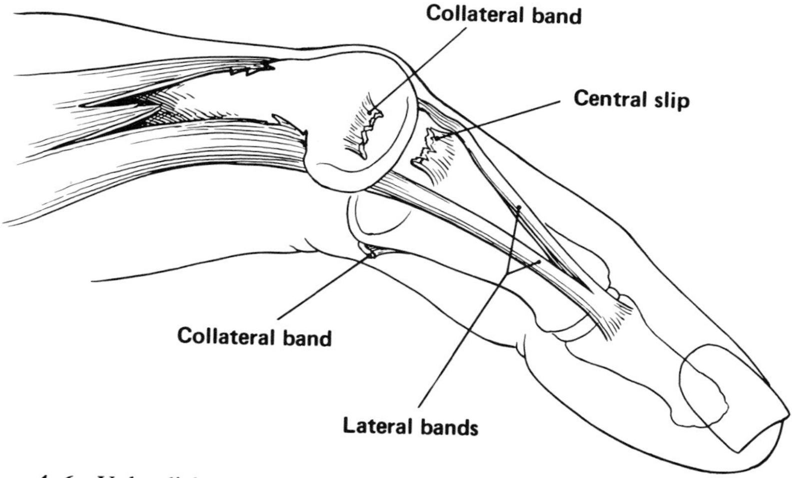

Figure 4–6 Volar dislocation with entrapment by the lateral band negating any attempts at closed reduction. Note the concomitant collateral ligament tear universally associated with this type of injury. (From McCue, F.C., Garroway, R.Y.: Sports injuries to the hand and wrist. In Schneider, R.C., Kennedy, J.C., Plant, M.L. (eds.): Sports Injuries: Mechanisms, Prevention and Treatment. Baltimore, Williams & Wilkins, 1985, p. 756.)

COLLATERAL LIGAMENT INJURIES

Collateral ligament injuries are quite common in most contact sports. The radial collateral ligament of the PIP joint is the most frequently injured, with tears occurring from the proximal attachment in the majority of cases. Collateral ligament injury is reported most often, but certainly not exclusively, in the index finger.[42] In McCue's series of 30 athletes with acute collateral ligamentous injuries, football was the most common activity, followed by wrestling, basketball, and baseball.[42] Collateral ligament tears are associated with partial or complete ruptures of the volar plate, depending upon the magnitude of the force applied. The mechanism of injury is an abduction or adduction force to the finger with the PIP joint held in extension. Examination reveals swelling and tenderness over the site of injury. As with other dislocations, both static and dynamic stability assessments are required. In differentiating a partial from a complete tear of the collateral ligament, one must be careful to avoid converting a partial tear into a complete rupture with too vigorous stressing. In complete ruptures instability is noted on clinical as well as radiographic stress testing (Fig. 4–7) with a local digital nerve block used as needed. Often, one of the collateral ligaments may be avulsed with a fragment of bone aiding the diagnosis. In general, sprains or partial ruptures are more common than complete ruptures.

Mild sprains of collateral ligaments are treated with splinting of the finger in a functional position until pain has subsided and range of motion is restored. This usually takes from 10 to 14 days. The athlete may be allowed to continue athletic competition by the use of a protec-

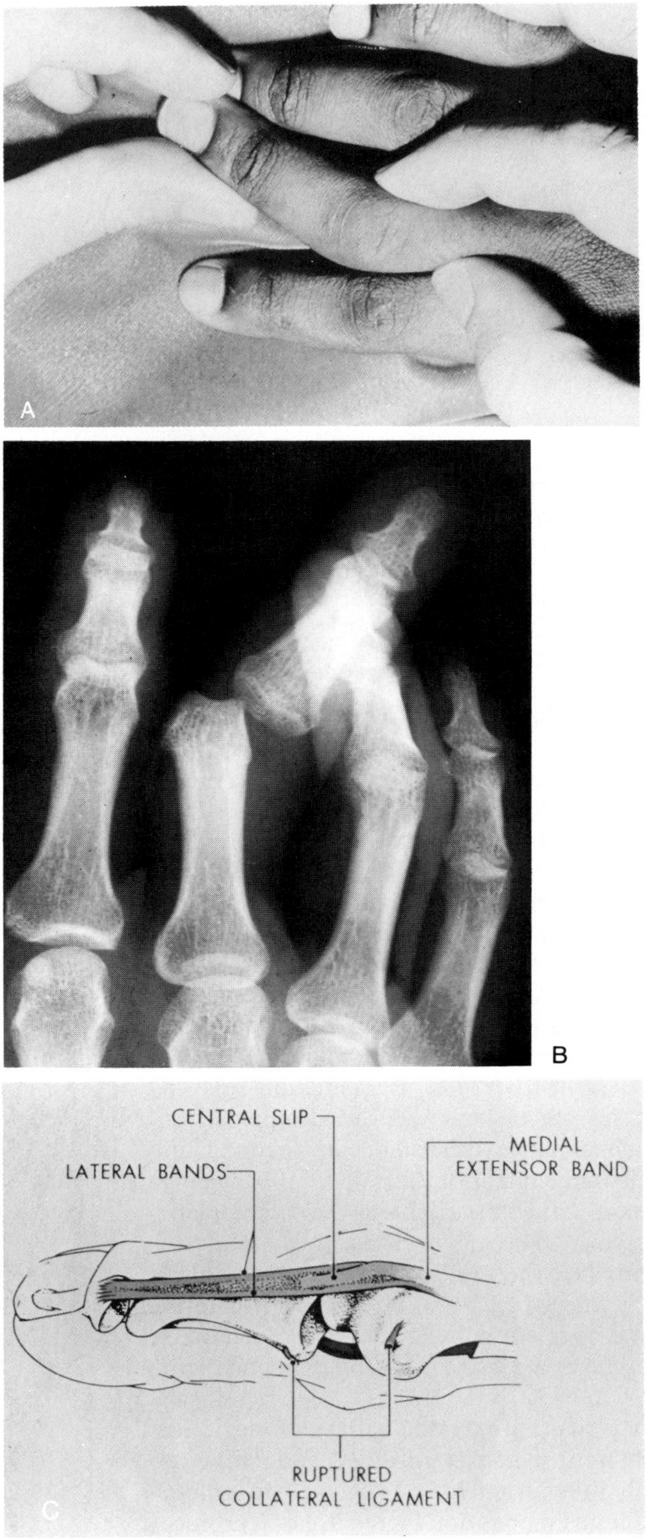

Figure 4–7 Clinical (*A*) and radiographic (*B*) findings in collateral ligament rupture. Note the diagrammatic representation (*C*) of the lateral dislocation with ruptured collateral ligament and (*not shown*) the partial tear of the volar plate from its distal attachments. (Parts *A* and *C* from: McCue, F.C., Garroway, R.Y.: Sports injuries to the hand and wrist. In Schneider, R.C., Kennedy, J.C., Plant, M.L. (eds.): Sports Injuries: Mechanisms, Prevention and Treatment. Baltimore, Williams & Wilkins, 1985, pp. 755 and 756. Part *B* from Poznanski, A.K.: The Hand in Radiologic Diagnosis. Philadelphia, W.B. Saunders Co., 1984, p. 685.)

tive splint as well as by buddy taping of the injured finger to an adjacent finger.

Injuries demonstrating laxity, but an incomplete tear of the ligament, should be immobilized with volar splinting in 30° of flexion. Active motion is instituted in 10 to 14 days with additional protective splinting for at least 3 weeks. Buddy taping to the adjacent finger should continue for an additional 4 to 6 weeks until full range of motion is obtained and tenderness has subsided; athletic participation is permitted during this period.

Controversy exists regarding the treatment of complete tears of collateral ligaments. Many authors advocate closed treatment, while McCue, Redler, Rodriguez, and others advocate open repair.[42, 49, 52] Again, the emphasis in operative repair is on enhancing adequate end-to-end healing and allowing for a minimal period of disability. Open treatment will allow the athlete to return to competition sooner, while closed treatment often leaves the patient with a swollen, tender joint that is unstable and susceptible to re-injury.

Open repair is performed, as in lateral dislocations of the PIP joint, through a midlateral incision. The most common proximal site of avulsion lends itself to repair by Bunnell's wire suture with 4-0 pull-out wire tied over a button on the opposite side of the finger. The joint is immobilized in 30° of flexion with a volar splint. The wire and splint may be removed at 3 weeks, and motion may be instituted. McCue reported excellent results and early return of function with this technique.[42]

BOUTONNIÈRE DEFORMITY

Untreated disruptions of the central slip of the extensor digitorum communis tendon over the PIP joint can result in a classic boutonnière deformity (Fig. 4–8). The injury can result from either a laceration of the dorsal PIP joint or a closed injury. In contact sports, such as football, closed injury is most often the result of forceful sudden flexion of the extended PIP joint. A volar PIP joint subluxation or dislocation may

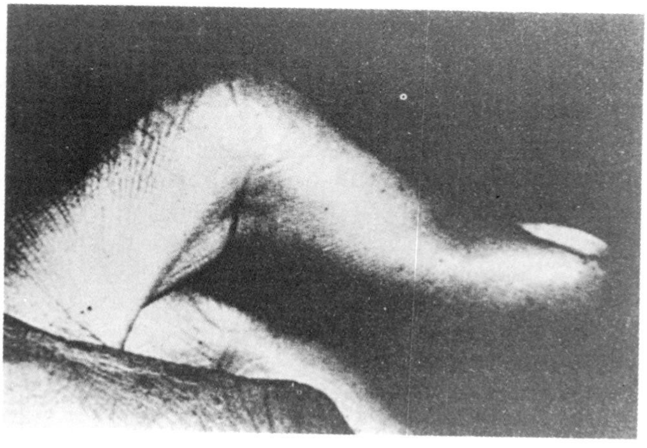

Figure 4–8 Classic boutonnière deformity showing hyperextension at the MCP and DIP with flexion of the PIP joint. (From McCue, F.C., Garroway, R.Y.: Sports injuries to the hand and wrist. In Schneider, R.C., Kennedy, J.C., Plant, M.L. (eds.): Sports Injuries: Mechanisms, Prevention and Treatment. Baltimore, Williams & Wilkins, 1985, p. 757.)

result in closed rupture of the central slip, avulsion fractures, or central slip attenuation injuries.[54, 57] Regardless of whether lacerated, attenuated, or ruptured, the triangular ligament is usually damaged, allowing the lateral bands to gradually migrate volarly. Classic boutonnière deformity is rarely seen acutely. One may note mild degrees of flexion deformity of 15 to 30° at the PIP joints. Most commonly, after acute injury, particularly with laceration, the patient is still able to extend the PIP joint quite adequately because the lateral bands are tightening over the dorsal aspect of the joint allowing extension. In closed injuries, diagnosis is much more difficult.[19, 34] The patient usually presents with generalized swelling of the PIP joint as well as pain and may or may not be able to extend the PIP joint. If there is less than 25° extension of the PIP joint, one should assume that a central slip rupture has occurred. The clinician must be astute enough to palpate over the central slip dorsally to elicit maximal tenderness, usually associated with central slip ruptures. If this important step is neglected, the physician may erroneously diagnose a soft-tissue contusion and splint with the PIP joint in flexion, which will cause the ruptured ends to separate and the lateral bands to spread. With lack of treatment or inappropriate treatment, the lateral bands will migrate volarly, usually within 10 to 21 days. Once they cross volarly to the flexion-extension axis of the PIP joint, they act as flexors. Secondary hyperextension changes occur in the MCP and DIP joints from overpull of the extensor mechanism in an attempt to extend the PIP joint. Initially, these deformities are quite supple, allowing conservative management, but secondary contractions will eventually develop in the soft tissues, as well as in the oblique retinacular ligaments, resulting in fixed classic boutonnière deformity. Roentgenograms are important to rule out fractures or avulsion fractures of the central slip.

Treatment

In order to correct these deformities, one has to re-establish the tendon balance over the joint, as well as the length relationships of the lateral band and central slip. Boutonnière deformities can be acute or chronic. Acute injuries are those noted up to 3 weeks after initial injury, while chronic injuries are present after 3 weeks, either from misdiagnosis or inappropriate treatment. For the most part, athletes are usually treated early in most well-supervised athletic programs. The closed acute central slip ruptures or attenuation injuries are usually devoid of secondary changes, the joints are supple, and the DIP joint has adequate flexion capabilities. This allows treatment by simple immobilization of the PIP joint in extension with the DIP joint free to allow for active flexion. Boyes utilizes a Bunnell type safety pin splint (Fig. 4–9), which offers three-point fixation.[4] An exercise program is started with active and passive flexion of the DIP joint, which tightens the lateral bands, preventing laxity in the triangular ligament complex and thus volar migration. It also prevents the ruptured central slip from retracting and allows maintenance of the central slip–lateral band length relationship. The splint is maintained for 5 to 6 weeks after which progres-

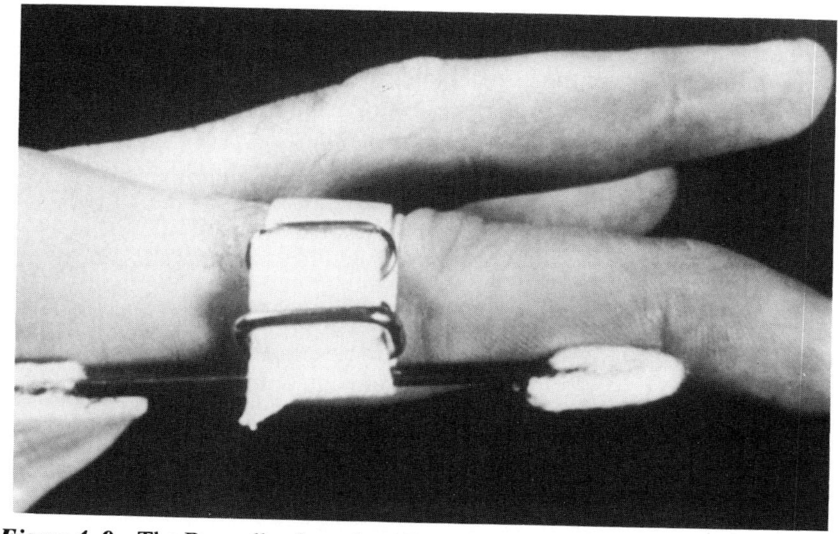

Figure 4–9 The Bunnell safety pin splint provides static three-point fixation to correct boutonnière deformities. (From McCue, F.C., Garroway, R.Y.: Sports Injuries to the Hand and Wrist. In Schneider, R.C., Kennedy, J.C., Plant, M.L. (eds.): Sports Injuries: Mechanisms, Prevention and Treatment. Baltimore, Williams & Wilkins, 1985, p. 759.)

sive exercises are instituted at the PIP joint level. Nighttime splinting is required for an additional 2 to 4 weeks.

Closed central slip ruptures seen more than 3 weeks postinjury usually present with more classic characteristics of the boutonnière deformity. These may still be treated conservatively as acute cases as long as the components of the boutonnière deformity are not fixed as contractures. Gradual active exercises are instituted with emphasis on recovery of PIP joint extension and DIP joint flexion. A combination of dynamic and static splinting can be utilized to achieve correction of the deformity. These measures are usually quite successful in most chronic boutonnière deformities, which are devoid of the soft-tissue fixed contractures of the volar plate, collateral ligaments, and flexor tendon sheath and intra-articular fibrosis. Full correction can take as long as 3 to 4 months in the more involved cases. Splinting should always be continued as long as one can see progressive improvements. It can be discontinued when recovery of full active PIP joint extension and full active DIP joint flexion is noted without recurrence of deformity. At this time, gradual active flexion exercises are instituted for the PIP joint.

Acute open lacerations of the central slip should be repaired surgically. Most of the time, the lacerations extend into the joint; consequently, irrigation and debridement are required. The tendon laceration can be repaired with Bunnell's suture with a 4-0 pull-out wire if no cuff of tendon is available distally or with a direct figure-of-eight nonabsorbable suture (e.g., 3-0 ticron) in cases in which there is significant cuff of tendon noted at the insertion site. Postoperative immobilization is continued with the PIP joint in extension allowing DIP joint flexion for 4 to 6 weeks. If there is loss of substance in the central slip, a reconstruction as described by Aiache, Barsky, and Weiner[3] should be performed over a dorsal incision over the PIP joint. The two medial longitudinal halves of the lateral bands are split for a distance of approximately 2 cm and are reattached centrally over the PIP joint.[30] Postoperatively, the wrist is splinted in extension, the MCP joint in 20° of flexion, and the PIP joint in extension for 3 weeks, after which exercises are instituted by the occupational therapist.

Avulsion fractures of the central slip were described earlier and can be treated conservatively with splinting for 3 to 4 weeks if displacement is less than 2 mm.

Surgical reconstruction for chronic boutonnière deformity is technically demanding and should be attempted only by surgeons well versed in hand surgery. Surgery is indicated in those patients with severely fixed deformities who fail to respond to conservative treatment. Regardless, all patients, no matter how severe their involvement, should undergo an extensive exercise program in addition to dynamic and static splinting. Even in the more severe chronic fixed deformities, some degree of correction is obtainable and significant loosening of the joints and improvement in skin tone can be achieved, which are absolute prerequisites to any surgical reconstruction.

VOLAR PLATE INJURIES

The volar plate is composed of a thick fibrocartilaginous tissue with a firm distal attachment to the proximal base of the middle phalanx. The proximal thin membranous portion tapers centrally and thickens laterally to attach to the proximal phalanx. The most common mechanism of injury is hyperextension forces on the extended PIP joint significant enough to disrupt the volar plate without causing complete dorsal dislocation. Isolated volar plate injuries are seen most commonly, but not exclusively, in contact sports, with football having the highest incidence. The two types of volar plate injuries are distal volar plate disruptions, which result in swan neck deformities, and proximal volar plate disruptions, which result in pseudo-boutonnière deformities. As a whole, these injuries are less common than dorsal dislocations because the hyperextension forces required for injury generally cause full dorsal dislocation at the PIP joint rather than the more limited volar plate injury. In McCue's series of 143 surgically treated PIP joint injuries seen from 1961 to 1968 at the University of Virginia, only five were isolated volar plate distal injuries and eight were proximal volar plate disruptions.[16] Both of these subgroups presented as chronic injuries, which implies that either the athlete did not seek medical attention or the injuries were misdiagnosed by either the trainer or the physician. With regard to the distal volar plate disruptions, all the athletes presented with greater than 15° of hyperextension at the PIP joint level with clinical symptomatology consisting of locking, catching, and discomfort at the PIP joint. With the proximal volar plate disruptions, all the athletes had flexion deformities of greater than 45° at the PIP joint with mild to moderate hyperextension deformity of the DIP joint. In both groups, there was a significant history of previous hyperextension injury to the PIP joint several months prior to presentation. When the volar plate tears distally, its check-rein function is destroyed and a hyperextension or swan neck deformity of the PIP joint will result. Proximal disruptions initially cause a flexion deformity, but if left untreated can result in pseudo-boutonnière deformities as described by McCue and associates.[42]

Acute volar plate injuries clinically present with a painful swollen PIP joint. Examination may reveal maximal tenderness at the volar plate. One should try to pinpoint tenderness to the distal or proximal volar plate area to distinguish the two types of injury. Distal disruption of the volar plate more commonly involves some degree of hyperextension deformity of the PIP joint and rarely may cause an actual swan neck deformity of the joint. The more proximal volar plate disruption rarely presents acutely with the pseudo-boutonnière deformity, since the deformity implies chronicity in its development. Most commonly, the patient with a proximal volar plate injury will present with a swollen PIP joint with tenderness as previously described and some mild flexion posture of the PIP joint.

Treatment

If a diagnosis of acute volar plate injury with hyperextension is considered, one should immobilize the PIP joint in 20 to 30° of flexion with a volar gutter splint for approximately 3 weeks. Occupational therapy is then started with active flexion and extension exercises. After the 4th week, the extension exercises are upgraded and passive stretching is begun if adequate extension has not been obtained. After the initial injury, the athlete can continue to participate with appropriate splinting of the digit. An additional 2 to 3 weeks of protective splinting by buddy taping is required until full pain-free motion is gained.

Late presentations of swan neck deformity and pseudo-boutonnière deformity present difficult management problems and may require surgical intervention. In swan neck deformities secondary to distal volar plate injuries, surgical treatment may be considered after exercise and splinting have failed. One must make an accurate diagnosis as to the etiology of the swan neck deformity. The differential diagnosis includes rheumatoid arthritis, flexor digitorum sublimis rupture, laxity in a grafted flexor digitorum profundus tendon, spastic conditions, mallet deformity of the DIP joint, and generalized systemic laxity. McCue and colleagues explored five recalcitrant swan neck deformities of the PIP joint that had symptomatic locking and catching and found distal disruptions of the volar plate in all five cases.[42] If significant contracture of the volar plate in the unreduced position is noted, direct repair may be attempted at the proximal base of the middle phalanx. Often, proximal elevation and release of the proximal volar plate will be required with a Freer elevator. In such cases, it would be wise to do a volar plate arthroplasty, attaching the volar plate to a cleft made at the base of the middle phalanx, using Bunnell's suturing technique with a 4-0 wire tied over a dorsal button with a pull-out wire, as described by Eaton.[16] If additional laxity or hyperextension deformity is still noted, McCue and associates recommend doing a Littler sublimis tenodesis by detaching one of the sublimis insertions proximally and reattaching it to the distal proximal phalangeal bone, thereby creating a sling effect.[31, 32, 42]

In chronic proximal volar plate injuries, a fixed flexion deformity of the PIP joint is characteristic with an associated mild hyperextension deformity of the DIP joint.[39] Unlike the true boutonnière deformity, the DIP flexion deformity is mild, and the patient retains the ability to actively flex the joint. Also, the pseudo-boutonnière deformity has been associated with proximal osteophyte and calcific spurring on the side of the injured volar plate in all reported cases.[39, 42] In their initial presentations, all of the chronic pseudo-boutonnière deformities were fixed deformities of greater than 45° degrees of flexion at the PIP joint that were recalcitrant to exercises and splinting. All required surgical correction. In 1975, McCue and associates reported on a larger number of pseudo-boutonnière deformities.[39] In this report, they were able to delineate two subgroups of patients depending on the initial degree of flexion deformity. Mild cases had PIP flexion deformities of less than 40°, slight radiographic changes, and no disability from the deformity. These cases are usually amenable to conservative treatment with a Bunnell safety pin splint (see Fig. 4–9), together with active and passive exercise of the DIP joint. Splinting should be discontinued only after the patient can actively extend the PIP joint and actively and fully flex the DIP joints. In the severe cases, the flexion deformity of the PIP joint was greater than 45°, did not respond to splinting, and in fact regressed in many cases in spite of splinting.

The radiographic changes include significant spurring and osteophyte formation.

Surgical treatment is warranted for the severe type of pseudo-boutonnière deformity, which is unresponsive to splinting and continues to progress in spite of it. Surgery is performed through a midlateral incision on the side of the osteophytic spur. Utilizing a rongeur and an air drill, the calcific spur or osteophyte is excised, the contracted accessory collateral ligaments are released, the contracted lateral band and oblique retinacular ligaments are also released, the proximal attachment of the volar plate is sharply incised along both lateral borders, and the proximal volar plate is released enough to establish sufficient mobility. Once full extension is obtained, the proximal attachment of the volar plate is sutured with fine nonabsorbable material. A transarticular 0.035 K-wire may be inserted for immobilization in extension if necessary. Postoperative immobilization with a volar splint allowing DIP flexion is continued for 3 weeks, at which time splinting and wiring are discontinued and active motion of the PIP joint is instituted. Athletic participation is allowed with additional splinting 3 to 4 weeks after the initial surgery. Additional protective splinting is continued for 4 to 6 weeks when not exercising. The results of surgically treated cases were all satisfactory.[39, 42]

Distal Interphalangeal Joint

Injuries of the distal interphalangeal (DIP) joint are common in contact sports, such as football, basketball, and baseball, and include dislocations, fracture-dislocations, extensor tendon injuries, and flexor digitorum profundi ruptures.

DISLOCATIONS

Dislocations of the DIP joint are usually dorsally displaced and may be complicated by an open injury. The mechanism of injury is hyperextension of the extended DIP joint. Because this dislocation is frequently easily reducible it is often "treated" by the patient or a teammate before the physician or trainer arrives. The joint is usually quite stable after reduction. As a part of the general examination, one should always check for additional damage to the collateral ligaments, as well as to the extensor or flexor tendon. The DIP joint is immobilized in extension after closed reduction in a volar or dorsal splint excluding the PIP joint. Athletic participation may be allowed early on with adequate splinting. It should be noted that in sporting activities that require good tactile sensibility and control, it may be more prudent to place the splint dorsally. Flexion exercises are begun after 3 weeks, and protective splinting is continued part-time for an additional 2 to 4 weeks until full range of motion is regained and tenderness has totally subsided. Associated open wounds obviously require initial treatment with open irrigation and debridement and are allowed to close by secondary intention.

INTRA-ARTICULAR FRACTURES

Intra-articular fractures of the DIP joint occur in the more aggressive contact sports from crush or axial forces. Fractures of the base of the DIP joint may be due to tendon avulsion fractures, dorsal or volar fracture-dislocations, or epiphyseal separations in children. Distal interphalangeal fractures are generally uncomplicated because there are no tendons spanning the fracture site and the phalanx is supported dorsally by the nail matrix and nail and volarly by the finger pulp.[8]

Fracture-dislocations or fracture-subluxations can occur volarly or dorsally. Volar fracture-dislocations usually are quite unstable, with the dorsal fragment attached to the extensor apparatus usually displaced. Open reduction and internal fixation can be performed with either 0.028 K-wires or Bunnell's suturing with 4-0 wire tied over a volar button with a pull-out wire.

Dorsal fracture-dislocations occur less frequently. They can be approached surgically in the manner described above, except that a midlateral incision rather than a dorsal approach is used. Postoperative immobilization of both types of DIP joint injuries is done in extension with volar or dorsal splinting for 3 to 4 weeks, at which time the K-wire or pull-out wires are removed. Occupational therapy is then instituted to gradually restore mobility. Athletic participation can be allowed after removal of internal fixation devices with appropriate splinting for protective purposes.

In most DIP fracture-subluxations and fracture-dislocations the displacement is severe enough to require surgical correction. However, in circumstances in which fracture fragments are undisplaced or displaced less than 2 mm or joint congruity is less than or equal to 2 mm of step-off, conservative treatment will give satisfactory results with volar or dorsal splinting for a period of 4 to 6 weeks. It must be remembered that these small joints are not weight-bearing joints and therefore are more tolerant of less than perfect anatomic fracture alignment. Epiphyseal fractures are discussed in the next section. Avulsion fractures of either the extensor apparatus or the flexor digitorum profundus are treated with tenodesis and are considered subsequently.

MALLET DEFORMITY

Mallet deformities of the DIP joint are one of the most common hand injuries seen in athletes and are especially common in the football receiver, the baseball catcher or fielder, and the basketball player.[1, 36] The mechanism of injury is a sudden forceful hyperflexion of the joint from an axial load to the extended DIP joint. The characteristic flexion drop deformity of the distal joint is referred to as mallet, or baseball finger. This deformity may result from several conditions, including extensor tendon attenuation, extensor tendon rupture, extensor tendon avulsion fractures, dorsal intra-articular fractures, and finally, Salter I epiphyseal disruptions of the DIP joint[34] (Fig. 4–10).

The most common of these injuries is rupture of the extensor tendon at its insertion into the distal tuft of the DIP joint.

Clinically, the patient presents with acute pain and tenderness dorsally with an obvious drop flexion deformity of the DIP joint. It is important to recognize the entity initially, so that proper treatment can be instituted. Delay in diagnosis and treatment can result in secondary contractures resulting in hyperextension deformities of the PIP joint by an over-compensated extensor mechanism with eventual swan neck deformity. If enough time elapses, this deformity can develop into a fixed static contracture making conservative management extremely difficult. Roentogenographic examination is imperative as a part of the general examination of this joint, as well as the PIP joint.[36]

Treatment

Stark, Boyes, and Wilson's classic series in 1962 was the first large group of patients with excellent results after treatment with either volar or dorsal splinting of the DIP joint in extension.[58] Smillie advocated casting and Lewin advocated metal splinting.[30, 55] The most frequently used immobilization devices are the simple aluminum splints that can be

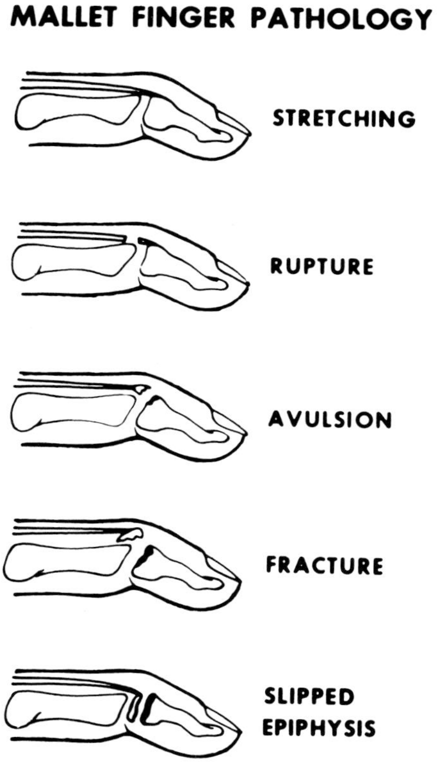

Figure 4–10 The five etiologies of the mallet deformity.

fashioned on the volar or dorsal side of the joint and the prefabricated stack splints (Fig. 4–11). Attenuation of the extensor tendon insertion, extensor tendon rupture insertion, and small avulsion chip fractures of the extensor tendon to the DIP joint can all be treated by either volar or dorsal splinting for 6 to 8 weeks. As previously mentioned, dorsal

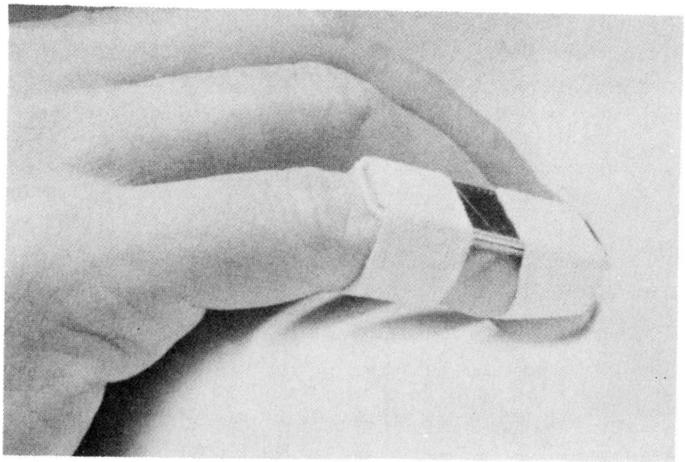

Figure 4–11 Static splints are well suited for treatment of mallet finger by creating controlled hyperextension at the DIP joint.

splinting allows better tactile control of the distal finger for athletes who are dependent on adequate fingertip sensation. It is important to avoid splinting in extreme hyperextension, as this may compromise vascularity or cause major skin slough. It is also important to educate the patient in removal and re-application of the splint for hygiene purposes, taking great care to avoid DIP joint flexion during cleansing of the digit or splint reapplication. Athletic competition may be allowed early on with adequate splinting of the digit. An additional 6 to 8 weeks of protected splinting is required until full range of motion is regained with occupational therapy. Conservative management with splinting has recently been advocated, even in chronic cases (up to 6 months postinjury) with good results.[36]

The results of surgical correction are unpredictable even in the best of hands and this modality should be restricted to those individuals with significant joint pain, functional disability, cosmetic deformity, or swan neck deformity resulting in altered function.

If the deformity is fixed and unresponsive to exercises and splinting, if joint surfaces are incongruent, or if significant degenerative changes are noted in the DIP joint, arthrodesis is indicated. If the flexion deformity can be passively corrected after exercises and splinting with adequate joint congruity, extensor tendon reconstruction may be feasible. Elliot has advocated three treatment methods: reefing of the attenuated tendon to take up the slack; excision of scar tissue from the ruptured ends with end-to-end repair; and the creation of a tendon slip from the surrounding tissues that can be advanced and inserted into the bone.[18] Problems with excess shortening can occur, either from overly vigorous resection of the scar tissue or too great a reefing. Only 2 to 3 mm of tendon resection or reefing is usually required in order to balance the extensor mechanism. Postoperative management is the same as for acute cases.

In children, Salter I epiphyseal injuries (see Fig. 4–10) present as mallet finger deformities. The mechanism of injury is the same as for the previously discussed cases. Usually, the injury can be adequately reduced by closed means. If stable enough, the joint can be immobilized as for other acute mallet fingers. If there is any question as to stability, a centrally placed transarticular 0.028 wire will provide adequate fixation. The wire is removed in 3 to 4 weeks and immobilization is continued as previously described.

FLEXOR DIGITORUM PROFUNDUS AVULSIONS

This injury, commonly referred to as "sweater" or "jersey" finger, is quite common in contact sports. The term describes the mechanism of injury, most often seen in tackling sports such as football or rugby: the finger is caught in the jersey of an opponent, forcing the actively contracting and flexing finger into extension. An avulsion of the flexor digitorum tendon insertion may occur with or without a chip fracture (Fig. 4–12). The injury may occur in any digit, although it is most commonly seen in the ring finger. The small finger frequently slips easily

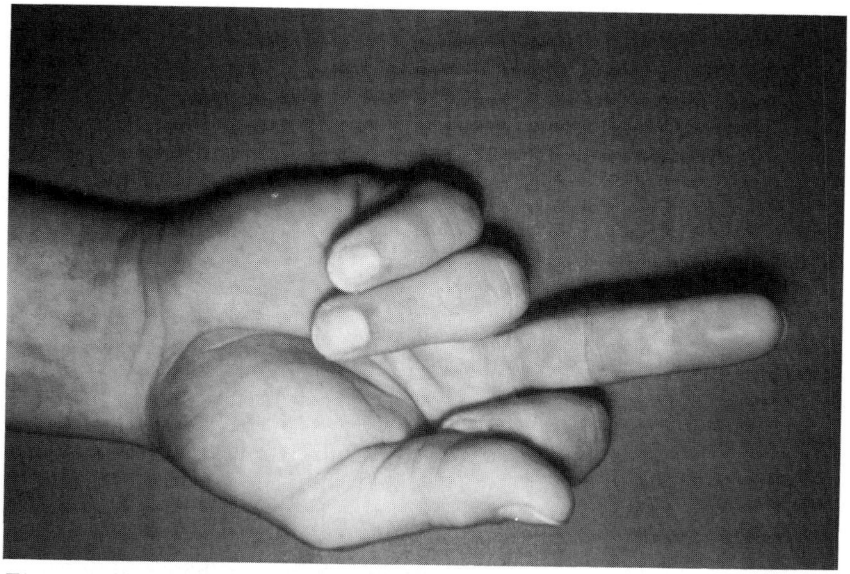

Figure 4–12 Clinical appearance of the "jersey" or "sweater" finger deformity secondary to a ruptured flexor digitorum profundus tendon of this football player's fourth finger.

from grasp during the act of clenching and fully flexes, thereby allowing all of the extrinsic force applied to the ulnar innervated deep finger flexors to be absorbed by the ring finger.[40] Unfortunately, the condition is often misdiagnosed or missed entirely. There is no consistent pattern of deformity, and often the lack of flexion at the DIP joint is ignored as merely secondary to soft-tissue contusion, swelling, and tenderness.[4, 6, 30]

Clinically, the patient initially experiences acute pain, but usually disregards the problem, since active flexion at the PIP joint level is possible with the intact flexor digitorum sublimi tendon. Roentgenograms must always be obtained as part of the evaluation to rule out associated fractures. Sometimes a tender mass may be palpable in the palm, signifying the distal portion of the avulsed tendon.

Three types of injury patterns are seen. The first is an avulsion fracture with part of a volar plate remaining attached to the fragment. This provides the best possible situation, since it tethers the avulsed tendon and prevents proximal retraction, thereby facilitating primary repair. The second type is an avulsion of the tendon itself with retraction to the level of the flexor sublimus hiatus. Further retraction is prevented by the vincula longus. Finally, complete avulsion with palmar retraction presents the worst of all possible situations.

In the first type described, the volar fracture fragment is usually large, enabling repair of the fracture with either 0.028 K-wires or Bunnell's 4-0 wire suture tied over a dorsal button with a pull-out wire. Immobilization of the PIP at 30°, the MPC at 45°, and the wrist at 30° of flexion decreases tensile forces at the fracture site. Immobilization in this degree of flexion is maintained for 3 weeks, at which time protected range of motion exercises are begun. The pull-out wires are removed at 3 to 4 weeks. Additional protected splinting is carried out for an additional 2 weeks until the fracture is fully healed.

In the second type of injury, the true tendinous injury, primary repair is usually possible if the patient is seen within the first 3 weeks. Postoperative immobilization is carried out in flexion of the PIP, MPC, and wrist as previously described for 3 weeks, during which active extension and passive flexion are performed through rubber band attachments to the nail beds. At 3 weeks, active protected flexion exercises are begun, and the rubber bands are discontinued. At 4 weeks, the dorsal splint is removed, and progressive exercises are continued. At 6 weeks, active resistive exercises can be instituted. However, if the injury is neglected, secondary tendon reconstruction with tendon graft may be required or a simple tenodesis of the DIP joint can be performed.

In cases in which the tendon has fully retracted into the palm, primary repair may be performed only within the first 7 to 10 days after injury, although secondary reconstruction may be required. Successful secondary reconstructions have been done by utilizing free tendon graft using either the palmaris longus, flexor sublimis of the small finger, or extensor tendons of the foot. In chronic cases, if the patient is seen within 3 weeks to several months, primary grafting may be feasible if the pulley system is still functional. However, if the pulley system is obliterated, a Hunter rod stage technique may be required followed by secondary grafting. Postoperative immobilization for primary grafting must be performed with the same degree of flexion previously described for primary tendon repairs for 3 weeks without rubber band mobilization. After the 3 weeks of immobilization, protected flexion exercises are begun. Protected splinting in a more functional position is then maintained for an additional 2 to 3 weeks until active resistive exercises are started at 6 weeks postsurgery.

Carpometacarpal Joint of the Thumb

ANATOMY

The carpometacarpal (CMC) joint of the thumb is formed by the base of the first metacarpal and the trapezium (Fig. 4–13). It is a biconcavoconvex joint in which the articular surfaces are a mirror image of the opposing articular space. The articular surface of the base of the first metacarpal has its concave surface in the anteroposterior plane and its convex surface in the lateral direction with the trapezium having a reverse arrangement of the articular surface, which is convex in the anteroposterior direction and concave from side to side.[47] This forms a saddle joint that permits only a certain form of motion, which is of particular importance because of its specialized function in opposition in combination with the motion of the MCP joint. It has been shown that the rotation around the longitudinal axis of the metacarpal takes place within a limited range of 15 to 20° passively or actively at termination of

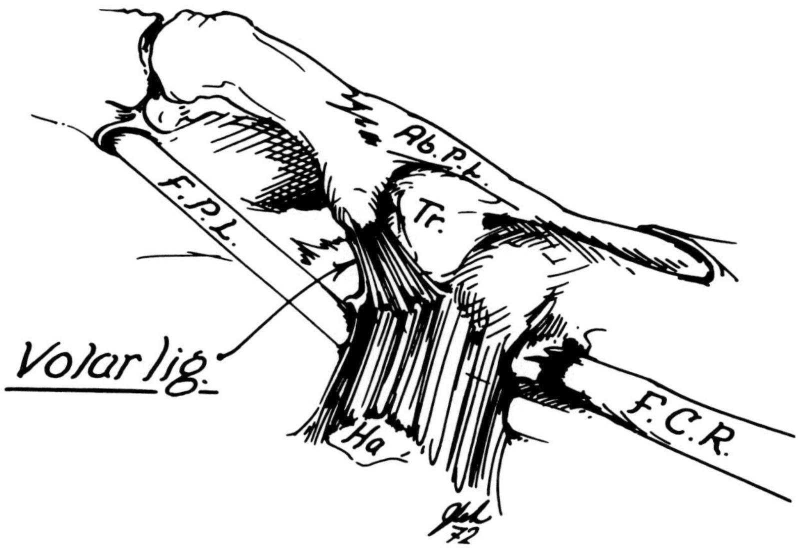

Figure 4–13 Anatomy of the CMC joint of the thumb. The volar ligament is the main stabilizer in the joint. (From Eaton, R.J., Littler, J.W.: Ligament reconstruction for the painful thumb carpometacarpal joint. J. Bone Joint Surg. 55A:1657, 1973.)

flexion at the metacarpal with rotation of the proximal phalanx also occurring. Theorists believe that opposition is a combined motion involving no rotation of the metacarpal around this longitudinal axis but a complex of flexion adduction.

The capsule surrounding the joint is lax, and the interarticular surfaces are not tightly bound together. The joint capsule has strategic areas of strength, which along with the contours of the bone, are the main forces in stabilization of the joint. The base of the first metacarpal shows a triangular beak in the neutral position oriented toward the ridge of the trapezium. These prominences are united by a strong volar ligament described in reference to the plane of the thumbnail; this is the single most important structure in maintaining carpometacarpal stability. A less prominent lateral ligament and a dorsal reinforcement of the capsule, along with the tendons of the thumb extensors and abductor pollicis longus, aid in soft tissue stabilization as well. In flexion and abduction of the thumb, the beak of the base of the first metacarpal fits into the area of the trapezium at the most distal point of the tubercle, while in abduction, extension, and traction, this beak is elevated and pulled away from the trapezium.

DISLOCATIONS

Complete traumatic dislocations of the CMC joint of the thumb are rarely seen.[9] Sprain or partial tears of the volar carpometacarpal ligament are much more common, although they are difficult to diagnose clinically because the patient often fails to seek medical attention.

Historically, very little has been written about this injury in the general orthopedic literature, with most reports dealing with the pathophysiology of chronic arthroses after trauma, rheumatoid arthritis, or idiopathic osteoarthritis of the basilar joint.[10, 17, 22, 28, 53] More recently, information has been obtained from anatomic and clinical studies of the basilar joint of the thumb.[9, 47]

Most commonly a fall on the outstretched hand results in hyperextension and/or hyperabduction forces across the volar aspect of the thumb metacarpal, damaging the volar ligamentous complex of the CMC joint (Figs. 4–14 and 4–15).[9] Clinically, the patient presents with a diffusely swollen basilar joint area with pain and inability to pinch in the fully dislocated cases. Standard anteroposterior and lateral roentgenograms are important to rule out joint pathology with associated fracture.

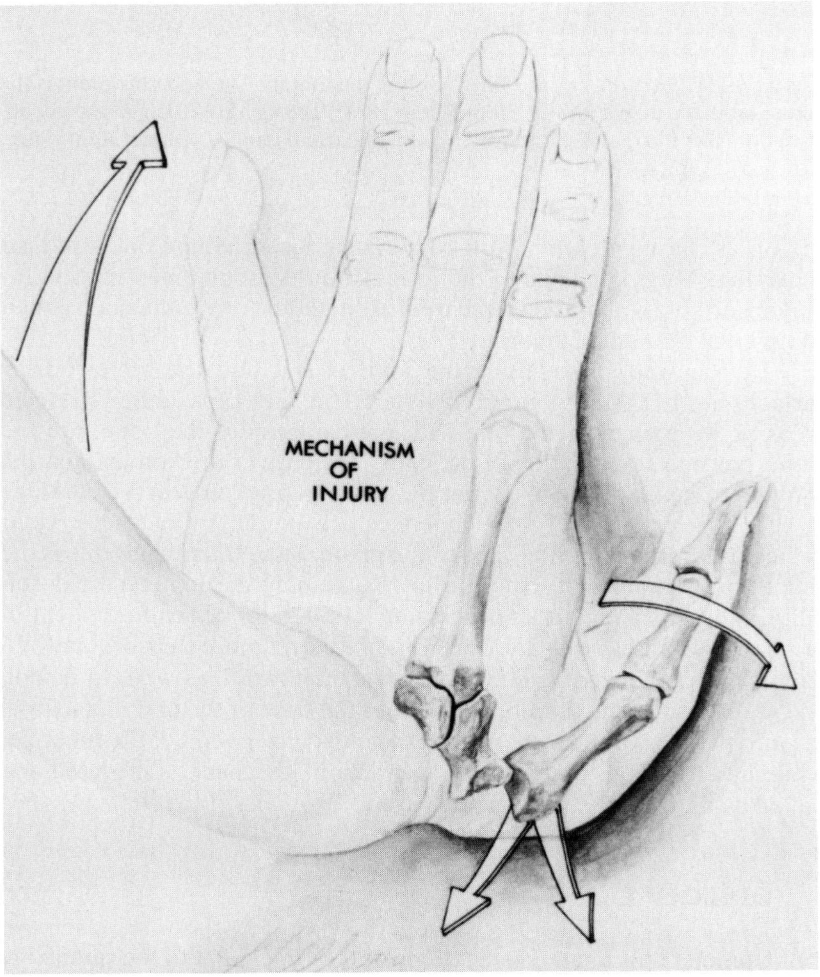

Figure 4–14 The most common mechanism described for CMC joint dislocation is a fall on the outstretched hand.

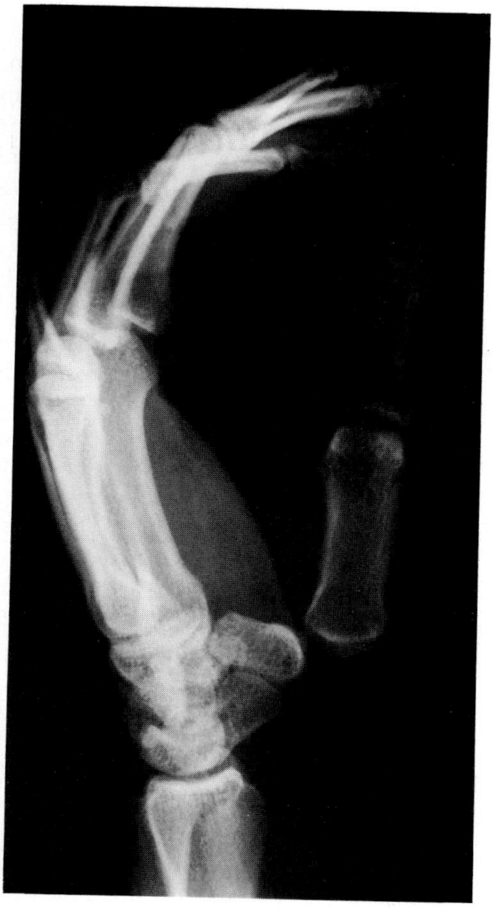

Figure 4–15 Roentgenogram of a CMC joint dislocation of the thumb.

Stress views may be required for injuries that appear reduced at the time of initial evaluation. The severity of the injury is dependent on the degree of ligamentous disruption and ranges from minor sprains to incomplete ruptures to complete ruptures of the volar ligament. Accordingly, varying clinical symptoms can be expected, depending on the degree of injury. Inappropriately administered treatment or lack of treatment will result in a vicious circle of ligamentous laxity and overall instability. Over time, this hypermobile state can result in a chronically painful joint and diminished hand function.[61]

Minor tears (1 to 2 mm) can be perpetuated by cyclical forces, causing hypermobility and eventually chronic arthrosis.[15, 61] Cooney and Chao in 1977 found the static compressive forces generated during pinch and strong grasp to be of the magnitude of 12 kg and 120 kg, respectively.[13] Because of these tremendous cyclical compressive forces, as well as uncalculated shear forces across a small surface area, it is necessary that absolute ligamentous stability be preserved after sprains, subluxations, or dislocations.[9]

Treatment

As previously noted, it is of paramount importance that all sprains of the carpometacarpal joint of the thumb have adequate treatment. Clinically, we cannot detect inconsequential trauma from minor sprains that may result in laxity. Patients with a history of hyperextension of the CMC joint of the thumb with tenderness at the same volar area and with or without evidence of instability radiographically should be treated in thumb spica immobilization for 4 to 6 weeks. The entire thumb, including the IP joint, should be immobilized in full palmar abduction.

Most authors suggest treatment for complete dislocation of the CMC joint of the thumb by closed reduction and long-arm thumb spica immobilization for 3 weeks, at which time the long-arm cast is converted to a short-arm thumb spica for an additional 3 weeks of immobilization. The cast is removed at 6 weeks and active exercises are begun.

Recently, Cabrera, Reyers, and Burkhalter have described a new pathophysiologic finding that seems to preclude conservative management of complete dislocations.[9] In their study, 25 percent of the eight cases presented, or 40 percent of the operated cases, in their series showed full dislocations of the carpometacarpal joint of the thumb with an intact volar ligament. This entity had not previously been described. The volar ligament remained attached to an ulnar volar periosteal cuff of tissue, allowing full dislocation through a dorsal radial rent in the capsule. Intraoperatively, significant capsuloligamentous laxity was noted when reduction was performed with the thumb in full palmar abduction, which is the only position obtainable after closed reduction and thumb spica casting. When adding full pronation to the thumb metacarpal as well as full palmar abduction, the capsuloligamentous structures became taut in those cases with intact volar ligament dislocations. This position could be maintained only by transarticular K-wire pinning. They also noted intraoperatively that all ruptured volar ligament dislocations had midsubstance tears and fraying, making surgical approximation problematic. They believe that in the subgroup of patients with intact volar ligament dislocations, healing would proceed with residual laxity that would culminate in chronic hypermobility if treatment were conservative. They also believe that if end-to-end approximation of the acute tears of the volar ligament is not surgically feasible, it certainly cannot be achieved by conservative means without residual laxity. They recommend open reduction of all acute dislocations with either K-wire transarticular fixation of the thumb metacarpal in full palmar abduction and full palmar pronation or an Eaton-Littler flexor carpi radialis extra-articular tenodesis for the volar ligament rupture dislocations.[15] A short arm cast should be maintained for 4 weeks, at which time cast and pins are removed, and active exercises are instituted. Protective splinting is performed for an additional 2 weeks. After 6 weeks, passive stretching exercises may be used to supplement active exercises.

Other authors advocate percutaneous K-wire pinning of the CMC joint of the thumb in unstable cases and reserve open reduction for unreducible cases or for patients in whom the joint reduction is inappropriate, suggesting interposition of soft-tissue or chondral fragments.

In some cases, open reduction is necessary for accurate approximation of the articular surfaces. It is certainly desirable to obtain complete anatomic reduction; however, less than this may be acceptable. In Bennett's fracture of the base of the thumb, metacarpal fixation of the metacarpal shaft to the trapezium will provide stability of the joint, even if some separation persists between the shaft and the volar fragment. This may be preferable to open reduction, which is not a completely innocuous procedure, especially if carried out by surgeons not thoroughly versed in the principles of surgery of the hand.

In these cases, a thumb spica cast or splint is worn for approximately 4 weeks, at which time the intra-articular joint transfixation pin is removed and active protected motion is begun. The remaining pins holding the fracture are left in place for a minimum of 6 to 8 weeks or longer if their presence is not causing pressure or impingement problems.

In late cases in which malunion is present, along with the persistent subluxation of the CMC joint or instability, reconstructive procedures may include wedge osteotomy at the base of the first metacarpal, fusion of the carpometacarpal joint, or Silastic interposition prosthesis.

Another type of intra-articular fracture is known as Rolando's fracture, which is a Y- to T-shaped fracture at the proximal end of the first metacarpal. The strong muscular pull at the flexors and extensors may force the fracture fragments apart over the wedge of the trapezium. Treatment will depend on the degree of comminution and displacement of the fracture fragments. Closed manipulation and a molded cast or splint may be the treatment of choice if the fragments are severely comminuted or if they are stable with relatively little displacement. If the fragments are large, the treatment of choice is precise open reduction and internal fixation in which the articular fragments are approximated and then reduced as a single stable fragment to the shaft. Motion is usually begun with protection at 3 to 4 weeks; protective splinting is continued from 5 to 6 weeks as indicated.

ULNAR COLLATERAL LIGAMENT INJURIES OF THE THUMB

The ulnar collateral ligament of the MCP joint of the thumb is prevalent in skiing and in sports that involve handling of objects in contact situations. Unfortunately, this injury is often overlooked in the acute stage, especially in the young poorly supervised athlete. Inadequately treated or untreated, complete tears of the ulnar collateral ligament result in instability of the MCP joint when it is stretched in abduction, which jeopardizes one of the most important functions of the hand—the thumb-index pinch. In most sports, normal thumb-index pinch is a vital functional necessity for performance on a competitive level. There is controversy over the proper method of treatment of this injury. Residual thumb-index pinch weakness and instability with resulting pain can occur following an inadequate course of conservative treatment.

Mechanism of Injury

The mechanism of injury is forced radial deviation. To appreciate how this injury occurs, it is necessary to understand the roles played by the different soft-tissue structures in stabilizing the normal MCP joint. The causative factor is usually forceful abduction but it can also be torsion, combined abduction and hyperextension, or more rarely, combined abduction and flexion.[41]

The adductor pollicis and its aponeurosis play an important role in active stabilization of the MCP joint against the forces tending to abduct the thumb but are of little or no assistance in passive resistance to abduction. It has been shown that if the adductor aponeurosis alone is severed, there is no change in lateral stability of the MCP joint. Complete severance of the ulnar collateral ligament, however, makes abnormal abduction possible, even if the adductor aponeurosis remains intact. During extension, the accessory ulnar collateral ligament is relaxed and the ulnar collateral ligament is under tension, and the reverse is true during full flexion. If the ulnar collateral ligament proper is severed and the accessory collateral ligament is left intact, the MCP joint will be stable in extension, but increased abduction will be possible when flexion is present in the joint; this increase will not be marked unless the accessory ligament has also been cut. Even with both ulnar collateral segments divided, the abnormal abduction mobility will be most apparent in flexion of the MCP joint, because in extension abduction is restricted to the volar plate and its capsular and ligamentous attachment.

Diagnosis

Rupture of the ulnar collateral ligament either partial or total, should be borne in mind in evaluating any injury to the MCP thumb joint in athletes. A functional disability in thumb-index pinch will frequently be present with instability, pain, and weakness when this injury has been overlooked or inadequately treated.

There is usually a history of force applied in the radial direction to the thumb. This occurs most commonly in skiing injuries, but it may also happen in any sport in which the outstretched fingers and spread thumb are used to grasp, guard opponents, handle objects such as balls and bats, or break a fall. The patient complains of pain and swelling in the thumb-index web space at the base of the thumb, and weakness in the thumb-index pinch is present.

In the acute injury, the following signs and symptoms are helpful in making the diagnosis. On physical examination, there is local tenderness over the ulnar collateral ligament and there is pain on the ulnar aspect with abduction stress. There may be some swelling along the ulnar side of the metacarpal head, which may be caused by the proximal displacement of the torn ligament or by the local hemorrhage. Weakness of thumb-index pinch occurs with both partial and complete ulnar ligament tears. Instability is marked in complete tears of the ulnar collateral ligament but may also be present to some degree with partial tears. Stability testing should be performed with the MCP joint held in both extension and flexion. A tear in the ulnar collateral ligament proper can be missed if joint stability is tested only in extension. If both proper and accessory collateral ligaments are torn completely and the joint is subjected to abduction stress, there will be marked radial play in the joint, as well as in flexion and supination of the phalanx (Fig. 4–18).

Roentgenograms Routine x-ray films of the hand should be obtained in all cases with stress views compared to the uninvolved side. Occasionally, the regular radiographic views will show an avulsion fracture from the base of the proximal phalanx with or without displacement of the fragment. This fragment is most commonly attached to the distal end of the collateral ligament.

Historical Review

There were few reports on injury to the collateral ligaments of the metocarpalphalangeal joint of the thumb prior to the articles of Moberg and Stener in 1953 and Strandell in 1959.[45, 60] The amount of published material has increased concurrently with the recognition of the functional importance of this injury.

Controversy continues over the proper method of treatment. Bunnell, in 1948, reported good results with 4 weeks of splinting in acute injury. In old injuries, he advised ligamentous reconstruction and reinforcement or arthrodesis. In 1955, Watson-Jones stressed the importance of adequate conservative protection to prevent lengthening of the ligament and recurrent instability of the joint.[62] Frykman and Johannson reported good results from surgical treatment in 1956, and in 1958 Wosnik stated that plaster immobilization by itself would not give satis-

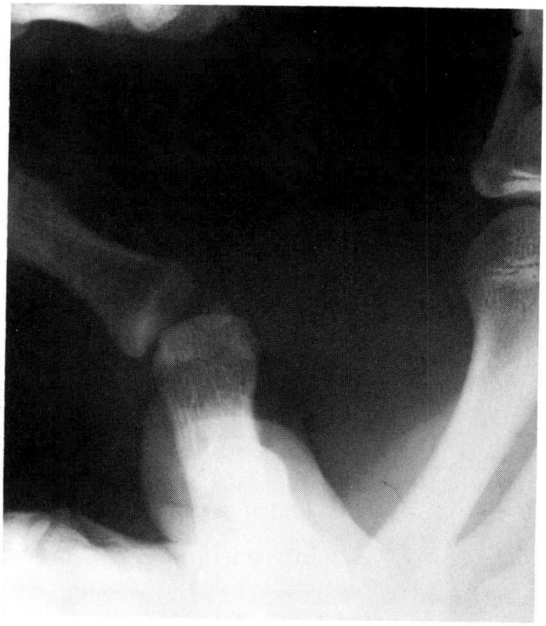

Figure 4–18 Radiographic stress testing of gamekeeper's thumb shows marked instability with the MP joint in flexion. (From Poznanski, A.K.: The Hand in Radiologic Diagnosis. Philadelphia, W.B. Saunders, 1984, p. 684.)

factory results in the majority of cases.[20, 63] Kaplan described two chronic cases of "gamekeeper's thumb" and performed experimental investigation in five specimens, including the defect that allowed radial subluxation of the thumb and ulnar displacement of the first metacarpal head, and found that the injury was not due to rupture of the ulnar collateral ligament but rather to disruption of the dorsal extensor apparatus between the adductor and extensor tendons and rupture of the dorsal capsule with secondary displacement of the extensor pollicis longus tendon to the radial side of the metacarpal head where it acted as a deforming force.[25, 26] In 1962, Stener pointed out the common occurrence of rupture of the ligament from its distal attachment at the base of the proximal phalanx with interposition of the adductor aponeurosis between the torn end of the ligament and its site of avulsion.[59] This so-called Stener lesion is commonly found in acute and chronic collateral ligament injuries. Kessler, in 1963, showed that the late instability of the MCP joint could be prevented by early diagnosis with the aid of stress radiographs and primary ligamentous repair.[27] In 1968, Coonrad and Goldner reported that ulnar or radial subluxation injuries should be treated with immediate immobilization for 4 weeks and that surgical repair should rarely be considered as an initial primary treatment.[14]

In 1972, the authors reported on 41 cases of surgical repair of complete tears of the ulnar collateral ligament in the MCP joint of the thumb, 16 of which were acute injuries and 25 chronic. The time interval from the injury to the day of surgery in the acute group was 9.8 days, and in the chronic group, the mean interval was 65 days. This represented the number of cases in a 10-year period from 1962 to 1972.[41] From 1972 to 1985, this series grew to 155 cases, of which 88 were acute injuries and 67 were chronic. The increase in acute injuries was due to the greater awareness of the condition, as well as to an increased number of ski injuries in our immediate geographic area. Our observations agree with those of Stener that tears of the ulnar collateral ligament occur in the distal attachment in a high percentage of cases. Overall, the best results were obtained in acute cases in which primary ligamentous repair was carried out. Although among cases treated within 9 weeks, the overall results were not significantly different, the percentage of good and excellent results decreased progressively when surgical treatment was further delayed. There were 11 cases in which replacement and reconstruction as augmentation with a free-graft was necessary in addition to repair of the remnants of the ligament, and in one case, fusion of the MCP joint was carried out due to degenerative changes. During this same period of time, there were 315 cases treated by closed immobilization for periods ranging from 3 to 5 weeks in the first 10 years from 1962 to 1972, and an additional 678 cases in the following 13 years, making a total of 993 cases treated by closed means.

Treatment

Interposition of the adductor aponeurosis cannot occur in partial rupture, even when the majority of the fibers are torn. These ligaments, even though stretched, will heal secondarily, contract, and shorten, and adequate protection will provide good results in the majority of cases. There is universal agreement that partial tears of the ulnar collateral ligament do not need surgical repair, except in the rare case in which a bony fragment is involved. These uncomplicated partial tears should be treated by a 3-week period of immobilization with the thumb in approximately 20° of flexion, after which protected exercise is begun for an additional 2 weeks in the thumb spica splint. Protection should continue until the soreness and swelling have abated and motion has been restored. However, the athlete may return to competition as soon as the pain is controlled so long as the thumb is protected by a thumb spica or a silicone or other soft cast or by taping the thumb in approximation to the hand.

Surgical indications for acute injuries include gross clinical instability, significant involvement of the articular surface, displacement and/or rotated fracture fragment and inability to reduce due to soft-tissue interposition. Surgical treatment of chronic injuries should be contemplated when the patient complains of pain, instability, and weakness in pinch.

When surgery is indicated, the ligament may be sutured to the base of the proximal phalanx using a pull-out wire. While volar subluxation is not as common as in the radiocollateral ligament injuries, repair of the dorsal capsule is important as is repair of the tear in the volar plate. When a large bone fragment is present, it may be reinserted and held with a pull-out suture or Kirschner wire. Small fragments can be excised and the ligament reattached with a pull-out wire into the defect. The approach is through a dorsal curvilinear incision that crosses the MCP joint and then runs distally along the midlateral ulnar aspect of the proximal phalanx. The distal end should lie volar enough to allow access to the base of the proximal phalanx where repair is carried out and to allow repair and advancement of the adductor pollicis. The sensory nerves and dorsal vein should be identified and protected. The extensor pollicis longus and its adductor aponeurosis are identified and, in the cases of a Stener lesion, may be observed along the proximal edge of the extensor hood. Incision is made through the adductor aponeurosis, paralleling the ulnar border of the extensor pollicis longus, which is reflected volarly to expose the MCP joint, including the adductor pollicis, and dorsally to free the extensor pollicis longus tendon.

The joint is exposed and examined, and the wound irrigated of clot and bony fragments. Repair is carried out as described previously depending on the pathology of injury. The ulnar portion of the volar plate is generally torn from the base of the proximal phalanx to a varying degree. This should be repaired with a mattress suture, along with the distal portion of the collateral ligament. A similar repair is carried out in the dorsal capsule to prevent volar subluxation as well as rotation of the joint. This repair is done in approximately 20° of flexion, and in certain selected cases, an intra-articular K-wire may be added for additional stabilization. The extensor hood is then repaired with interrupted sutures and the wound closed. The thumb is mobilized in the appropriate position with a compression bulky dressing and volar plaster splint, which is changed in 10 to 14 days, the sutures are removed, and a snug-fitting thumb spica is applied, leaving the IP joint free. Active motion exercises prevent adherence of the extensor mechanism. Gentle exercise is begun at 3 to 4 weeks, with protection for 5 weeks in normal activity and for at least 3 months following surgery when the patient is engaged in competition (Fig. 4–19).

CHRONIC ULNAR COLLATERAL LIGAMENT INJURIES

The surgical approach for reconstruction in the chronic injury is the same as in the acute case. The Stener lesion and tear in the collateral ligament are more difficult to isolate. The possibility of direct repair diminishes with time. In many cases, reconstruction of the ligament from the remnant of scarred capsule and ligament is possible with reattachment to the base of the proximal phalanx with the joint in 15° of flexion. In all chronic injuries, we have advanced a slip of the adductor pollicis from its insertion into the ulnar sesamoid dorsally and distally, in addition to the reconstruction. In the majority of cases, these two components of reconstruction are adequate to give functional stability. However, in those cases in which the remaining scarred remnants are not capable of giving adequate ulnar stability, reinforcement with a tendon transfer or free graft is indicated.

In our experience, this procedure consists of the following steps. The scarred remnant of the capsule and collateral ligament is reconstructed and a slip of the adductor pollicis is transferred dorsally and distally, as described. In addition, a free graft utilizing the palmaris longus or a tendon slip of the abductor pollicis longus is left attached to its insertion at the base of the first metacarpal. A drill hole is made parallel to the joint just proximal to the flare, and the graft is passed from the radial side to the ulnar dorsal aspect of the distal end of the first metacarpal. It is then passed distally and volarly, along with the reconstructed remnants, to a volar drill hole at the base of the proximal phalanx and then passed from the ulnar side to exit radially and then sutured on to itself or attached to the radial collateral ligament. Care must be taken to place the joint in 15 to 20° of flexion or motion will be lost. Dorsal capsular repair to alleviate volar subluxation and K-wire

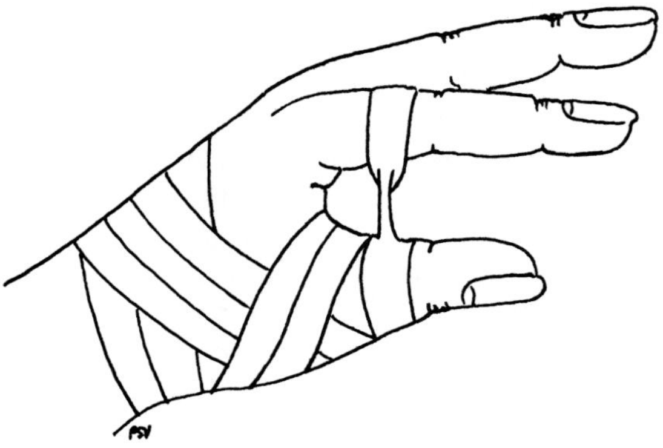

Figure 4–19 This check-rein method of taping of the thumb can be used in prophylactic as well as postoperative management of ulnar collateral ligament injuries of the thumb MP joint. (From Gieck, J.H., Mayer, V.: Protective splinting for the hanc and wrist. Clin. Sports Med. 5:801, 1986.)

fixation in the prescribed position may be carried out as indicated. Closure and immobilization are done as described previously for partial and acute reconstructions.

In summary, the mechanism of injury and functional impairment vary with the sport and the specific position played by the athlete. In specific situations, we feel that temporary taping and splinting may be utilized to allow continued athletic participation and delay surgery until a more opportune time without jeopardizing the final surgical result. The method of taping depends on the positional and sports needs of the athlete and should be used until discomfort has subsided and motion in the thumb has been restored.

RADIAL COLLATERAL LIGAMENT INJURIES

Injury of the radial collateral ligament in the MCP joint of the thumb is much less common than that of the ulnar collateral ligament. Although pinch is not involved to the same significant degree, disability and functional loss can be severe if treatment is delayed or inadequate.

The mechanism of radial collateral ligament injury is forced adduction and torsion on the flexed MP joint with avulsion from the base of the proximal phalanx more frequent than from the metacarpal head.

Volar subluxation in this injury appears to be more common than ulnar involvement and is often the initial diagnostic finding. Injury to the dorsal capsule is predominant, as the stress is one of pronation and ulnar deviation. The volar subluxation is visible both clinically and on lateral radiographic views and is an indication for surgical repair.

Treatment is similar to that for ulnar side injuries. Immobilization is the treatment of choice in partial tears. There is no interposition of the aponeurosis as on the ulnar side, so complete tears may heal more readily radially. Surgical repair gives a more predictable result in complete lesions especially when associated with ulnar shift and volar subluxation. The principles of repair and of postoperative care are similar to those for ulnar side injuries.

INTERPHALANGEAL FRACTURES

Condylar fractures of the proximal phalanx of the thumb can result from torque or crush injury to the IP joint area. Condylar fractures can be singular, bicondylar, or comminuted. Fractures that are nondisplaced or minimally displaced (less than 1 to 2 mm) can be treated conservatively in a thumb spica cast for a period of 4 to 6 weeks. Again, as with all hand fractures, attention must be directed to angular and rotational deformities. This may be more difficult in the thumb than in the fingers because of the lack of reference points. By the same token, the thumb is much more forgiving of minor degrees of deformity, since its tremendous mobility allows adequate compensation.

Surgical options include closed reduction with percutaneous K-wire pinning for condylar fractures, parallel K-wire pinning after open reduction with or without diagonal pinning or suturing for bicondylar fractures, and open reduction and K-wire pinning of comminuted poorly aligned proximal phalangeal head fractures that have large fragments. As in finger fractures, care must be taken to avoid damaging the blood supply to the condylar fragment at the level of the collateral ligament attachment by too vigorous a dissection. It should also be stressed that when confronting a severely comminuted fracture of the condyles, it may be more prudent to attempt closed reduction and splinting or casting for 2 to 3 weeks followed by early therapy.

Postoperative management includes a well-molded thumb spica cast that includes the IP joint for a period of 3 to 4 weeks, after which the K-wires may be removed. Occupational therapy is instituted with progressive flexion and extension exercises of all the thumb joints, as well as protective splinting for an additional 2 weeks.

Injuries of the IP joint of the thumb most commonly result from crush injuries, since significant torque stresses usually bypass the IP joint and more frequently damage the MCP joint. Regardless, fracture-subluxations and fracture-dislocations of the distal tuft are seen and should be handled in the same way as finger DIP joint injuries.

Extensor and flexor tendon ruptures and avulsion fractures may be seen in the IP joint but they are rare. The mechanisms of injury and management are quite similar to those already described for the finger DIP joint. The extensor rupture will result in a swan neck deformity if sufficient time elapses between injury and treatment. The flexor pollicis longus avulsions present a significant problem if the tendon rupture is not recognized during the first 3 weeks postinjury. The complex fiber osseous pulley system to the thumb, as well as the precarious blood supply to the flexor pollicis longus, which can be damaged if allowed to retract into the forearm, adds to the difficulty of surgical management.

REFERENCES

1. Abouna, J.M., Brown, H.: The treatment of mallet finger: the results in a series of 148 consecutive cases and a review of the literature. Am. J. Surg. 55:653, 1968.
2. Agee, J.M.: Unstable fracture dislocations of the proximal interphalangeal joint of the fingers: A preliminary report of a new treatment technique. J. Hand Surg. 3:336, 1978.
3. Aiache, A., Barsky, A.J., Weiner, D.L.: Prevention of boutonniere deformity. Plast. Reconstr. Surg. 46:164, 1970.
4. Boyes, J.H.: Operative Technique in Surgery of the Hand. AAOS Instructional Course Lecture, Vol. 9, 1952.
5. Boyes, J.H. (ed.): Bunnell's Surgery of the Hand, 5th ed. Philadelphia, J.B. Lippincott, 1972, pp. 439–442, 616–618.
6. Boyes, J.H., Wilson, J.N., Smith, J.W.: Flexor tendon ruptures in the forearm and hand. J. Bone Joint Surg. 42A:637, 1960.
7. Bunnell, S: Surgery of the Hand, 4th ed. Philadelphia, J.B. Lippincott, 1964.
8. Burton, R.I., Eaton, R.G.: Common hand injuries in the athlete. Orthop. Clin. North Am. 4:809, 1973.
9. Cabrera, J.M., Reyers, F., Burkhalter, W.: Acute traumatic dislocation of the basilar joint of the thumb. A report of eight cases. Submitted for publication, J. Bone Joint Surg. [Am.] 1986.

10. Chao, K.O.: Translocation of the abductor pollicis longus tendon. A treatment for chronic subluxation of the thumb carpometacarpal joint. J. Bone Joint Surg. 52A:1166, 1970.
11. Cleland, A.: On the cutaneous ligaments of the phalanges. J. Anat. Physiol. 12:526, 1978.
12. Contis, R.M.: Treatment of injuries of the proximal interphalangeal joints of the fingers. Curr. Pract. Orthop. Surg. 2:125, 1964.
13. Cooney, W.P., Chao, E.V.: Biomechanical analysis of static forces in the thumb during hand function. J. Bone Joint Surg. 59A:27, 1977.
14. Coonrad, R.W., Oldner, J.L.: A study of the pathological findings and treatment in soft tissue injuries of the thumb metacarpophalangeal joints with a clinical study of the normal range of motion in one thousand thumbs and a study of post mortem findings of ligamentous structures relating to function. J. Bone Joint Surg. 50A:439, 1968.
15. Eaton, R.G., Littler, T.W.: Ligament reconstruction for the painful thumb carpometacarpal joint. J. Bone Joint Surg. 55A:1655, 1973.
16. Eaton, R.G., Mallerich, M.M.: Volar plate arthroplasty for the proximal interphalangeal joint. A ten year review. J. Hand Surg. 5:260, 1980.
17. Eggers, G.W.N.: Chronic dislocation of the base of the metacarpal of the thumb. J. Bone Joint Surg. 27:500, 1945.
18. Elliot, R.A., Jr.: Injuries to the extensor mechanism of the hand. Orthop. Clin. North Am. 1:335, 1970.
19. Flynn, J.E.: Acute trauma to the hand. Clin. Orthop. 13:124, 1959.
20. Frykman, G., Johannson, O.: Surgical repair of rupture of the ulnar collateral ligament of the metacarpophalangeal joint of the thumb. Acta Chir. Scand. 112:58, 1956.
21. Green, D.P., Terry, G.C.: Complex dislocation of the metacarpophalangeal joint. J. Bone Joint Surg. 85A:1481, 1973.
22. Jensen, J.S.: Operative treatment of chronic subluxation of the first carpometacarpal joint. Hand 7:269, 1975.
23. Kaplan, E.B.: Functional and Surgical Anatomy of the Hand. Philadelphia, J.B. Lippincott, 1953.
24. Kaplan, E.B.: Dorsal dislocations of the metacarpophalangeal joint of the index finger. J. Bone Joint Surg. 39A:1081, 1957.
25. Kaplan, E.B.: Lateral subluxation of the metacarpophalangeal joint of the thumb: Experimental study. Bull. Hosp. Joint Dis. 21:200, 1960.
26. Kaplan, E.B.: The Pathology and treatment of radial subluxation of the thumb with ulnar displacement of the head of the first metacarpal. J. Bone Joint Surg. 43A:541, 1961.
27. Kessler, I: Chronic subluxation of the metacarpophalangeal joint of the thumb. J. Bone Joint Surg. 45B:805, 1963.
28. Kestler, O.C.: Recurrent dislocation of the first carpometacarpal joint repaired by functional tenodesis. J. Bone Joint Surg. 28:858, 1946.
29. Landsmeer, J.M.F.: The anatomy of the dorsal aponeurosis of the human finger and its functional significance. Anat. Rec. 104:31, 1949.
30. Lewin, P.: A simple splint for baseball finger. J.A.M.A. 85:1059, 1925.
31. Littler, J.W.: The Hand and Wrist. In Howorth, M.B. (ed.): A Textbook of Orthopaedics. Philadelphia, W.B. Saunders, 1952, p. 284.
32. Littler, J.W.: The finger extension mechanism. Surg. Clin. North Am. 47:415, 1967.
33. MacElfrish, E., Dobyns, J., O'Brien, E.: Management of fracture dislocation of the proximal interphalangeal joints by extension-block splinting. J. Bone Joint Surg. 54A:1705, 1972.
34. McCue, F.C., Abbott, J.L.: The treatment of mallet finger and boutonniere deformities. Va. Med. 94:623, 1967.
35. McCue, F.C., Andrews, J.R., Hakala, M.W.: The coach's finger. Am. J. Sports Med. 2:270, 1974.
36. McCue, F.C., Baugher, W.H., Bourland, W.L., et al.: Hand injuries in athletes. Surg. Rounds 1:8, 1978.
37. McCue, F.C., Baugher, W.H., Bourland, W.L., et al.: Hand injuries in athletes. Surg. Rounds 2:24, 1979.

38. McCue, F.C., Baugher, W.H., Kulund, D.N., et al.: Hand and wrist injuries in the athlete. Am. J. Sports Med. 7:275, 1979.
39. McCue, F.C., Honner, R., Gieck, J., et al.: A pseudo-boutonniere deformity. Hand 7:166, 1975.
40. McCue, F.C., Garroway, R.Y.: Sports injuries to the hand and wrist. In Schneider, R.C., Kennedy, J.C., Plant, M.L. (eds.): Sports Injuries: Mechanisms, Prevention and Treatment. Baltimore, Williams & Wilkins, 1985, p. 743.
41. McCue, F.C., Hakala, M.W., Andrews, J.R., et al.: Ulnar collateral ligament injuries of the thumb in athletes. Am. J. Sports Med. 2(2):70–80, 1975.
42. McCue, F.C., Honner, R., Johnson, M.E., et al.: Athletic injuries of the proximal interphalangeal joint requiring surgical treatment. J. Bone Joint Surg. 52A:937, 1970.
43. McLaughlin, H.L.: Complex "locked" dislocation of the metacarpophalangeal joints. J. Trauma, 5:682, 1965.
44. Milford, L.W., Jr.: Retaining Ligaments of the Digits of the Hand: Gross and Microscopic Anatomic Study. Philadelphia, W.B. Saunders, 1968.
45. Moberg, E., Stener, B.: Injuries to the ligaments of the thumb and fingers: Diagnosis, treatment and prognosis. Acta Chir. Scand. 106:166, 1953.
46. Murphy, A.F., Stark, H.H.: Closed dislocation of the metacarpophalangeal joint of the index finger. J. Bone Joint Surg. 49:1599, 1967.
47. Napier, J.R.: Form and function of the carpometacarpal joint of the thumb. J. Anat. 89:3, 1955.
48. Pulvertaft, R.G.: Repair of severed tendons in the hand. In Rob, C., Smith, R., eds.: Operative Surgery, Vol. 6. London, Butterworth's, 1958, p. 31.
49. Redler, I., Williams, J.T.: Rupture of a collateral ligament of the proximal interphalangeal joint of the finger. Analysis of 18 cases. J. Bone Joint Surg. 49A:332, 1967.
50. Riordan, D.C.: Fractures about the hand. South. Med. J. 50:637, 1957.
51. Robertson, R.C., Cawley, J.J., Faris, H.M.: Treatment of fracture-dislocation of the interphalangeal joints of the hand. J. Bone Joint Surg. 28:68, 1946.
52. Rodriguez, A.L.: Injuries to the collateral ligaments of the proximal interphalangeal joints. Hand 5:55, 1973.
53. Slocum, D.M.: Stabilization of the articulation of the greater multangular and the first metacarpal. J. Bone Joint Surg. 25A:626, 1943.
54. Sonter, W.A.: The boutonniere deformity. A review of 101 patients with division of the central slip of the extensor expansion of the fingers. J. Bone Joint Surg. 49B:710, 1967.
55. Smillie, I.S.: Mallet finger. Br. J. Surg. 24:439, 1937.
56. Smith, R.J.: Balance and kinetics of the fingers under normal and pathological conditions. Clin. Orthop. 104:95, 1974.
57. Spinner, M., Choi, B.Y.: Anterior dislocations of the proximal interphalangeal joint. J. Bone Joint Surg. 52A, 7:1329, 1979.
58. Stark, H.H., Boyes, J.H. and Wilson, J.N.: Mallet finger. J. Bone Joint Surg. 44A:1061, 1962.
59. Stener, B.: Displacement of the ruptured ulnar collateral ligament of the metacarpophalangeal joint of the thumb. A clinical and anatomical study. J. Bone Joint Surg. 44B:869, 1962.
60. Strandell, G.: Total Rupture of the ulnar collateral ligament of the metacarpophalangeal joint of the thumb. Results of surgery in 35 Cases. Acta Chir. Scand. 118:72, 1959.
61. Sultro, C.J.: Hypermobility of bones due to "overstrengthened" capsular and ligamentous tissues. A cause for recurrent intra-articular effusions. Surgery 21:67, 1947.
62. Watson-Jones, R.: Fractures and Joint Injuries, 3rd ed. London, E. and S. Livingston, 1955.
63. Wosnick, H.: Die Greschlossenln Bandverlet Zunger des Dawmengrund Gelenlis. Hefte Zur Unfallneilkundk 56:45, 1958.

CHAPTER

5

Collateral Ligament Injuries of the Thumb Metacarpophalangeal Joint

Robert J. Neviaser, M.D.

Injuries to the collateral ligaments of the thumb metacarpophalangeal joint are common in athletes. Some of the sports in which they occur are skiing, football, baseball, softball, rugby, and volleyball.

Anatomy

The metacarpophalangeal (MCP) joint of the thumb is supported by a group of ligaments and the joint capsule. To a certain extent the intrinsic muscles of the thumb also contribute to stability of this joint. The ligaments include the radial and ulnar collateral and accessory collateral ligaments and the volar plate. The collateral ligaments run from slightly dorsal on the metacarpal neck to a more volar attachment on the base of the proximal phalanx. Immediately palmar to these structures lie the accessory collateral ligaments, and on the volar surface of the joint is the tough, fibrocartilaginous volar plate. Two sesamoids are within the plate, blending with the adductor pollicis tendon as it inserts into the plate.

Joint Function

This is a diarthrodial joint that has a hingelike action. It functions primarily in the flexion-extension plane, although there is some abduction and adduction. It has been demonstrated that there is a great variation in motion in this joint. Flexion may be as little as 0° or as much as 100° with the average being 75°.[1] Extension varies from 0° to 90° with an average of 20°. Normal abduction and adduction can be as high as 20° but average approximately 10°. The joint is most lax in 15 to 20° of flexion, while the collateral ligaments are most taut in full flexion.

Mechanism of Injury

The direction of the force applied to the thumb determines the nature of the injury. The two collateral structures that can be injured are the ulnar collateral complex and the radial collateral complex. These two structures are referred to as ligament complexes, since the rupture does not occur through the isolated proper collateral ligament alone but rather involves the dorsal capsule, the volar capsule, and the accessory collateral ligament of the injured side as well. For the injury to occur on the ulnar side, the thumb must be forced into flexion, radial deviation, and pronation. To occur on the radial side, the thumb must be deviated into flexion, ulnar deviation, and supination.

One of the most common athletic injuries to the thumb MCP joint is the ski pole injury. The traditional method of holding the straps and pole is to loop the strap around the wrist, pass it through the palm, and out the thumb web. This causes the strap to lie against the ulnar side of the thumb so that during a fall the strap places a tremendous radial deviation, flexion, and pronation force on the thumb, rupturing the ulnar collateral complex. Sports that involve a ball moving with some speed, such as basketball, football, and volleyball, produce various ligament injuries. The thumb can also be caught on another player's jersey or struck by the body or extremity of someone else. A fall is another common type of injury.

Pathologic Anatomy

As implied earlier, a rupture of the collateral ligament comprises more than that phrase connotes. In the case of ulnar or radial collateral ligament injuries, the proper ligament tears along with the corresponding accessory collateral ligament and the dorsal and the volar plate on the affected side (Fig. 5–1). The site of detachment is almost always the base of the proximal phalanx, and fragments of avulsed bone can be found here.

Diagnosis

As with most injuries, the diagnosis can usually be established through a careful history and thorough physical examination. In this age of sophisticated technology, the simple fact is that the ligament injuries to the thumb can be correctly diagnosed nearly every time by listening to the patient and examining the thumb. Not only can the specific ligament injury be established, but the severity can also be determined in this manner.

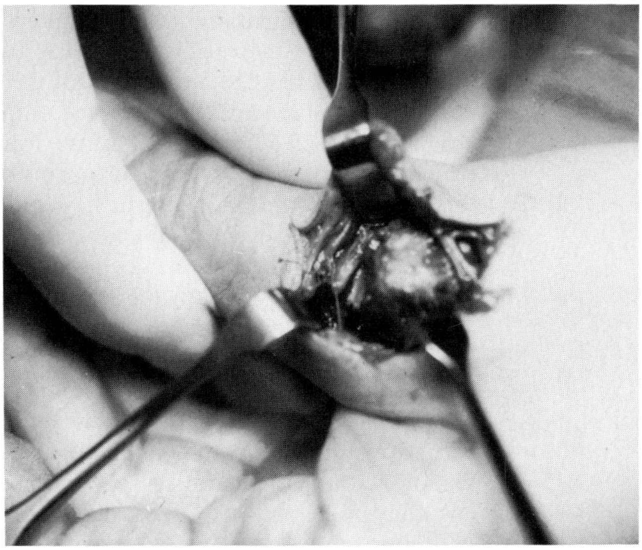

Figure 5–1 This intraoperative photograph reveals the extent of the capsular disruption in an ulnar side injury. In addition to the collateral ligament, the dorsal capsule, the accessory collateral ligament, and the volar plate are torn.

For the acute injury, the patient will usually be able to relate the mechanism of injury, if asked. He or she will state that the thumb was struck with a ball or was caught in the strap of the ski pole and was bent backward or pulled to the side.[7] For the chronic injury, the patient may not be able to recall the original mechanism of injury but can often describe the functional deficit. With ulnar side laxity, there is often difficulty in pinching activities (Fig. 5–2), such as turning a key in a lock. With laxity on the radial side, the thumb will give way during keyboard work or while doing pushups.

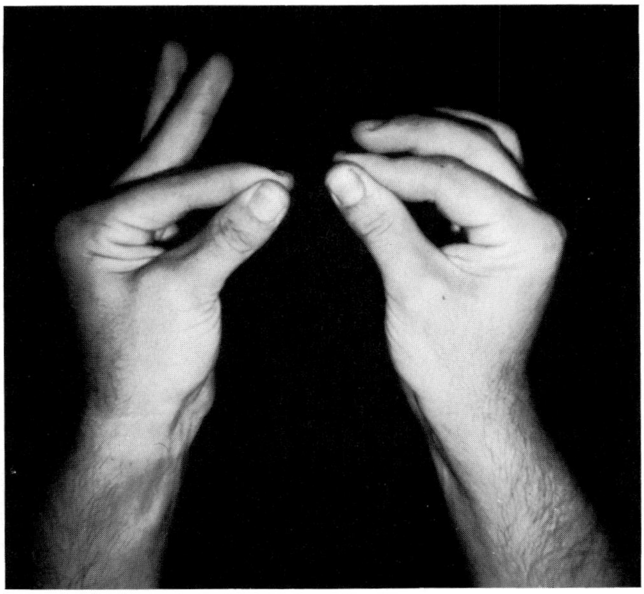

Figure 5–2 With an ulnar side injury, pinching functions are weakened due to instability, as seen in the left thumb in this patient.

When examining the acutely injured thumb, the examiner must perform the testing thoroughly but gently. After looking for obvious deformity, one palpates the attachment of the important ligaments. The most common site of tenderness is the base of the proximal phalanx where these structures attach. The stressing of the ligaments is the key to determining which ligament is injured as well as how severely. The examiner must do this in a very gentle manner or the test will be so painful that an assessment of the degree of injury will not be possible. The patient's metacarpal shaft is grasped and stabilized between the examiner's thumb and index finger with the latter supported by the long finger. The patient's thumb is grasped with the examiner's other hand between the same three digits. In order to check the collateral ligaments one applies a radial or ulnar deviating force to the thumb (Fig. 5–3). It has been suggested that this be done with the metacarpal phalangeal joint fully flexed,[5] but this is rarely possible in a recently injured thumb. It is practical to test the ligaments in as much flexion as the patient can reasonably tolerate without compromising the accuracy of the diagnosis. Although there are different guidelines concerning the degree of laxity that indicates a completely torn ligament, most observers consider between 20 and 30° of increased laxity when compared with the normal thumb as representing a pathologic state. One can also judge by the "feel" of the joint. If there is a definite end-point on stress, the ligament is not completely torn.

It is appropriate to obtain radiographs of the injured thumb. Occasionally there is a small avulsion fracture from the base of the proximal phalanx on the injured side. Rarely, there will be a large fracture fragment that represents more than a ligament injury. With rupture of the radial collateral ligament the phalanx may rest in an ulnarly deviated position due to the strong unopposed pull of the adductor pollicis (Fig. 5–4*A* and *B*).

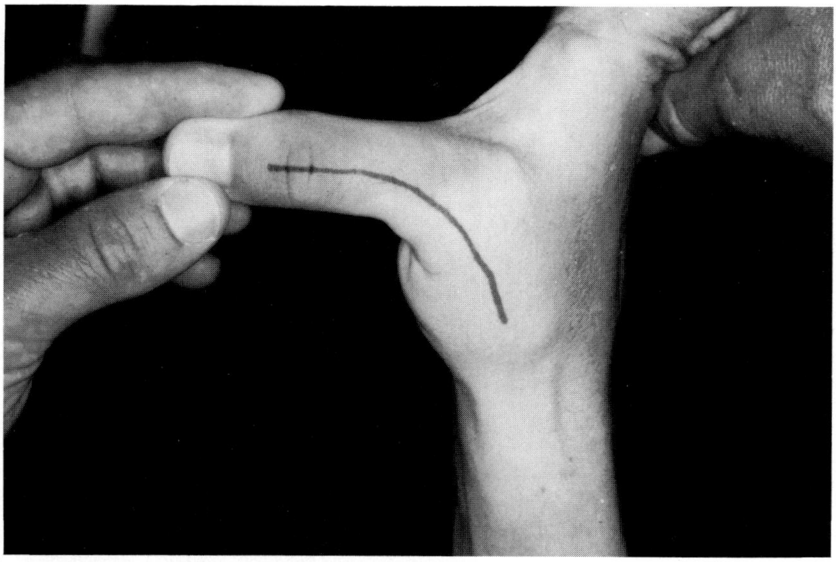

Figure 5–3 A dramatic demonstration of a complete rupture of the ulnar collateral ligament.

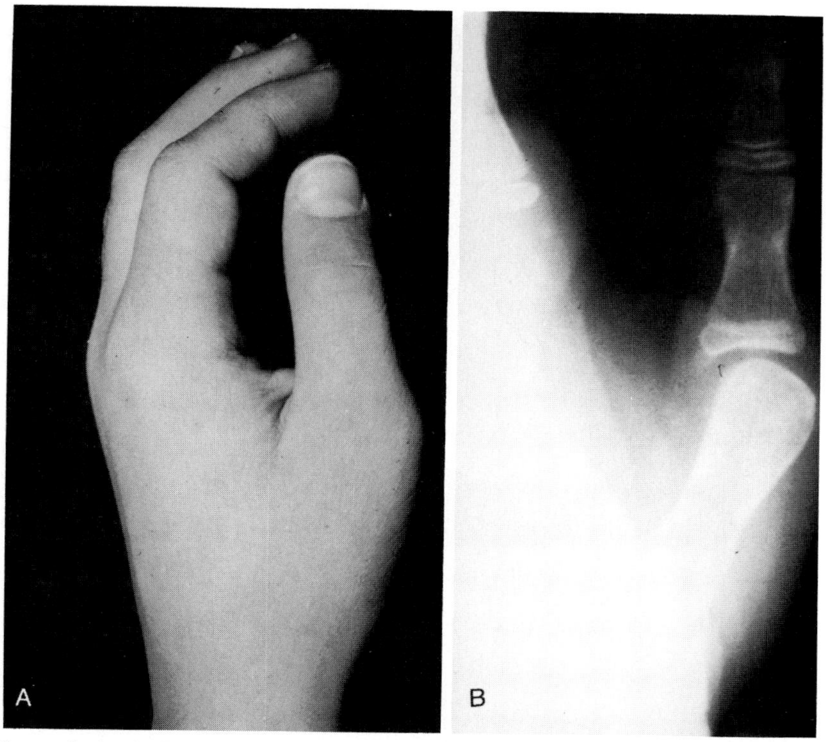

Figure 5–4 *A,* Resting ulnar angulation of the thumb with a radial collateral ligament rupture. The unopposed adductor pollicis pulls the thumb into this position. *B,* Radiographic confirmation of the clinical picture.

There is some difference of opinion on the value of stress films in general and in the presence of an avulsion fracture in particular. In most cases the physical examination will be sufficient to establish the correct diagnosis and the degree of injury. In the unusual instance when the diagnosis is in doubt, a stress radiograph can be taken. In the acutely injured thumb local anesthesia is often needed. The thumb is grasped by the examiner and stress is applied as it is for the clinical examination (Fig. 5–5). Most observers caution against taking a stress film in the presence of an avulsion fracture, especially an undisplaced one. They note that a displaced fracture means that the end of the ligament is displaced as well and that if the fracture is undisplaced, the end of the ligament is too. In fact, they advise that the thumb not even be stressed for the purposes of examination if there is an avulsion fracture. Unfortunately the ligament is not always attached to the avulsed fragment of bone, so gentle stressing is important to the assessment of the degree of instability and should be done, avulsion fracture or not (Fig. 5–6).

There has been some interest in arthrography of the metacarpophalangeal joint of the thumb as a means of telling not only whether the ligament is torn, but, of greater importance, where the tear lies. This study takes considerable experience to interpret correctly and has not gained much popularity.

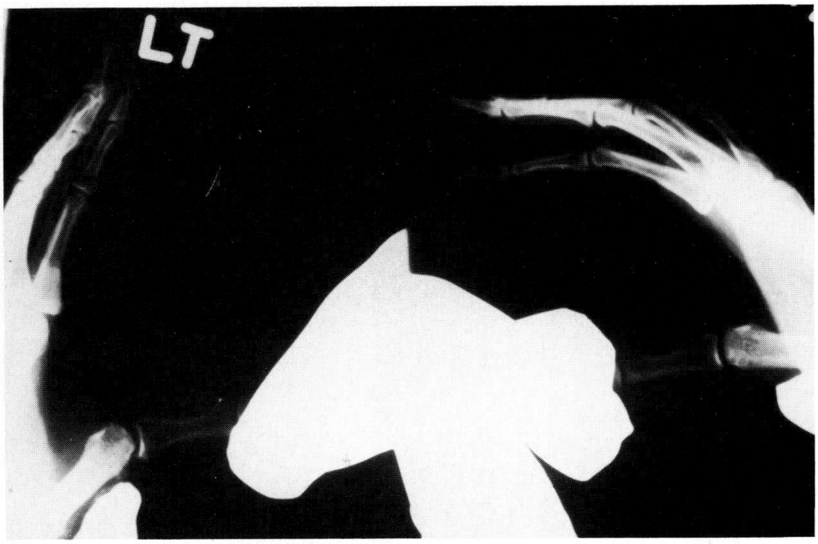

Figure 5–5 A stress view showing the instability of the left thumb.

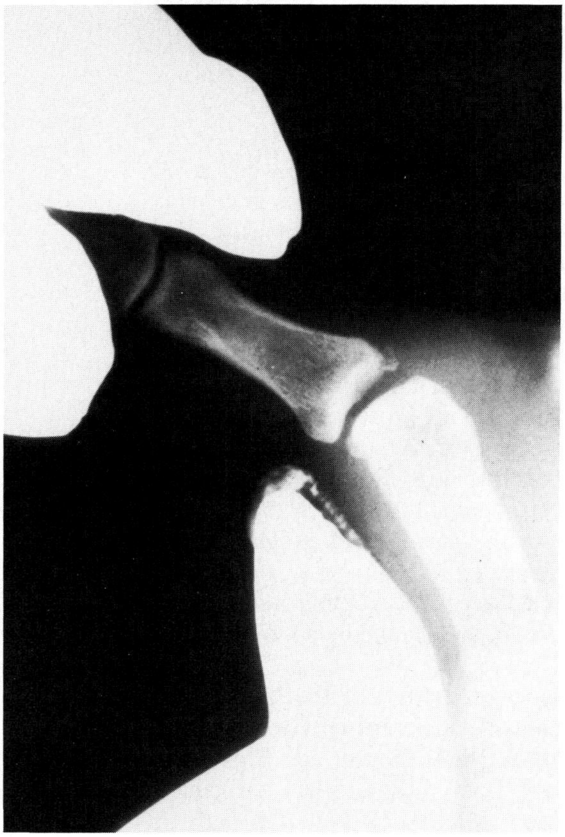

Figure 5–6 Stress view of an avulsion fracture. Note that the fracture moves with the phalanx, indicating that the fragment is not attached to the ligament, which has torn its phalangeal attachment.

Treatment

Incomplete and complete injuries are treated differently. The incomplete tear with good residual stability is managed by initial immobilization. For injury to the collateral ligament (either radial or ulnar), the thumb should be immobilized in a thumb spica plaster. The length of immobilization is determined by the severity of the reaction and the degree of incomplete laxity. The less the degree of reaction and laxity, the shorter the period of splinting. The time may be as short as a few days, but should be no longer than 3 weeks. Rehabilitation is usually rapid and the return to the sport is dependent on the activity involved. If the thumb is at significant risk for re-injury, a removable splint of a heat-malleable synthetic material that hardens on cooling can be used. Taping the thumb is a less secure means of protecting it.

The following discussion of the management of complete injuries emphasizes operative treatment, which provides the potential for the best functional outcome for the reasons presented below. In the professional or high-level amateur athlete, circumstances may dictate delaying the acute repair and performing a late reconstruction after the season is over. The thumb can be protected with taping, padding, or splinting during practice or competition.

ACUTE COMPLETE INJURIES

If the ulnar collateral ligament is considered to be completely ruptured, most observers recommend early repair. Closed treatment has certain risks of failure. Stener[6] has shown that three things can happen to the torn end of the ligament. It can rest adjacent to its original site of attachment and will therefore heal with good residual stability. It can also fold back on itself, with the interposed adductor aponeurosis lying between the end of the ligament and its site of attachment, and fail to heal with adequate stability. Finally it can pop completely outside of the adductor aponeurosis with the latter lying between the ligament and the bone, preventing healing. Two of these circumstances will result in a persistently unstable MCP joint.

Since there is no consistently reliable way to determine where the end of the ruptured ligament is, surgical repair is the more reliable form of treatment. The repair can be done through a straight or chevron incision (Fig. 5–7) over the dorsolateral aspect of the joint. There is a consistent sensory branch that must be recognized and protected. The adductor aponeurosis is detached from the extensor pollicis longus and reflected for later repair. An incision is made at the dorsal edge of the ulnar collateral ligament, and with a probe the ligament is inspected to determine where it is detached. The most common location is from the proximal phalanx. The ligament is stretched to length, and the site of reattachment selected. If, as usual, there is an adequate stump distally, the two portions are sewn together. If the distal stump cannot hold a suture securely, the phalanx is roughened, a hole is drilled across the phalanx (larger on the ulnar side), and the ligament is pulled into the hole with a pull-out suture that is tied

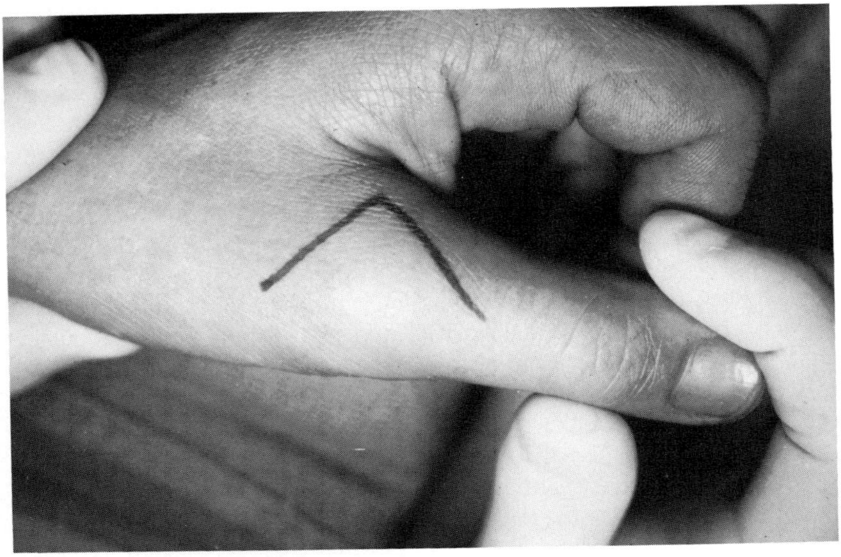

Figure 5–7 The chevron incision.

externally to keep the repair taut during the healing process. Other structures, such as the dorsal capsule and the volar plate, should be repaired to the extent necessary. The adductor aponeurosis is reattached to the extensor mechanism and the skin closed.

For the acutely ruptured radial collateral ligament, the approach is the same. The ligament is approached from the radial side using a dorsal radial or a radial chevron incision. The abductor aponeurosis is reflected and the torn ligament freed. The same surgical steps for repair are used as discussed for the ulnar collateral ligament.

CHRONIC COMPLETE INJURIES

Chronic injuries are best treated surgically for optimal functional restoration. Before the operation is discussed with the patient, a radiograph should be obtained. If there is evidence of posttraumatic arthrosis, an arthrodesis of the metacarpophalangeal joint is the preferred procedure, regardless of the underlying ligamentous injury. If, however, there is no arthrosis, reconstructive procedures can be used.

Although there are many reconstructive procedures described for chronic ulnar collateral ligament laxity, the following is widely used and has proven successful over the past 20 years.[2, 4] The surgical approach is the same as that for exposure of the acute injury. After reflecting the adductor aponeurosis, the scarred remnant of the collateral ligament is dissected out. Care is taken not to transect the ligament at any point until the site of ligamentous detachment is determined. As mentioned earlier, the rupture usually occurs from the proximal phalanx. The ligament is freed as much as possible. The main tendon of the adductor pollicis tendon is isolated as it inserts into the volar plate and the sesamoid and is detached with as much length as possible. A hole is drilled from ulnar to radial in the midaxial line of the proximal phalanx at a point just less than a centimeter from the joint, which corresponds approximately to the base of the metaphyseal flare. The ulnar hole is enlarged to accommodate the end of the adductor tendon. The ligament is then imbricated slightly and sutured in a pants-over-vest style to the distal remnant at the base of the distal phalanx, creating a passive restraint to radial stress and rendering the joint stable. A criss-cross pull-out suture is passed through the end of the tendon and through the hole in the phalanx with a straight needle to exit through the skin on the radial side of the thumb. The needle and suture are passed through a piece of sponge rubber and a button and pulled up snugly so that the end of the tendon is brought into the ulnar hole in the phalanx (Fig. 5–8). When the tendon fits securely in the hole, the suture is tied with some tension over the sponge rubber and button. The adductor aponeurosis is repaired and the skin closed. The repair is protected with a thumb spica plaster for 4 weeks, at which point the pull-out suture is removed and rehabilitation is started.

The procedure for chronic injuries to the radial side is a mirror image of the one just described.[2,3] The approach is the same as that for the acute injuries. Once the scarred ligament is dissected out (with the same precautions as on the ulnar side), the tendon of the abductor pollicis brevis is isolated and detached with as much length as possible. The hole is drilled in the phalanx from radial to ulnar and the radial side enlarged to accept the tendon. The radial collateral ligament is imbricated to restore passive joint stability, and the tendon is passed through the phalangeal hole on a straight needle and through the skin on the ulnar side as well as a piece of sponge rubber and a button (Fig. 5–9). The suture is pulled up so that the tendon fits snugly in the hole and is tied over the sponge rubber and button with enough tension to keep the tendon securely in the hole. The abductor aponeurosis is reattached and the skin closed. Immobilization in a thumb spica plaster is continued for 4 weeks before rehabilitation is started.

REHABILITATION

Early rehabilitation consists exclusively of motion exercises. Strengthening, especially power pinch, is avoided for 8 weeks from surgery. This is true regardless of the nature of the repair (i.e., direct repair for the acute rupture or reconstruction for the chronic tear).

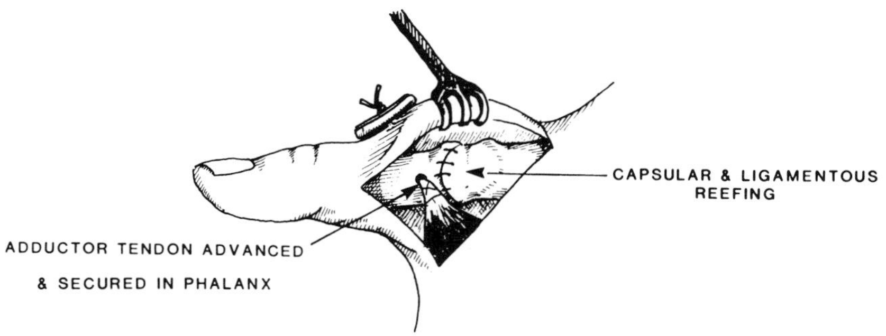

Figure 5–8 Diagramatic representation of the adductor advancement after capsular plication for chronic ulnar collateral ligament laxity.

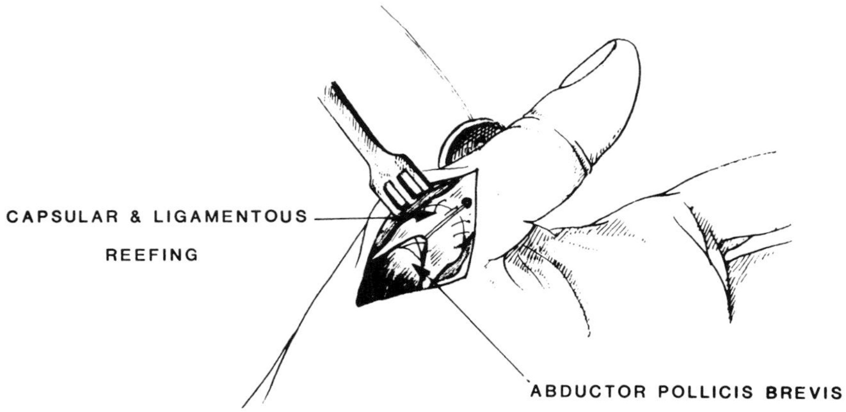

Figure 5–9 Diagram of the abductor advancement associated with capsular reefing for chronic radial collateral ligament ruptures.

Return to athletics is dependent on the nature of the sport, the degree of injury, and the treatment. For the incomplete tear treated by splinting, a rapid return can be anticipated, even as soon as a week or two, if the thumb is subject to re-injury. If the thumb is not at risk, or a removable splint is allowed, the player can resume the sport at once or whenever it is convenient.

With surgically treated complete ruptures (acute or chronic) in the nondominant hand for sports that are primarily one-handed or are not stressful to the injured thumb, return may be permitted in 6 to 8 weeks, unless the use of a removable splint is permitted and will not inhibit performance. Under those conditions, the competitor can often return in 2 to 3 weeks. In sports in which the thumb is at significant risk of re-injury, even with a protective splint, return should be delayed for as long as 8 to 12 weeks.

Conclusion

Injuries of the collateral ligaments of the thumb metacarpophalangeal joint are common and demand careful evaluation and appropriate treatment. Although incomplete injuries are handled nonoperatively, complete ruptures are best repaired or reconstructed, since persistent laxity can result in functional impairment and arthrosis.

REFERENCES

1. Coonrad, R.W., Goldner, J.L.: A study of the pathological findings and treatment in soft tissue injury of the thumb metacarpophalangeal joint. J. Bone Joint Surg. 50A:439, 1968.
2. Neviaser, R.J.: Dislocations and ligamentous injuries of the digits. In Chapman, M.W., ed.: Operative Orthopaedics. Philadelphia, J.B. Lippincott, 1988, p. 1199.
3. Neviaser, R.J., Adams, J.P.: Complications of treatment of injuries to the hand. In Epps, C.H., ed.: Complications in Orthopaedic Surgery. Philadelphia, J.B. Lippincott, 1978, p. 366.

4. Neviaser, R.J., Wilson, J.N., Lievano, A.: Rupture of the ulnar collateral ligament of the thumb (gamekeeper's thumb). J. Bone Joint Surg., 53A:1357, 1971.
5. Palmer, A.K., Louis, D.S.: Assessing ulnar instability of the metacarpophalangeal joint of the thumb. J. Hand Surg., 3:542, 1978.
6. Stener, B.: Displacement of the ruptured ulnar collateral ligament of the metacarpophalangeal joint of the thumb. J. Bone Joint Surg., 44B:869, 1962.
7. Smith, R.J.: Post-traumatic instability of the metacarpophalangeal joint of the thumb. J. Bone Joint Surg., 59A:14, 1977.

CHAPTER

6

Soft Tissue Injuries of the Wrist

Julio Taleisnik, M.D.

Injuries to the athlete's wrist are similar to those sustained in industry or as a consequence of recreational or other occupational activities. What makes them to some extent unique, are their steadily increasing frequency and the difficulties involved in returning the athlete to competition. The increasingly young age of participants is causing demands on the musculotendinous apparatus that surpass normal anatomic and physiologic parameters. As an example, the skeletally immature wrists of young competitive gymnasts are the source of baffling, disabling overuse syndromes that frequently lead to withdrawal from this sport. Greater competitiveness, at levels that appear to never peak, is also the source of potential musculoskeletal problems. It is difficult to place a limit on human physical achievement. In 1934, University of California coach Brutus Hamilton predicted what he believed would be the ultimate performances in track and field: 50.40 seconds in the 400-meter hurdles (the world record is now more than 3 seconds lower), 6′11″ in the high jump (the world record is already almost a foot higher), and 15′1″ in the pole vault (the world record is now over 19′8″).[6] In the upper extremity, these factors have resulted in an ever-increasing number of athletes temporarily or permanently disabled by injuries to the wrist, this most vulnerable of joints.

Greater also is the spectrum of treatable wrist unjuries, now including conditions that were unknown or extremely rare just a few years ago, such as the impaction syndromes, the occult ganglions, and the more subtle forms of carpal instability. The "sprained wrist" has changed from a diagnostic wastebasket for painful wrists to a very limited diagnosis, arrived at only *after* other entities have been ruled out by thorough clinical, radiographic, and special examinations. True sprains present few clinical signs, negative radiographic and special findings, and total resolution of symptoms, without recurrence, after a period of immobilization. Therefore, sprains may be thought of as a diagnosis at one end of a spectrum of conditions that at the other end includes the major fractures, dislocations, and fracture-dislocations, a concept advanced by Destot in 1923.[10] This discussion will be limited to soft tissue injuries that involve more joint disruption than sprains but less than fractures and dislocations. Also excluded are extra-articular causes of pain in the area of the wrist, such as tendinitis, tendon subluxations, and nerve compressions.

Mechanism of Injury

Soft tissue injuries to the wrist may result from single trauma or from repetitive stresses, predominantly angulatory loads applied to the wrist in dorsiflexion. The final outcome of a single load applied to the wrist (collision injury), depends on the following factors.

The Characteristics of the Injury Force These include its point of application, magnitude, rate of loading and direction.[17, 18]

The Position of the Hand at Impact This includes further angulation and rotation as loading progresses.[17, 42, 47] Most sports injuries follow compressive loading of the wrist in some degree of dorsiflexion.[21] Rotation, either of the forearm or of the wrist itself, is frequently present, either in addition to pure dorsiflexion, palmarflexion, or radial or ulnar deviation or as a primary mechanism in injuries to the distal radioulnar joint and to the ulnar carpal column. Mayfield and colleagues[26] produced sequential carpal dislocations in cadaver specimens of wrists subjected to extension, ulnar deviation, and intercarpal supination. The initial result was a scapholunate dissociation. Subsequent stages produced actual carpal dislocations. There is also enough clinical evidence to suggest that loading on the ulnar side of the carpus, with carpal hyperpronation, results in triquetrolunate injury.[45]

The Relative Strength of Carpal Bones and Ligaments Biologic or genetic ligamentous laxity is often seen in athletes[19, 40] and is frequently augmented by strenuous stretching exercises. This "joint hypermobility" may result in ligamentous elongation or partial or complete tears following a single tension loading of the wrist (collision injuries) that may have otherwise produced a fracture or a fracture-dislocation.[41] Ligamentous laxity also predisposes to cumulative joint injury following repetitive stresses (overuse injuries). In addition to this difference in ligament behavior between different subjects, it has been suggested that there is a qualitative difference in yield strength within ligaments of any given person, the weakest being those on the radial and palmar quadrants of the wrist.[25] The scapholunate interosseous ligament and the radioscaphoid portion of the radioscaphocapitate ligament have shown a qualitatively greater degree of elongation prior to failure. Furthermore, recent publications demonstrate that within the scapholunate ligamentous complex itself, yield strength of the palmar portion is approximately twice that of the dorsal portion.[24] Viscoelasticity may therefore play a significant role and may explain the presence of clinically detectable instabilities without a radiographic, arthrogaphic, or surgically demonstrable ligamentous tear. This quality may also explain why some carpal instabilities not seen in initial roentgenograms become demonstrable in radiographs obtained weeks, months, or even years after the original injury.

Occult Dorsal Carpal Ganglion

DIAGNOSIS

Ganglions, usually dorsal, constitute the most frequent soft tissue tumors of the wrist. The dorsal wrist ganglion originates consistently from the dorsal scapholunate ligament and is the extra-articular manifestation of a continuous duct system that connects it with the scapholunate joint.[1] A history of specific trauma may be elicited in approximately 15 percent of patients with clinically apparent ganglions.[1] Such a history of trauma is, however, frequently missing in patients with occult ganglions[15]; these may form, instead, in response to chronic stress.[1, 37] In our experience, an inverse relationship seems to exist between the size of the ganglion and the symptoms it produces: smaller, tense ganglions are more uncomfortable and tender than the larger, softer cysts. In some patients, the appearance of the palpable lump is preceded by a few days or weeks of discomfort and pain, which is suddenly relieved when the cystic mass becomes more obvious.

The occult dorsal carpal ganglion probably represents a variant in which intraligamentous, smaller cysts may be seen on microscopic examination of the excised capsule in the area where the capsule adheres to the dorsal scapholunate ligament (Fig. 6–1). Less frequently, these areas of mucinous degeneration coalesce into a single, bigger, tense cyst that never enlarges enough to become visible or palpable. These occult ganglions produce chronic wrist pain, sometimes constant, sometimes present only after activities.[37] There is localized tenderness, and maximal aggravation of pain during palmarflexion.[37] There may be limitation of motion, and weakness of grip. Routine radiographic studies and arthrograms are of no diagnostic value. Published series using radionuclide bone imaging have not included occult ganglions among the diagnoses.[39] The diagnosis is essentially one of exclusion and should be suspected in patients under the age of 35.[37] It is supported by relief of symptoms following very localized anesthetic injections into the scapholunate joint under radiographic control. It is not confirmed, however, until direct visualization of the joint, which may be done through an arthroscope, or at times until microscopic examination of the excised specimen is performed.

TREATMENT

Treatment consists of an excision of the area of the dorsal capsule centered over the scapholunate joint, together with a V-shaped portion including the dorsal 10 percent of the scapholunate ligament (Fig. 6–2).[37] Results are generally satisfactory, with eventual return to competition in

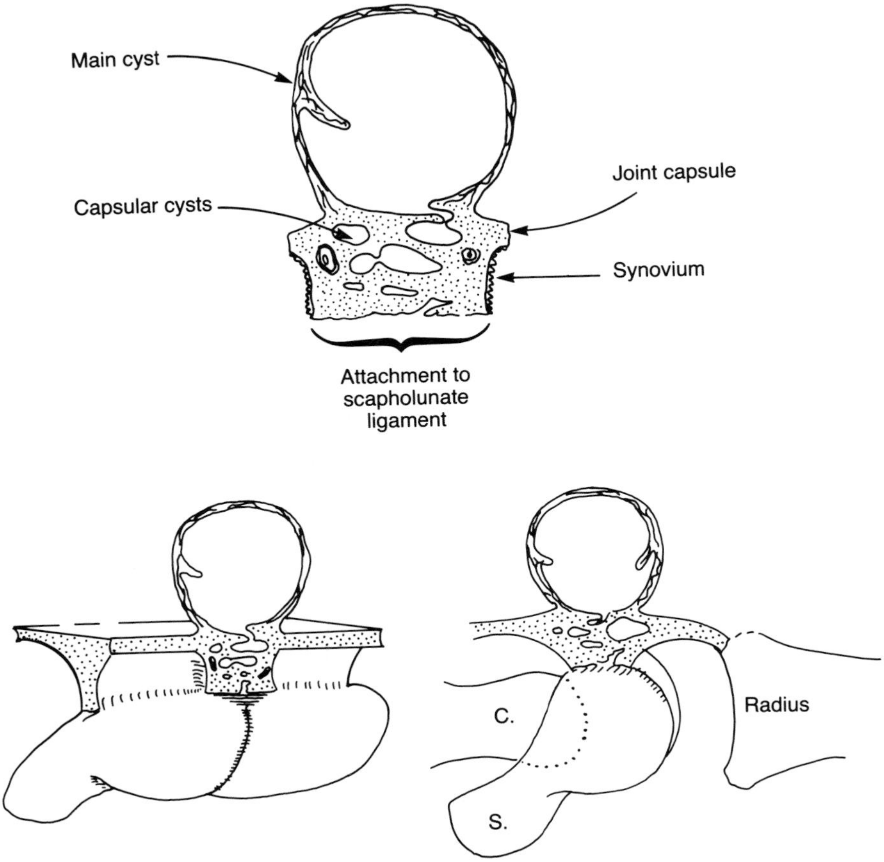

Figure 6–1 *A,* Composite illustration of a pathologic specimen showing the main cyst and capsular cysts within the connective tissue of the joint capsule. Intercommunications between cysts and lumen are shown. Note opened capsular cysts resting on scapholunate ligament. *B,* Coronal section of the dorsal ganglion, shown in situ, resting on the scapholunate ligament. *C,* Sagittal section of the same specimen shown in situ. (From Angelides, A.C., Wallace, P.G.: The dorsal ganglion of the wrist: Its pathogenesis, gross and microscopic anatomy, and surgical treatment. J. Hand Surg. 1:228, 1976.)

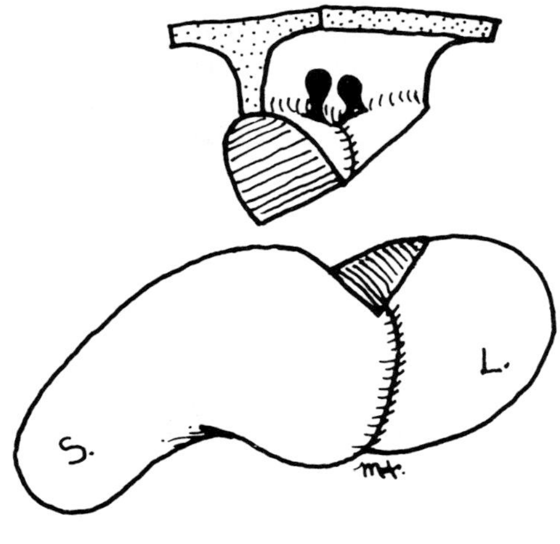

Figure 6–2 Complete excision of the capsular attachments to the scapholunate ligament is assured by wedge resection of the dorsal 10 percent (or less) of the ligament. Alternatively, the scapholunate ligament may be cleaned with a small rongeur. This drawing has been purposely exaggerated to better show the method of resection. (From Sanders, W.E.: The occult dorsal carpal ganglion. J. Hand Surg. 10B:257, 1985.)

most cases. In some patients, when the scapholunate ligament appears normal, the point of a no. 11 scalpel blade can be inserted in the ligament, just proximal to the dorsal scapholunate ridge, leading to a small collection of clear ganglion jelly, which may be further emptied out with a tiny curette.[15]

Dorsal Impaction Syndromes

DIAGNOSIS

Repetitive loading of the wrist in maximum dorsiflexion may lead to chronic dorsal pain syndromes. According to Linscheid and Dobyns, shear forces are created in compressed contact areas, which may result in injuries ranging from localized synovitis to actual osteocartilaginous fractures.[21] This is a frequent occurrence in gymnasts, who learn to think of their dorsal wrist pain as an unavoidable consequence of the sport rather than as an injury.[3] There is pain and point tenderness, usually on the central mid-dorsal area of the wrist, at the projection of the lunocapitate joint.

TREATMENT

Surgical exploration in these patients may disclose nothing but very localized, hypertrophic synovitis, a condition that has been named "meniscoid of the wrist."[36] When allowed to progress, cartilaginous and bony changes may develop, including the formation of a hypertrophic ridge of the dorsal rim of the scaphoid or along the dorsal border of the lunate as it impinges against the neck of the capitate in dorsiflexion. Most of these patients are successfully treated by restricting wrist hyperextension, by strengthening of wrist flexors,[3] and by the judicious use of local injections of steroids. When these fail, immobilization and cessation of aggravating activities for 4 to 6 weeks should be tried, followed by gradual return to the sport. Recurrence of symptoms, inability to perform, and chronic wrist pain present after menial activities and at rest obligate the athlete and the physician to decide between abandoning the sport and operative intervention. Surgical treatment consists of limited synovectomy and cheilotomy of hypertrophic ridges and bony margins shown to impinge during passive dorsiflexion of the wrist under direct visualization. Although these operations do not necessarily succeed in returning the athlete to sports, they are frequently successful in relieving the constant pain, allowing at least the comfortable use of the wrist for less strenuous activities.

Carpal Instability

Carpal instability in athletes may be seen following collision injuries during basketball or football. It is relatively frequent in tennis players and can result from falls or motorcycle accidents. The resulting carpal abnormalities may be suspected clinically and demonstrated in routine radiographs by the abnormal alignment of carpal bones. These have been called *static* forms of carpal instability (Fig. 6–3*A*).[43, 44] There is a group of patients with unstable carpi whose routine radiographic studies are within normal limits but who can voluntarily change carpal alignment and return to normal. These patients exhibit a *dynamic* form of instability (Fig. 6–3*B*). Within this group should also be included those patients whose instability is reproducible by manipulation only, all other ancillary tests, with the possible exception of bone scans, being normal. Like the static types, these more subtle forms may be the result of single impact loading, although they can occur after repetitive stresses, such as in gymnastics and weight lifting. Dynamic instabilities are frequently secondary to destabilization of the midcarpal joint. The most common carpal collapse is secondary to ligamentous disruption between scaphoid and lunate, followed by that between lunate and triquetrum, and by the dynamic midcarpal instabilities. Ulnar translocations are rarely seen as a consequence of sports injuries; they usually follow major collision trauma, such as is seen in motorcycle accidents. Carpal instabilities secondary to malunions of fractures of the distal radius are beyond the scope of this chapter.

SCAPHOLUNATE DISSOCIATION

Diagnosis This instability is secondary to the loss of support to the proximal pole of the scaphoid through rupture or elongation of its ligamentous restraints. Usually, these young athletes show excessive midcarpal laxity of the uninjured wrist and hypermobility of other joints.[19, 40] Scaphoid instability may be static, in which case radiographic studies are diagnostic, or dynamic, in which the scaphoid is made unstable by either the patient or by manipulation by the examining physician, a maneuver described by Watson (Fig. 6–4).[51] For this test, the patient's elbow rests on his or her lap, and the forearm is pronated. The examiner's opposite hand takes the patient's wrist into full ulnar deviation. In this position the scaphoid is aligned longitudinally. Next, the patient's hand is radially deviated while the examiner's ipsilateral thumb presses against the distal pole of the scaphoid in an attempt to prevent it from palmarflexing. When the scaphoid is unstable, this maneuver will force the dorsal pole to sublux, and the patient's pain is reproduced. Clinical examination may also disclose tenderness and localized swelling on the dorsoradial aspect of the wrist.

The diagnosis of the static forms, and of the voluntary recurrent subluxations of the scaphoid, is established by appropriate radiographic projections, including anteroposterior views with the hand and forearm in supination (Fig. 6–5*A*), lateral views (Fig. 6–5*B*) and, for the voluntary dynamic subluxations, radiographs obtained *after* the patient has produced the scaphoid collapse (Fig. 6–6). The classic sign is a gap between scaphoid and lunate that is wider than in the normal wrist. The distal pole of the perpendicular scaphoid is seen end-on—the cortical "ring" sign (Fig. 6–5*A*).[2, 9] The lateral projection shows the scaphoid aligned with its longitudinal axis perpendicular to that of the radius,[12] and the lunate in dorsiflexion (Fig. 6–5*B*).[22, 23] The normal scapholunate angle ranges from

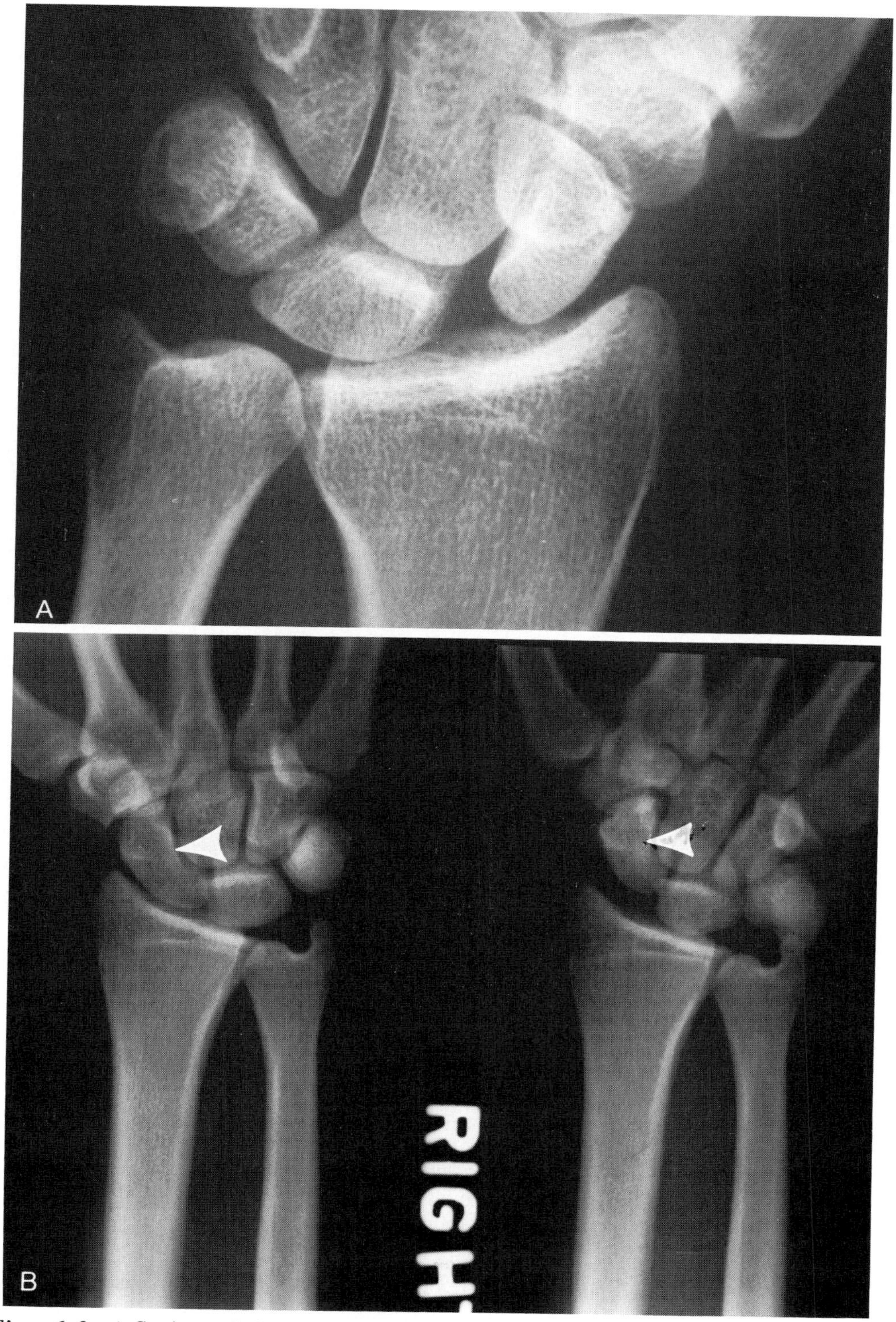

Figure 6–3 *A*, Static scapholunate instability. There is perpendicularization of the scaphoid, seen end-on, palmar flexed. Notice the increased gap between scaphoid and lunate. *B*, Dynamic scapholunate instability. The arrows point to the change of position of the scaphoid in radiographs obtained before and after the patient actively subluxated his scaphoid.

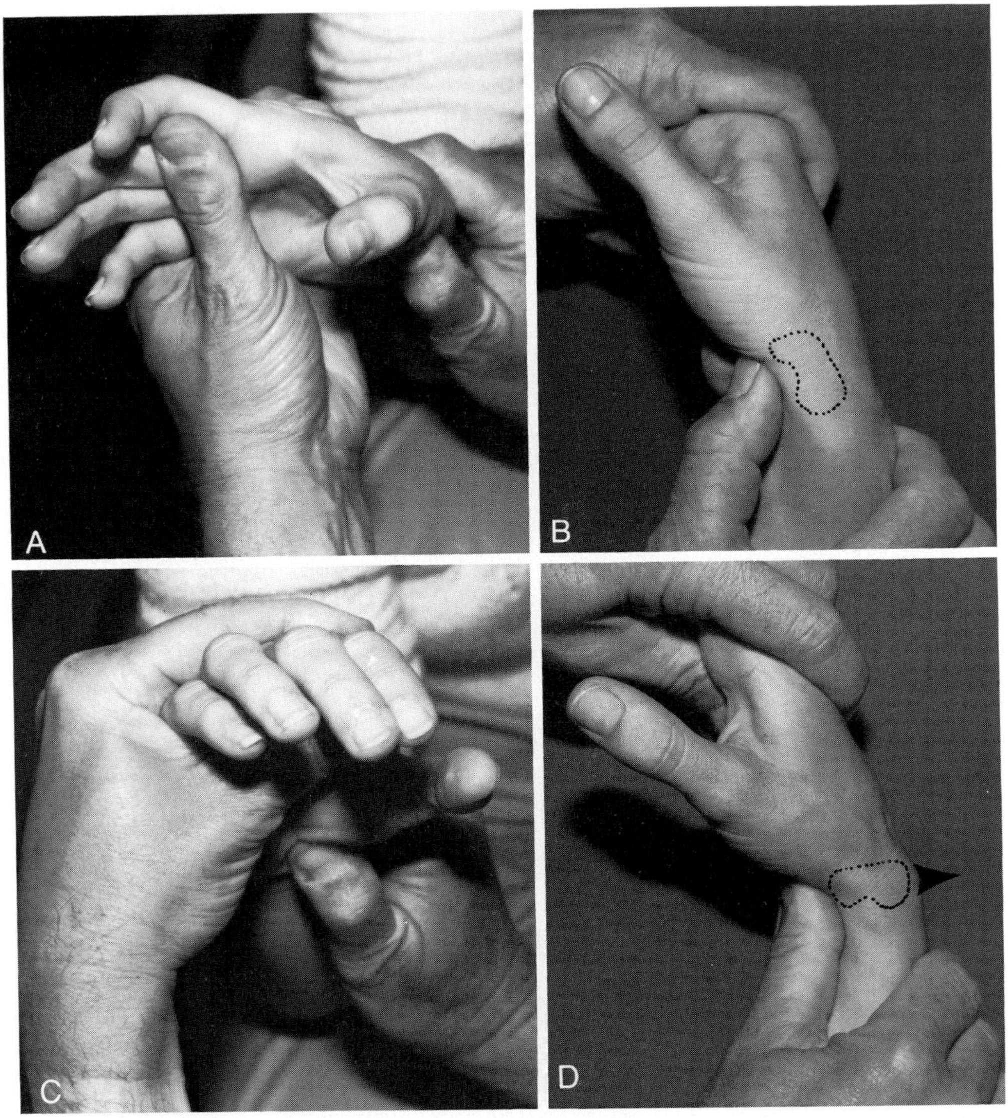

Figure 6–4 Clinical test for instability of the scaphoid, described by Dr. H.K. Watson, Hartford, Connecticut. *A,* The patient's elbow rests on his lap and the forearm is pronated. *B,* The hand is brought into ulnar deviation and pressure is applied to the distal pole of the scaphoid (*dotted line*). *C,* Next the hand is radially deviated while pressure is maintained on the distal pole of the scaphoid, in an attempt to prevent normal palmar flexion. *D,* When the scaphoid is unstable, its proximal pole is forced to subluxate dorsally (*arrow*), a maneuver that is accompanied by pain. (From Taleisnik, J.: The Wrist. New York, Churchill Livingstone, 1985.)

30 to 60°; angles greater than 70° are a clear indication of scapholunate dissociation.[11] Normally, the long axis of the scaphoid and a line drawn tangential to the palmar flare of the distal radius are closely parallel to each other. When the scaphoid is subluxated in palmar flexion, these lines converge at an acute angle.[42] The volar cortical outlines of the scaphoid and of the radial styloid, normally shaped as a C or as a wide bracket

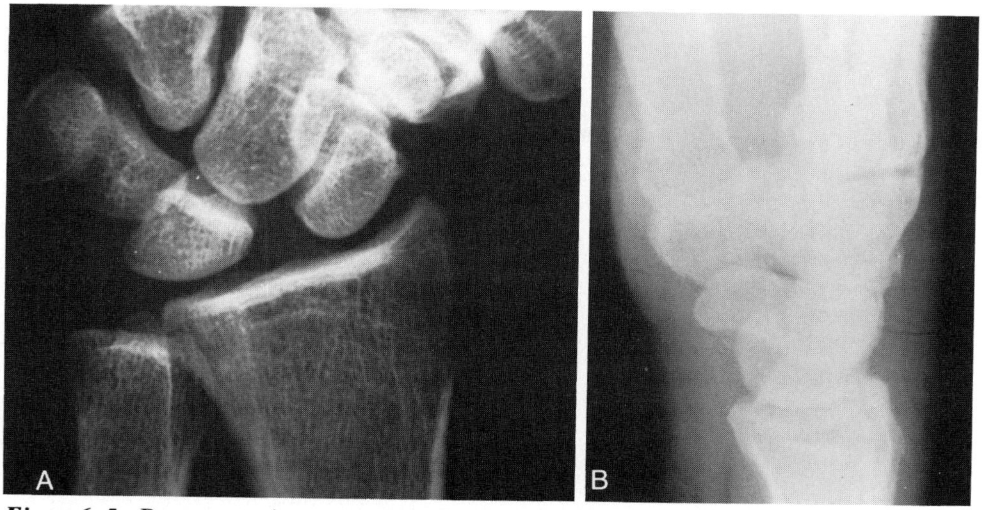

Figure 6–5 Posteroanterior (*A*) and lateral (*B*) radiographs of scapholunate dissociation.

opened anteriorly, collapse into a sharp V when the scaphoid is subluxated (Fig. 6–7).[14, 42] Cineradiography, arthrography, arthroscopy, and isotope scanning may be of help in those cases in which the diagnosis is strongly suggested by the history of injury and clinical findings but cannot be demonstrated with routine radiographic techniques (Fig. 6–8).

Treatment Manipulation and closed pinning under cineradiographic control may succeed in correcting fresh scapholunate dissociations within the first 3 or 4 weeks following injury. Reduction is accomplished by dorsiflexing the wrist until scapholunate alignment is restored, followed by fixation with multiple 0.045 Kirschner wires introduced across the scaphoid into the capitate and lunate. Care should be exercised not to traverse the radiocarpal space with any of the pins. Postoperatively the wrist is immobilized in palmar flexion at the radiocarpal joint level, with the forearm in pronation, to relax the involved palmar radiocarpal ligaments.[34, 45]

In most cases surgical visualization of the torn ligaments using a dorsal approach, and occasionally a palmar approach as well, and their repair, protected by internal fixation with Kirschner wires, is more reliable for the management of these injuries in athletes. This is followed by immobilization as discussed. For the chronic scapholunate dissociations, particularly in very young athletes whose epiphyses are still open, an attempt should be made at ligament repair, augmented by a dorsal capsuloligamentodesis as described by Blatt (Fig. 6–9).[4] This technique requires fashioning a dorsal capsular flap, left attached proximally to the radius, which is inserted distally into a groove carved on the reduced scaphoid, beyond its axis of rotation. The purpose of this flap is to tether the distal pole dorsally, keeping it from subluxating in a palmar direction. For the skeletally mature, when ligamentous repair and capsulodesis are not possible, I prefer a limited arthrodesis to the trapezium and trapezoid for the stabilization of the scaphoid, a technique popularized by Watson and Hempton (Fig. 6–10).[50]

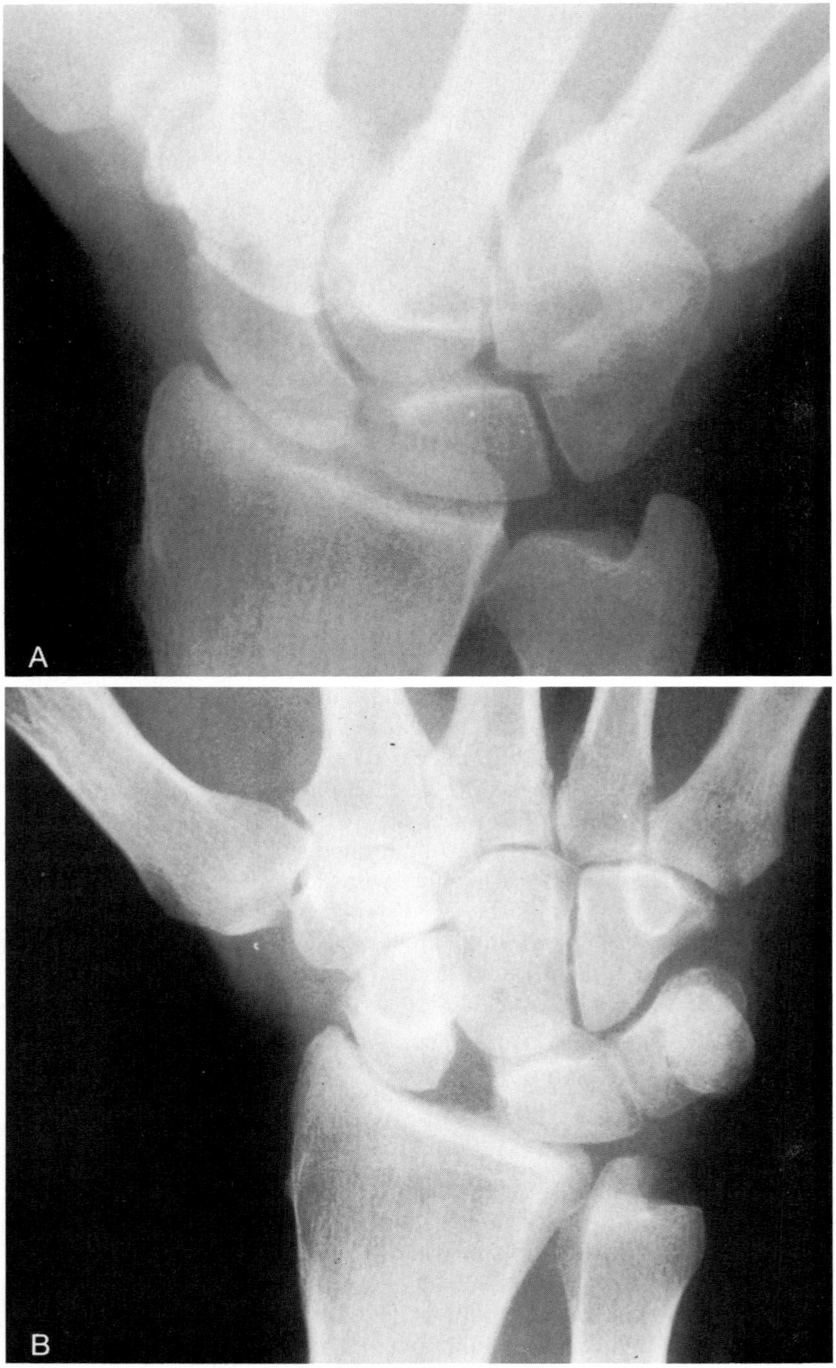

Figure 6–6 Dynamic scapholunate dissociation. Normal alignment (*A*) and dissociation actively produced by the patient (*B*).

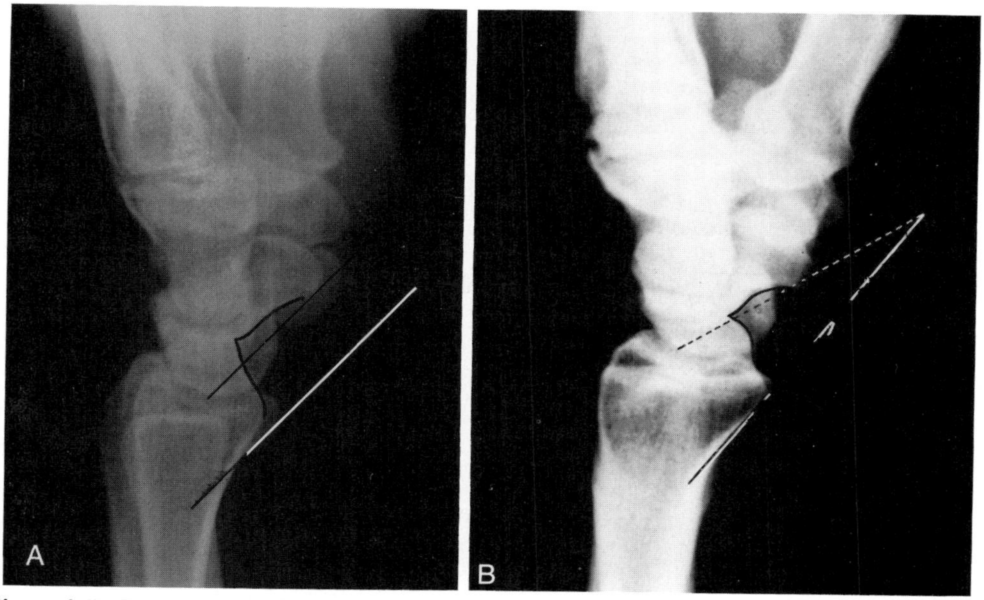

Figure 6–7 Lateral view of normal wrist (*A*) and of wrist with scapholunate dissociation (*B*). *A*, Longitudinal axis of scaphoid and line drawn tangential to the palmar flare of distal radius are nearly parallel. Palmar outlines of scaphoid and radial styloid form a C or bracket. *B*, Axis of scaphoid and line along flare of distal radius intersect at an acute angle. The palmar scaphoid-radial styloid outline is collapsed into a V. (From Taleisnik, J.: The Wrist. New York, Churchill Livingstone, 1985.)

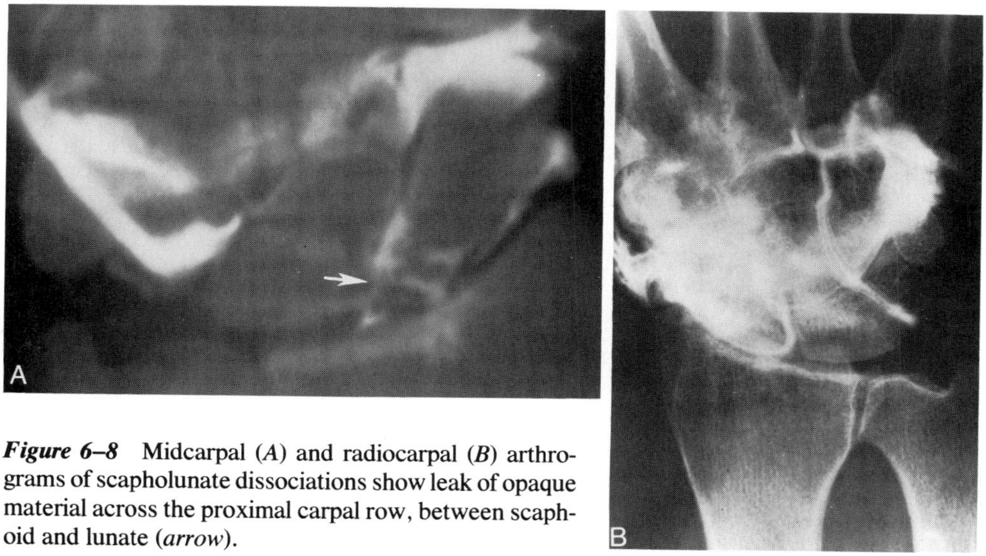

Figure 6–8 Midcarpal (*A*) and radiocarpal (*B*) arthrograms of scapholunate dissociations show leak of opaque material across the proximal carpal row, between scaphoid and lunate (*arrow*).

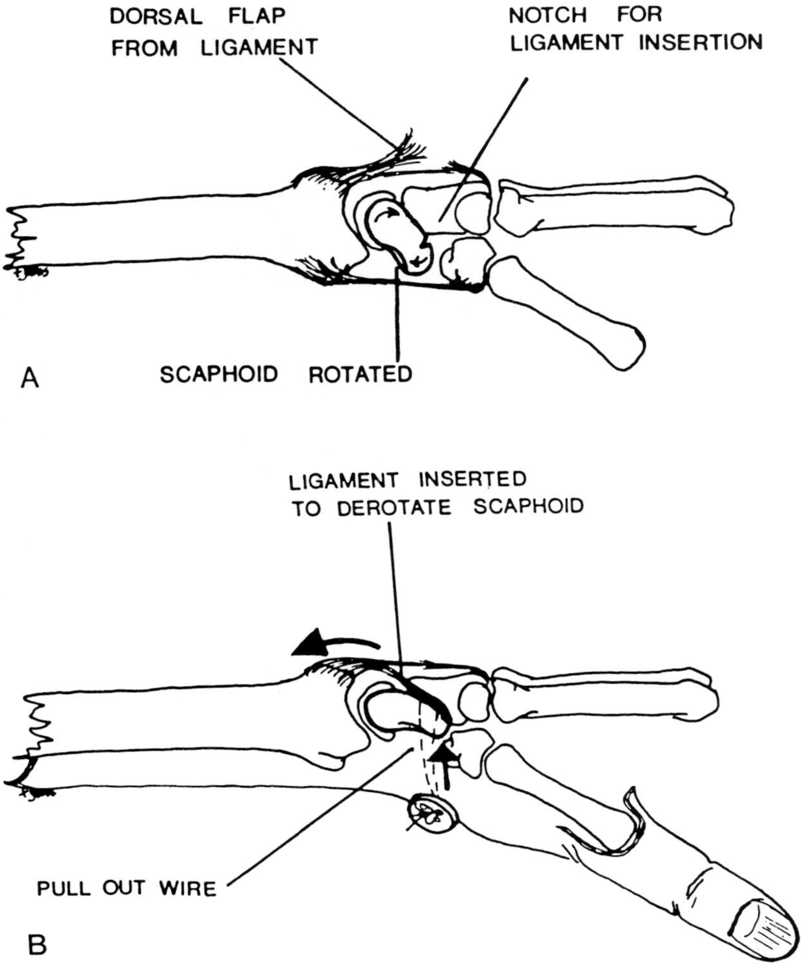

Figure 6–9 Graphic representation of the technique of dorsal capsulodesis. *A*, A proximal based ligamentous flap is developed from the dorsal wrist capsule. A notch for the ligament insertion is created in the dorsal cortex of the distal pole of the scaphoid, distal to the midaxis of rotation. *B*, The scaphoid has been derotated and the ligament inserted with a pull-out wire suture. (From Blatt, G.: Capsulodesis in reconstructive hand surgery. Hand Clin. North Am. 3:81, 1987.)

TRIQUETROLUNATE INSTABILITY

Diagnosis Just as in scapholunate dissociations, a whole spectrum of injuries to the lunotriquetral ligaments is possible, from true sprains to partial tears or complete tears without carpal malalignment to static volar intercalated segment instability (VISI) deformities.[21, 35] I have never seen a full-blown VISI deformity following an athletic injury. In all the other stages of lunotriquetral instability, the patient's main complaint is pain on the dorsoulnar side of the carpus, and the common finding is localized tenderness at the lunotriquetral projection. The lunotriquetral bal-

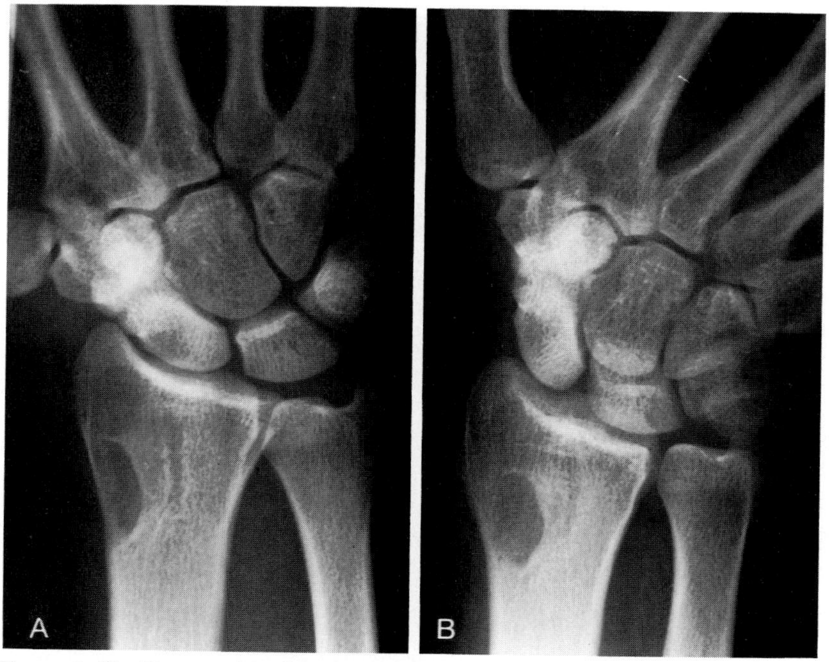

Figure 6–10 Range of radial (*A*) and ulnar (*B*) deviation following scapho-trapezium-trapezoid arthrodesis for scapholunate dissociation. (From Taleisnik, J.: The Wrist. New York, Churchill Livingstone, 1985.)

lottement test, in which the examiner supports the lunate between the thumb and index finger of one hand while displacing the triquetrum with the other, reproduces the patient's pain.[35] Localized injections of an anesthetic into the lunotriquetral space should relieve symptoms and, in those patients with grip weakness, restore or improve strength. Routine radiographs are diagnostic only in those advanced cases with established VISI deformity. Otherwise, tears of the lunotriquetral ligament may be demonstrated by arthrographic studies. Midcarpal arthrography is particularly helpful in these cases, for it may demonstrate even incomplete tears (Fig. 6–11).[49] An additional injection of opaque material into the radiocarpal space may be needed to rule out simultaneous injury to the triangular fibrocartilage. Indeed, the association of lunotriquetral instability, perforation or tear of the triangular fibrocartilage, and an ulna plus variant is frequent, particularly in chronic cases. Such is the case with gymnasts, in whom ulnar wrist pain is common and is consistently associated with ulna plus variants.

The importance of the relationship between carpal injury and ulnar variant was strongly suggested by the experimental studies of Oreck, Gillespie, and Youm.[29] These investigators induced injuries to the ulnar side of the wrist and found the expected damage to ulnar structures but also an unexpected number of scapholunate tears. There was an inverse relationship between these and the ulnar ligament injuries and an apparent correlation with ulnar variance, suggesting that ulnar variance affects the final location of injury, with ulnar minus variance leading to radial axis

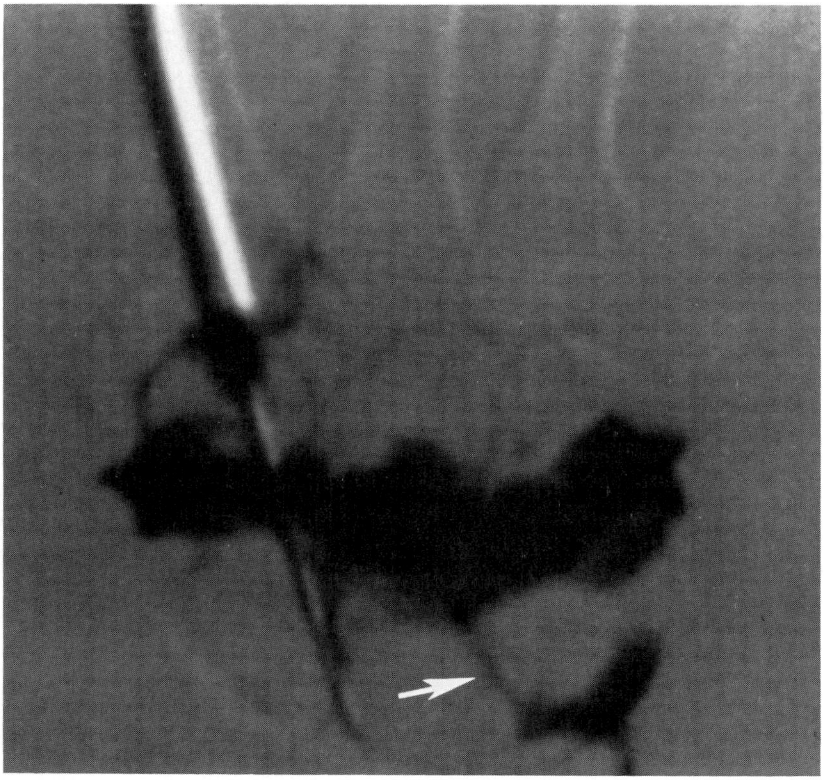

Figure 6–11 Midcarpal arthrogram shows the leak of opaque material between lunate and triquetrum (*arrow*).

injury and ulna neutral or plus variants to ulnar axis injury. For those patients with ulnar pain and an undetermined diagnosis, bone scans and arthroscopy may be needed to demonstrate lunotriquetral pathology.

Treatment For the acute injury, and for chronic cases that have not been previously treated, when there is no demonstrable tear, an injection of a steroid preparation followed by above-elbow plaster immobilization will prove rewarding in a large number of patients. Even in the presence of incomplete tears this approach should be considered first. When disabling pain continues, operation may be the only alternative, if the athlete is determined to return to his or her sport. If possible, an attempt should be made at repairing the lunotriquetral ligament, particularly in fresh injuries after failure of immobilization. When there is an ulna plus variant, especially if a perforation of the triangular fibrocartilage is present, ulnar shortening is the procedure of choice. My experience with lunotriquetral arthrodesis has not been uniformly satisfactory.

ULNAR TRANSLOCATION

Diagnosis This is a rare injury in the athlete. It is the result of a violent impact, beyond that found in most sports, with the possible exception of motorcycle or car racing. Traumatic ulnar translocation is possible only after a massive tear of *all* radiocarpal ligamentous support, dorsal and palmar, usually from the radius. This allows the carpus to slide along the incline of the articular surface of the distal radius in an ulnar direction (Fig. 6–12). There is severe swelling and loss of motion. The diagnosis is established by radiographic examination, which will demonstrate the abnormal translation of the carpus and, in some cases, a scapholunate diastasis produced by the ulnar displacement of the lunate and not by a subluxation of the scaphoid. An abnormal rotation of the proximal carpus may also be present, usually into palmar flexion (Fig. 6–13).

Treatment Soon after injury, surgical exploration routinely discloses a massive capsular tear, dorsal and palmar, from the radius. Frequently, an unsuspected scapholunate ligamentous tear is present. I no longer believe that reattachment of the capsule to the radius is the treatment of choice, even for fresh injuries.[45] Should the surgeon succeed in a stable relocation of the carpus in its normal position through capsular reattachment alone, this will be accomplished at the expense of a severe loss of motion. More frequently, translocation will recur soon after internal fixation and plaster immobilization are discontinued. Experience with the treatment of ulnar translocation in the arthritic wrist[7,43] has shown that relocation of the carpus and maintenance of reduction by radiolunate arthrodesis is a more reliable technique, conducive to a more stable and pain-free wrist with satisfactory preservation of motion (Fig. 6–14). This is a more reliable operation, allowing the athlete to return to stressful use of the wrist when full range of motion is not a prerequisite to satisfactory performance.

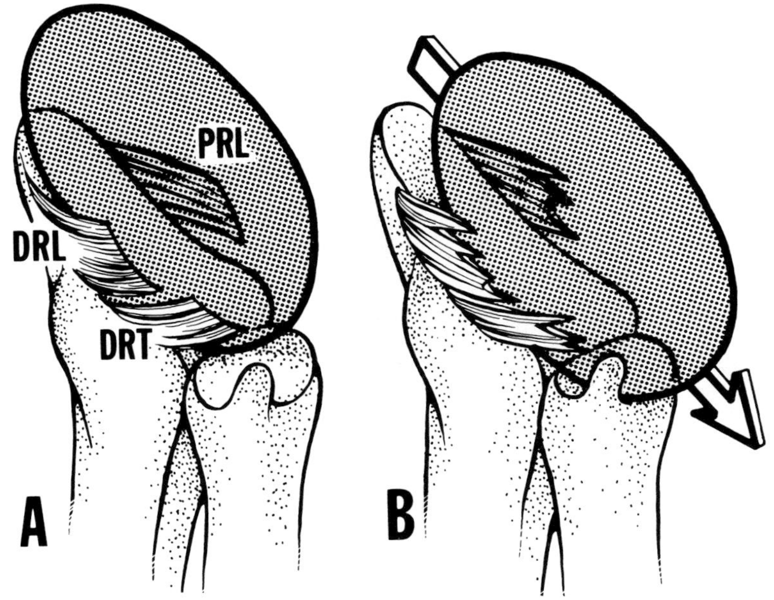

Figure 6–12 *A,* Radiocarpal ligamentous apparatus keeps carpus against ulnar slope of distal radius. PRL, palmar radiolunate ligament; DRL, dorsal radiolunate ligament; DRT, dorsal radiotriquetral ligament. *B,* Without this support, the carpus tends to slide in an ulnar direction, down the incline of the articular surface of the distal radius. (From Taleisnik, J.: The Wrist. New York, Churchill Livingstone, 1985.)

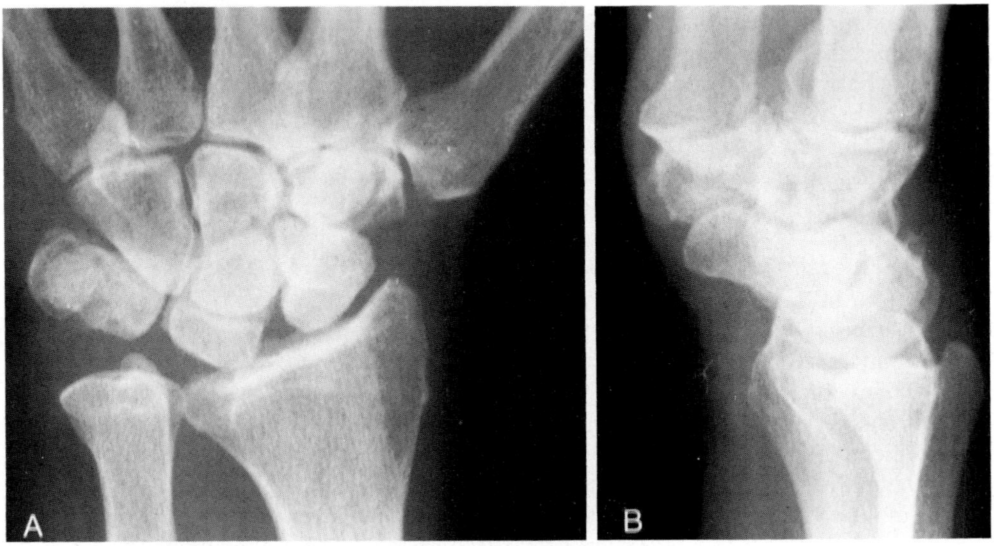

Figure 6–13 Anteroposterior (*A*) and lateral (*B*) radiographs of wrist with ulnar translocation and palmar flexion volar intercalated segment instability (VISI) of the proximal carpal row. (From Taleisnik, J.: The Wrist. New York, Churchill Livingstone, 1985.)

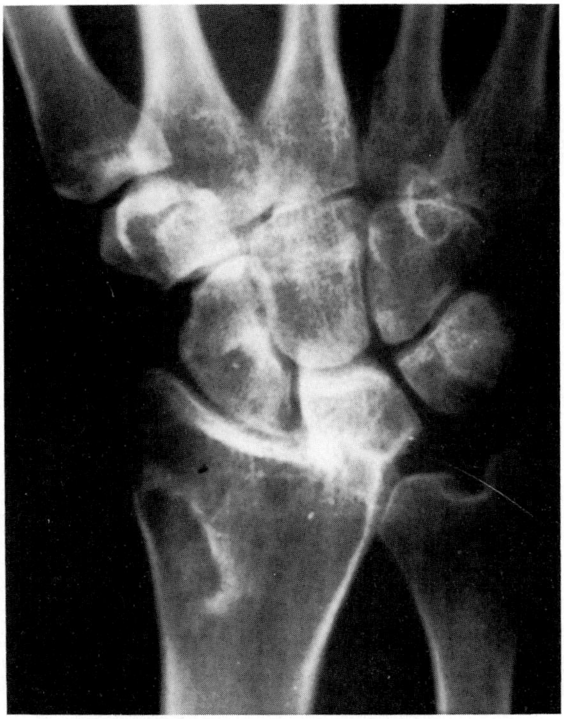

Figure 6–14 Radiolunate fusion successfully anchors the carpus in its reduced position in relation to the radius.

Ulnocarpal and Distal Radioulnar Joints

Soft tissue injuries involving the distal radioulnar joint *without* distal radioulnar subluxation or dislocation are rare. Chondromalacia of the ulnar head, a source of disability in many athletes with complaints of pain localized to the distal radioulnar joint, is beyond the scope of this discussion. The main soft tissue injury in this region involves the triangular fibrocartilage.

TRIANGULAR FIBROCARTILAGE INJURY

Injury to the triangular fibrocartilage (TFC) may result in perforations, usually degenerative, and in avulsions.[32] The TFC is a stabilizer of the distal radioulnar joint (DRUJ). It is also part of the ulnocarpal complex, which completes with the radius an articular surface for the carpal condyle and supports the ulnar carpal column.

In a study of cadaver wrists, Mikic reported regressive changes in the TFC that were related to age.[27] Degenerative changes of the TFC were first seen in the third decade of life, the youngest specimen with such changes being that of a 27-year-old. Mikic disregarded biomechanical, metabolic, and traumatic factors, although he accepted trauma as a probable added factor in discs that had already started to degenerate, and mentioned a solitary case of a perforated disc without degeneration in an uremic subject. In my experience, however, aside from the obvious pernicious effect of synovitis (e.g., in rheumatoid arthritis), degenerative changes may be seen in a much younger population, in relation to anatomic and occupational factors. From the anatomic standpoint, the thickness of the TFC is important and is in turn related to the ulnar variance. In ulna plus wrists, the center of the TFC is thinner.[33] In these wrists, once degenerative perforation or tear of the TFC occurs, lunotriquetral tears may ensue. Regarding occupational factors, youngsters with ulna plus variants involved in sports requiring repetitive loading of the wrist in ulnar deviation, are subject to degenerative changes of the TFC similar to those seen in the older population. In effect, I believe that it is the relationship among the anatomy, the characteristics of the stress placed on the wrist, and its duration that determine the presence and the age of onset of degenerative perforation of the TFC.

The second type of injury to the TFC is traumatic avulsion, usually from the ulna. Acute avulsions result in dislocation or subluxation of the distal ulna in relation to the radius.

Diagnosis Perforations or tears of the TFC are a cause of pain on the ulnar side of the wrist, frequently aggravated by forearm rotation. In these patients, the immediate differential diagnosis should be established between involvement of the distal radioulnar joint and injury to the structures within the ulnocarpal space, predominantly the TFC. In the latter, the DRUJ is entirely silent to manipulation and nontender.[46] Injury to the TFC is suspected when there is tenderness and crepitus between the ulna and the triquetrum.[21] It is further proven by the presence of a positive ulna variant in radiographs and by arthrographic demonstration of communication between the radiocarpal and distal radioulnar joints, particularly if the tear is through the thick portion of the disc and the patient is under 30. Arthroscopy may prove to be the ultimate diagnostic tool in these patients.

Patients with TFC avulsions resulting in dislocation of the distal radioulnar joint are easier to diagnose clinically and radiographically because of the obvious abnormal displacement of the distal ulna in relation to the radius (Fig. 6–15). For the more subtle forms of subluxation, a computed tomographic scan is of great help in evaluating distal radioulnar congruency (Fig. 6–16).[32]

Treatment For the acute injury without dislocation or subluxation and for those patients with several weeks of pain who have not had a trial at adequate treatment, immobilization in a long arm plaster cast, usually with the forearm in neutral rotation, should be tried initially. This should continue for a minimum of 4 and preferably 6 weeks, and be followed by a gradual return to activities, with intermittent support provided by above-elbow splinting. An injection of a steroid preparation into the ulnocarpal space immediately prior to the application of plaster is frequently helpful. Operative treatment should be considered only when the patient is still unable to return to his or her sport and is disabled for other activities as well and when nonsurgical management has failed to relieve symptoms or the condition has become chronic. I believe that the surgical choices for the torn or degenerative TFC are reduced to debridement of localized defects[28, 31, 32] or decompression of the ulnocarpal space, through either ulnar shortening (Fig. 6–17*A* and *B*),[20] distal radioulnar joint excisional hemiarthroplasty (Fig. 6–17*C*),[5] or the Kapandji procedure (Fig. 6–17*D*).[13, 38] Repair of tears may also be considered, particularly if localized within the periphery of the disc and in conjunction with ulnar recession.

Studies of the blood supply to the TFC demonstrate vascularity in the outer 15 to 20 percent of the disc only.[48] These findings suggest that tears of the TFC within the peripheral vascular zone have the potential to heal if repaired and may explain the frequency of relief of symptoms following nonsurgical treatment by prolonged immobilization. In my opinion, exci-

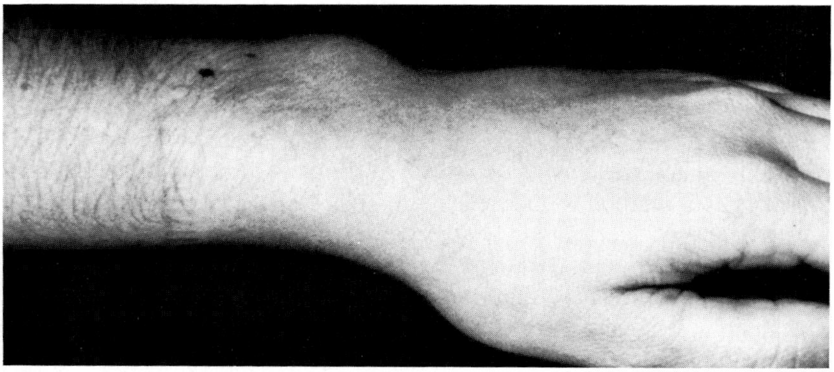

Figure 6–15 Subluxation of the distal radioulnar joint, with the ulna dorsal, is clinically apparent.

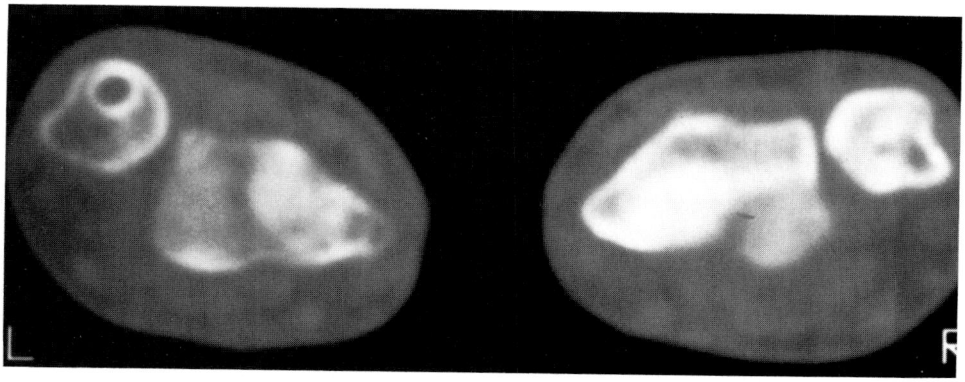

Figure 6–16 CT scan demonstrates subluxation of the distal radioulnar joint, with the ulna dorsal (*left*).

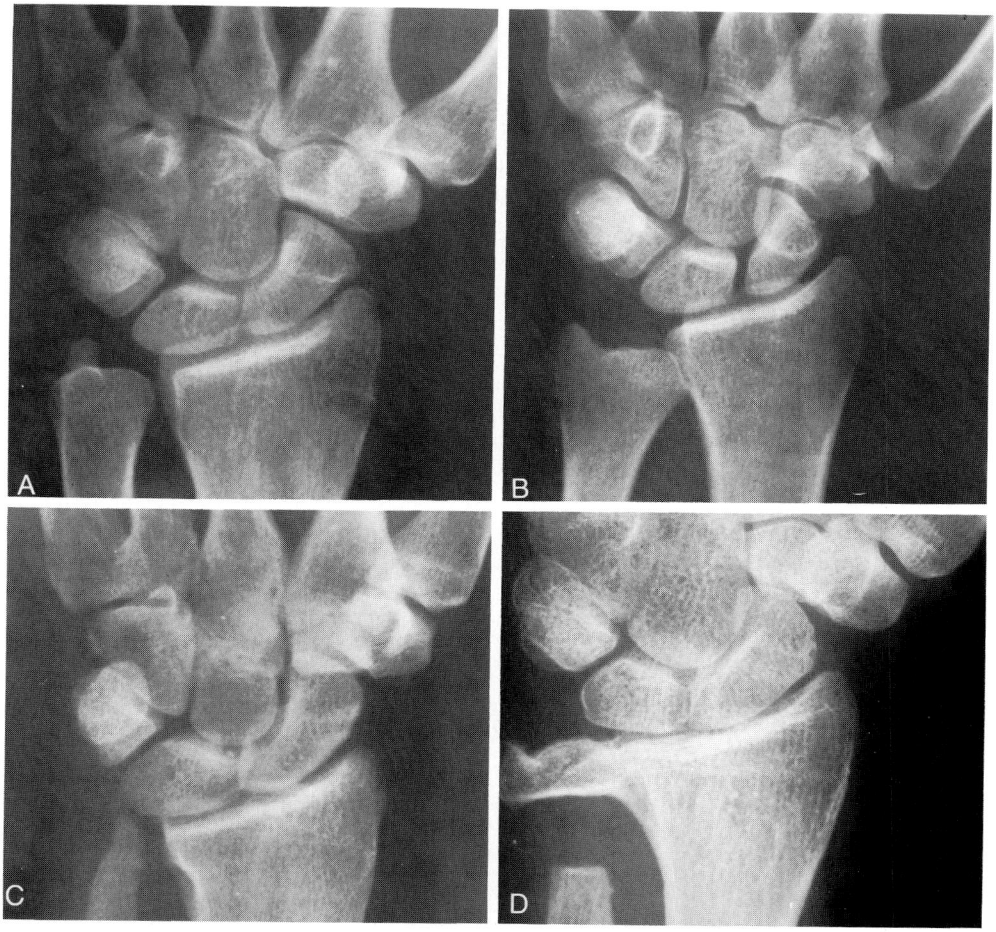

Figure 6–17 Preoperative (*A*) and postoperative (*B*) radiographs after ulnar shortening in patient with perforation of the triangular fibrocartilage and lunotriquetral dissociation proven arthrographically. Example of hemiresection-interposition arthroplasty of the distal radioulnar joint (*C*) and of a Sauve-Kapandji procedure (*D*).

sion of the TFC and the Darrach operation should be avoided in the treatment of these younger, more vigorous individuals. Factors to consider in selecting the procedure are the condition of the articular surface of the ulnar head; the presence of an ulna plus variant; the extent, nature, and location of the TFC defect; and the presence of associated carpal problems (e.g., lunotriquetral dissociation).

For the athlete with a long-standing or degenerative tear of the TFC and an ulna plus or even a zero variant, ulnar shortening is the procedure of choice and should be considered in preference to other techniques whenever possible. This type of decompression of the ulnocarpal space can be expected to succeed when the distal radioulnar joint is uninvolved and may restore stability to an associated lunotriquetral instability through longitudinal tightening of ulnocarpal constraints.

When the ulna variant is negative, debridement of the TFC defect may succeed in relieving pain. This debridement is limited to excision of loose cartilaginous tags or degenerative perforations of the TFC without interfering with the support portions of the TFC complex. Load transmission is not altered as long as the larger defect that results is limited to an area involving no more than the central third of the TFC.

Acute avulsions resulting in distal radioulnar instability, subluxation, or dislocation are successfully managed by above-elbow immobilization with the forearm in the position of stability or reduction. When instability persists after an adequate initial nonoperative treatment, and in neglected or untreated cases, restoration of support by reattachment of the TFC has been proposed,[16] a technique with which I have had very limited experience.

REFERENCES

1. Angelides, A.C., Wallace, P.F.: The dorsal ganglion of the wrist: Its pathogenesis, gross and microscopic anatomy, and surgical treatment. J. Hand Surg. 1:228, 1976.
2. Armstrong, G.W.D.: Rotational subluxation of the scaphoid. Can. J. Surg. 11:306, 1968.
3. Aronen, J.G.: Problems of the upper extremity in gymnasts. Clin. Sports Med. 4:61, 1985.
4. Blatt, G.: Capsulodesis in reconstructive hand surgery: dorsal capsulodesis for the unstable scaphoid and volar capsulodesis following excision of the distal ulna. Hand Clin. 3:81, 1987.
5. Bowers, W.H.: Distal radioulnar joint arthroplasty. The hemiresection-interposition technique. J. Hand Surg. 10A:169, 1985.
6. Cart, J.: The upper limits. *Los Angeles Times,* June 8, 1986, Part III, p. 3.
7. Chamay, A., Della Santa, D., Vilaseca, A.: L'arthrodèse radiolunaire facteur de stabilite du poignet rhumatoîde. Ann. Chir. 2:5, 1983.
8. Darrow, J.C., Linscheid, R.L., Dobyns, J.H. et al.: Distal ulnar recession for disorders of the distal radioulnar joint. J. Hand Surg. 10:482, 1985.
9. Demos, T.C.: Radiologic case study: Painful wrist. Orthopaedics 1:151, 1978.
10. Destot, E.: Traumatismes du Poignet et Rayons X. Paris, Masson et Cie, 1923.
11. Dobyns, J.H., Linscheid, R.L., Chao, E.Y.S., et al.: Traumatic instability of the wrist. Am. Acad. Orthop. Surgeons Instruc. Course Lect. 24:182, 1975.
12. England, J.P.S.: Subluxation of the carpal scaphoid. Proc. R. Soc. Med. 63:581, 1970.
13. Gonçalves, D.: Correction of disorders of the distal radioulnar joint by artificial pseudarthrosis of the ulna. J. Bone Joint Surg. 56B:462, 1974.
14. Green, D.P.: Carpal dislocation. In Green, D.P., ed.: Operative Hand Surgery, Vol. I. New York, Churchill Livingstone, 1982.
15. Gunther, S.F.: Dorsal wrist pain and the occult scapholunate ganglion. J. Hand Surg. 10A:697, 1985.

16. Hagert, C.-G.: The distal radioulnar joint. Hand Clin. 3:41, 1987.
17. Jeanne, L.A., Mouchet, A.: Les lesions traumatiques fermeès du poignet. 28th Congrès Français de Chirurgie, 1919.
18. Johnson, R.P.: The acutely injured wrist and its residuals. Clin. Orthop. 149:33, 1980.
19. Kirk, J.A., Ansell, B.M., Bywaters, E.G.L.: The hypermobility syndrome. Rheum. Dis. 26:419, 1967.
20. Linscheid, R.L.: Ulnar lengthening and shortening. Hand Clin. 3:69, 1987.
21. Linscheid, R.L., Dobyns, J.H.: Athletic injuries of the wrist. Clin. Orthop. 198:141, 1985.
22. Linscheid, R.L., Dobyns, J.H., Beabout, J.W., et al.: Traumatic instability of the wrist. J. Bone Joint Surg. 54A:1612, 1972.
23. Linscheid, R.L., Dobyns, J.H., Beckenbaugh, R.D. et al.: Instability patterns of the wrist. J. Hand Surg. 8:682, 1983.
24. Logan, S.E., Nowak, M.D., Gould, P.L., et al.: Biomechanical behavior of the scapholunate ligament. Biomed. Sci. Instrum. 22:81, 1986.
25. Mayfield, J.K., Johnson, R.P., Kilcoyne, R.K.: The ligaments of the human wrist and their functional significance. Anat. Rec. 186:417, 1976.
26. Mayfield, J.K., Johnson, R.P., Kilcoyne, R.K.: Carpal dislocations: Pathomechanics and progressive perilunar instability. J. Hand Surg. 5:226, 1980.
27. Mikic, Z.D.: Age changes in the triangular fibrocartilage of the wrist joint. J. Anat. 126:367, 1978.
28. Neviaser, R.J., Palmer, A.K.: Traumatic perforation of the articular disc of the triangular fibrocartilage complex of the wrist. Bull. Hosp. Joint Dis. 44:376, 1984.
29. Oreck, S.L., Gillespie, T., Youm, Y.: Patterns of injury in experimentally induced ulnar side wrist injuries. Orthop. Trans. 10:201, 1986.
30. Palmer, A.K.: The distal radioulnar joint. Orthop. Clin. North Am. 15:321, 1984.
31. Palmer, A.K.: Triangular fibrocartilage complex abnormalities. AAOS Symposium. Orthop. Today 4:11, 1985.
32. Palmer, A.K.: The distal radioulnar joint. Hand Clin. 3:31, 1987.
33. Palmer, A.K., Glisson, R.R., Werner, F.W.: Relationship between ulnar variance and triangular fibrocartilage complex thickness. J. Hand Surg. 9A:681, 1984.
34. Rask, M.R.: Carponavicular subluxation: Report of a case treated with percutaneous pins. Orthopedics 2:134, 1979.
35. Reagan, D.S., Linscheid, R.L., Dobyns, J.H.: Lunotriquetral sprains. J. Hand Surg. 9A:502, 1984.
36. Redler, I.: Meniscoid of the wrist. Clin Orthop 88:138, 1972.
37. Sanders, W.F.: The occult dorsal carpal ganglion. J. Hand Surg. 10B:257, 1985.
38. Sauve, and Kapandji: Nouvelle technique de traitement chirurgical des luxations recidivantes isolees de l'extremite inferieure du cubitus. J Chirurgie 47:589, 1936.
39. Stein, F., Miale, A., Jr., Stein, A.: Enhanced diagnosis of hand and wrist disorders by triple phase radionuclide bone imaging. Bull. Hosp. Joint Dis. 44:477, 1984.
40. Sutro, C.J.: Hypermobility of bones due to "overlengthened" capsular and ligamentous tissues. Surgery 21:67, 1947.
41. Taleisnik, J.: The ligaments of the wrist. J. Hand Surg. 1:110, 1976.
42. Taleisnik, J.: Wrist: Anatomy, function and injury. Am. Acad. Orthop. Surg. Instruct Course Lect 27:61, 1978.
43. Taleisnik, J.: Post-traumatic carpal instability. Clin. Orthop. 149:73, 1980.
44. Taleisnik, J.: Carpal instability. Symposium. Contemp. Orthop. 4:107, 1982.
45. Taleisnik, J.: The Wrist. New York, Churchill Livingstone, 1985.
46. Taleisnik, J.: Pain on the ulnar side of the wrist. Hand Clin. 3:51, 1987.
47. Tanz, S.S.: Rotation effect in lunar and perilunar dislocations. Clin. Orthop. 57:147, 1968.
48. Thiru-Pathi, R.G., Ferlic, D.C., Clayton, M.L., et al.: Arterial anatomy of the triangular fibrocartilage of the wrist and its surgical significance. J. Hand Surg. 11A:258, 1986.
49. Tirman, R.M., Weber, E.R., Snyder, L.L., et al.: Midcarpal wrist arthrography for detection of tears of the scapholunate and lunotriquetral ligaments. A.J.R. 144:107, 1985.
50. Watson, H.K., Hempton, R.F.: Limited wrist arthrodesis. I. The triscaphoid joint. J. Hand Surg. 5:320, 1980.
51. Watson, H.K.: Personal communication, 1982.

CHAPTER

7

Management of Extra-articular Fractures of the Phalanges and Metacarpals

Hill Hastings, II, M.D.

The 27 major bones composing the intercalated osseous structure of the hand are particularly prone to injury during athletic endeavors. Fortunately, the energy absorption by the hand is usually low, the fracture pattern relatively simple, and the soft tissues minimally involved. Nevertheless, significant playing time can be lost, and even simple fractures can lead to impairment of digital performance with malunion, joint stiffness, and tendon adhesions.

With the increasing emphasis on fitness, competitive demands of athletes, and financial concerns in treating professional athletes, the treatment process becomes subject to a myriad of concerns that complicate decision making. The treating physician may be pressured into choosing a more aggressive means of treatment over a more conservative and equally predictable treatment in an attempt to shorten the disability time. At other times the patient may refuse the preferred method of treatment in deference to a less involved and less predictable method offering shorter disability time. The correct choice of treatment will depend upon experience and a comprehensive understanding of fractures of the hand and the potential problems characteristic to each fracture. The physician must have command of a variety of treatment methods to tailor to the individual situation to achieve the most predictable complication-free rate of fracture union and earliest return to athletic play. The physician should be cognizant of complex issues that enter into this decision-making process and, as perhaps the most independent party involved, should make sure that the proper course of treatment is chosen for both the patient's athletic career and future hand performance.

This chapter addresses the treatment of the most common extra-articular fractures of the metacarpals and phalanges. Emphasis is given to treatment methods we have found in experience with over 2200 tubular bone fractures of the hand to be effective, to be relatively straightforward to perform, and to permit the most rapid return to athletic activity.

Mechanism of Injury

Nonepiphyseal injuries occur through torque, angular forces, compressive forces, or a direct blow to the metacarpal or phalanx. The most common mechanisms for epiphyseal fractures are avulsion, shear, and compressive loading of the epiphyseal plate. In each of the metacarpals and phalanges there are common recurring fracture patterns that relate to each bone's relative susceptibility to these mechanisms. For example, metacarpals have concave palmar surfaces that contribute to the longitudinal arch of the hand. Compressive loads to the metacarpal head result in fracture through its weakest point—the subcapital region proximal to the head.[23] Volar cortical comminution and the volar shortening forces of the intrinsic muscles and flexor tendons invariably lead to dorsal angulation (Fig. 7–1). The phalanges are relatively protected from such axially directed forces through the ability of the metacarpophalangeal (MCP) and

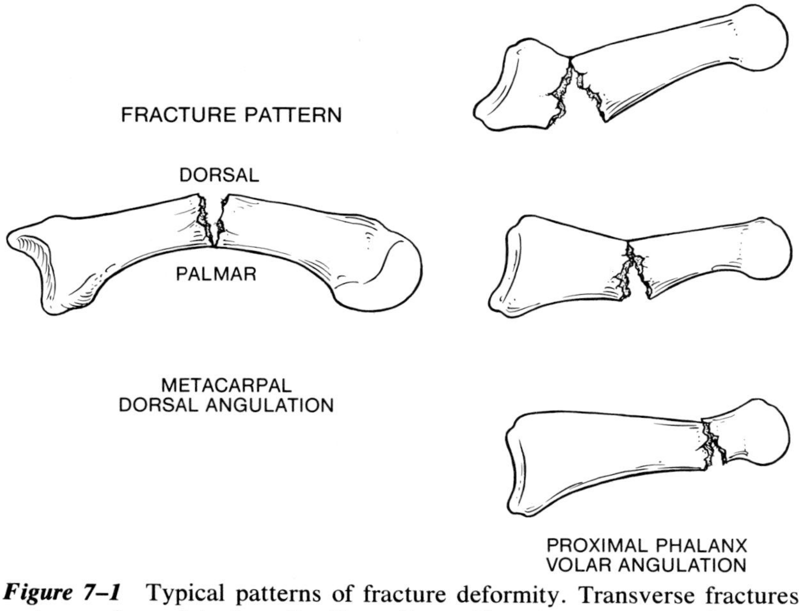

Figure 7–1 Typical patterns of fracture deformity. Transverse fractures of metacarpal angulate dorsally. Regardless of location, transverse fractures of proximal phalanx angulate volarly.

interphalangeal (IP) joints to collapse into extension or flexion. Direct blows or dorsally directed forces to the proximal phalanx lead to transverse fractures, which typically angulate volarly through volar flexion influence of the interossei on the proximal fragment and extension of the distal fragment through the extensor mechanism (Fig. 7–1). The middle phalanx is relatively protected from injury through its short length and force-absorbing adjacent IP joints. Fractures proximal to the insertion of the flexor digitorum superficialis angulate dorsally (Fig. 7–2*A*), and those distal to the flexor digitorum superficialis insertion angulate volarly (Fig. 7–2*B*). Extra-articular fractures of the distal phalanx are invariably caused by crushing forces that lead to longitudinal and comminuted or transverse fracture patterns.

The hand can be injured in almost any position in athletic endeavors, and a review of fracture patterns unique to each sport is not of treatment significance. Most hand injuries occur in sports involving throwing and catching, such as football, baseball, and basketball, where the inertial forces of the ball striking the hand or digit produce angular or rotational movements. Basketball injuries most commonly center on the proximal interphalangeal (PIP) joint, whereas baseball injuries most frequently involve the distal interphalangeal (DIP) joint. Crush injuries are more likely to occur in contact sports, such as football, where the digit of a player may be stepped upon and crushed by the cleated shoe of an opponent.

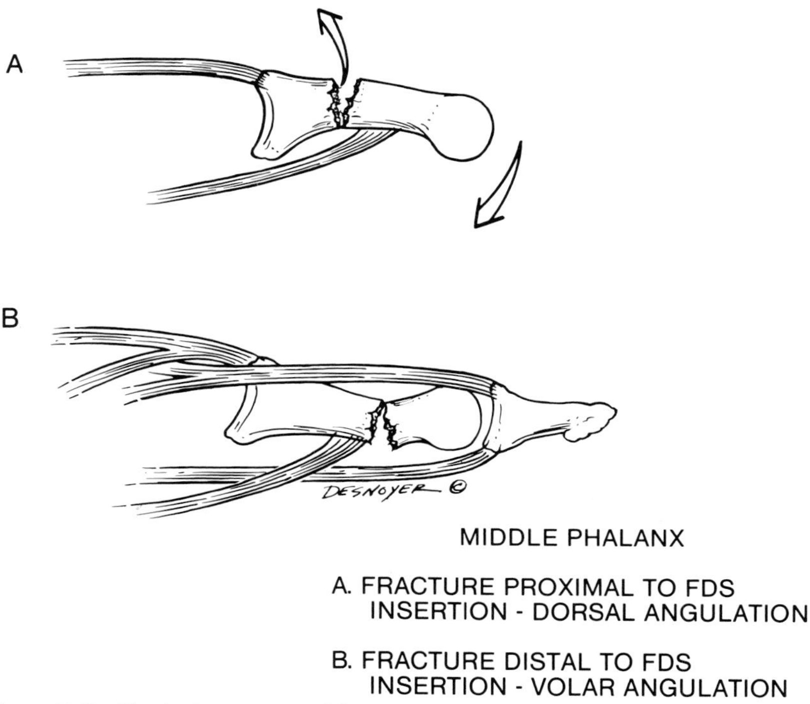

Figure 7–2 Typical patterns of fracture deformity seen in middle phalanx. Transverse fractures proximal to flexor digitorum superficialis (FDS) insertion angulate dorsally. Transverse fractures distal to flexor digitorum superficialis insertion angulate volarly.

While most sports have adopted safety regulations, these are often circumvented. For example, protective gloves are required in lacrosse, but injuries continue to be seen when individuals cut out the fingertips and palm of the glove for improved stick handling. Also, equipment designed to protect the head, neck, and shoulders often causes injury to digits. The thumb MCP joint is unusually susceptible to injury in Alpine skiing, where it accounts for more than 40 percent of the injuries to the upper extremity and 9 to 10 percent of all skiing injuries.[10] While ski pole grips with breakaway straps offer protection to the shoulder, angular as well as axially directed forces to the thumb still render it excessively susceptible to injury at the MCP and carpometacarpal (CMC) joints.

Initial Evaluation in the Athletic Arena

Critical information can be obtained by careful observation of the individual at the time of injury. Angulation and displacement are most apparent at injury prior to application of an immobilization splint. The direction and extent of deformity should be noted and may provide useful information on the stability or instability of the fracture. Proper emergency care by means of splint immobilization provides comfort and minimizes subsequent soft tissue swelling, which interferes with correct positioning of injured joints and reduction of fracture fragments. While the application of ice packs to acute injuries is usually helpful, it can injure the digits and should be used only at or proximal to the metacarpal level. Prior to transport, open injuries should be covered with an occlusive, sterile dressing to prevent infection. Reduction on the playing field should not be attempted unless deformity is so excessive that it prevents application of a splint.

Physical Examination

The physician should not only focus on the obvious but should also carefully document neurovascular status and extensor and flexor tendon function. Fractures with significant soft tissue swelling and angular displacement deformity are relatively easy to diagnose. The major pitfalls occur with oblique or spiral fractures that create displacement in planes and are difficult to recognize. Careful examination is required to avoid overlooking rotational malalignment. Identification of local swelling, tenderness, or both early after injury is most helpful. Remember that subtle amounts of malrotation are difficult to visualize in a position of digital extension but are readily visible in a position of flexion. Every fracture of the metacarpal or distal phalanges should be examined in a position of full digital flexion to rule out rotational malalignment. Acceptance of patient discomfort as an excuse for an incomplete examination will result in an initially happy patient and physician but later an embarrassed physician and angry patient. Rotational malalignment of the small finger is difficult to evaluate; in mild flexion, it normally crowds the ring finger. Some guid-

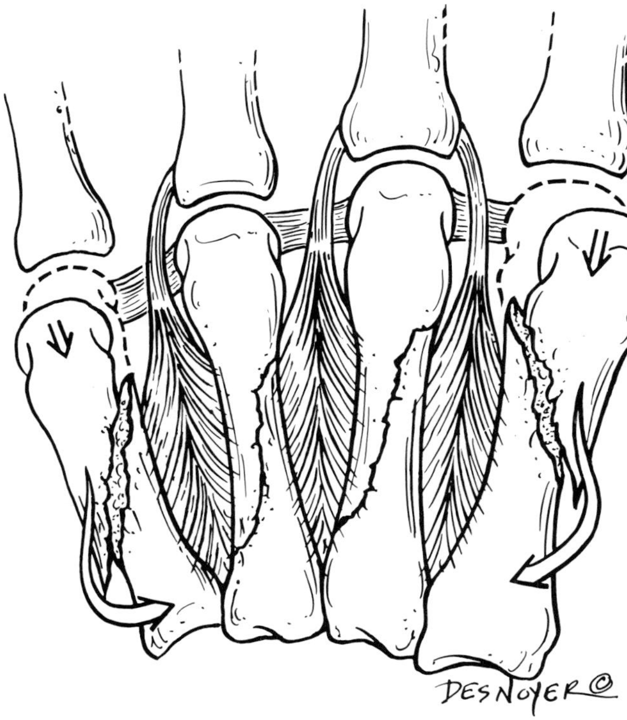

Figure 7–6 Spiral fractures of the metacarpals tend to be most unstable in the border digits, where only one side of the metacarpal is supported by a deep intermetacarpal ligament.

forces applied to the proximal phalanx and transmitted to the metacarpal through the collateral ligaments of the MCP joint. These fractures occur from tension.[14] Because of the obliquity of a spiral fracture, any significant shortening of the metacarpal caused by the compressive forces of the extrinsic and intrinsic muscle tendon units may lead to malrotation (see Fig. 7–6). When simultaneous axial loading, torsional loading, and angulation occur, an oblique fracture results.[2] Shortening of oblique fractures

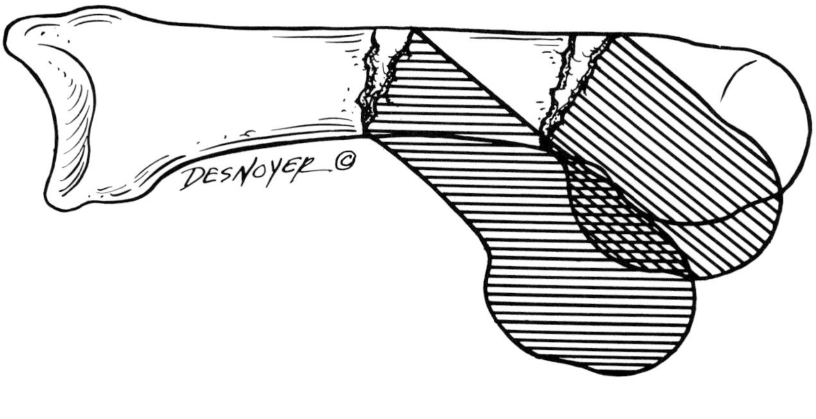

THE MORE PROXIMAL THE FRACTURE,
THE GREATER THE PALMAR PROMINENCE.

Figure 7–7 Effect of fracture level on metacarpal head displacement.

can lead to rotational malalignment, but less frequently than with spiral fractures.[6]

METACARPAL NECK FRACTURES

The most common fractures of the metacarpals are those involving the distal metaphysis or neck of the ring and small digits. The dorsal angulation that occurs is commonly associated with volar comminution. Fractures close to the joint, even with significant angulation, may not cause deformity other than loss of the dorsal prominence of the metacarpal head. Equivalent angulation through fractures proximally lead to deformity of the metacarpal head characterized by an absent dorsal knuckle contour of the metacarpal head and reciprocal volar prominence of the metacarpal head within the palm (see Fig. 7–7). This is well tolerated in the small metacarpal, in which 30° of flexion and extension at the CMC joint allows for the metacarpal to extend and move away from distal palmar pressure. The ring metacarpal with 15° of flexion and extension at the carpometacarpal joint similarly tolerates an angular fracture deformity. Since the index and middle metacarpals have little to no carpometacarpal joint motion, no significant angulation can be accepted.

Treatment will depend upon three main considerations. *First,* because the mode of bony failure in subcapital fractures of the metacarpal is that of dorsal tension and volar compression, there is some degree of volar comminution. The tendency of a fracture to settle following reduction depends upon the amount of volar comminution and compression; most fractures will settle back close to the original angulated position. *Second,* the decision whether to accept the position as is or reduce the fracture will depend upon the function of the digit in its prereduced alignment. Is there a rotational abnormality? Is there excessive prominence of the metacarpal head in the palm? Any dorsal angulation of index or middle metacarpal fractures will lead to volar prominence of the metacarpal head in the palm. No angulation greater than 15° can be accepted in metacarpal neck fractures of the index and middle finger, but greater amounts can be accepted in the ring and small metacarpals (up to 50° to 70° if close to the joint). The more distal the fracture, the better tolerated any amount of angulation, and the more proximal the fracture, the less tolerance of angulation. *Finally* and most importantly, is the angulation significant enough to cause clawing of the fractured digit? The likelihood of clawing following a metacarpal neck fracture does not correlate with the amount of angulation. Rather, it depends on the amount of metacarpal *shortening* that weakens the intrinsic muscles. *Angulation*, in addition to weakening the intrinsic muscles, results in a MCP joint that appears to be extended when, in fact, it is hyperextended. Marked MCP joint hyperextension can render the central tendon inefficient in extending the PIP joint (Fig. 7–8). Despite the amount of angulation, if the patient can fully extend the digit without an extensor lag at the PIP joint, closed treatment is indicated. For the ring and small digits, angulatory deformities at the fracture of less than 40° are accepted and immobilized. Fractures with greater than 40° of angulation should be reduced and immobilized. If the examination reveals rotational problems

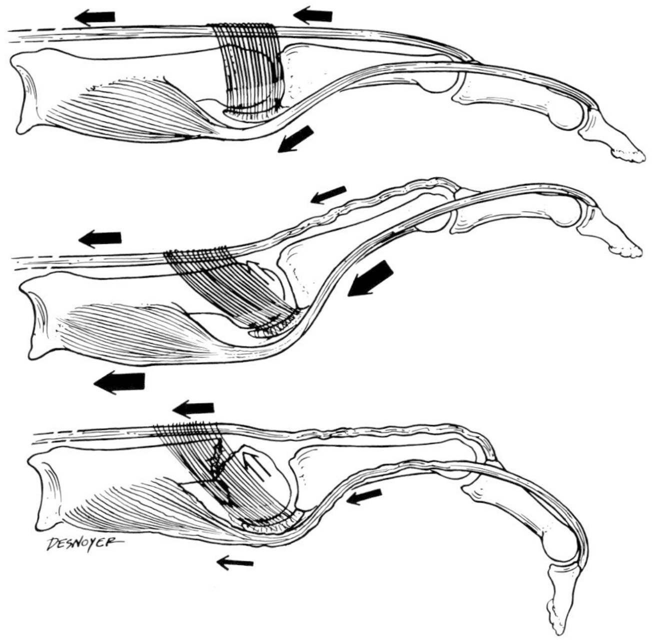

Figure 7–8 Mechanism of clawing with severely angulated and foreshortened metacarpal neck fracture. As the metacarpal neck fracture falls into marked dorsal angulation, extreme MCP hyperextension is required to achieve clinical neutral extension of the digit. In the hyperextended MCP position, the common extensor tendon is lax and does not provide adequate extensor force at the PIP joint.

or excessive volar prominence to the metacarpal head and/or a clawing tendency, closed reduction should be supplemented by internal fixation to maintain the reduction and prevent a gradual settling postreduction.

The closed reduction maneuver has been described by Jahss (Fig. 7–9).[18] Reduction is achieved first by disimpacting the fracture by digital traction. The MCP and PIP joints are then both fully flexed. Dorsally directed pressure is applied along the shaft of the proximal phalanx through the PIP joint, and volarly directed pressure is supplied by another digit placed directly over the dorsal apex of the fracture. The fracture is immobilized with a short arm gutter splint holding the wrist in neutral position to tighten and allow the dorsal extensor mechanism to act as a tension band for the fracture. The MCP joint is fully flexed, and the interphalangeal joints are extended. The splint is continued for 10 to 14 days, followed by initiation of active range of motion. When progressive angulation or redisplacement of the second and third metacarpals is of greater concern, follow-up radiographs at 5 to 7 days are mandatory. Reduction loss with dorsal angulation can still be corrected at that point, but with further delay, correction will likely require manipulative force or osteotomy/refracture.

When reduction has been lost, repeat closed reduction and internal fixation are necessary. This can be carried out by placement of a transmetacarpal Kirschner wire (K-wire) proximal and distal to the fracture to prevent the proximal shaft from displacing dorsally and the metacarpal head from displacing volarly (Fig. 7–10). Oblique cross K-wires across the fracture can be inserted through the collateral ligament recess. Alternatively, several intermedullary K-wires or pins can be placed down the shaft of the metacarpal as an internal splint (see Fig. 7–10). The latter method is most suitable for the second and fifth metacarpals.

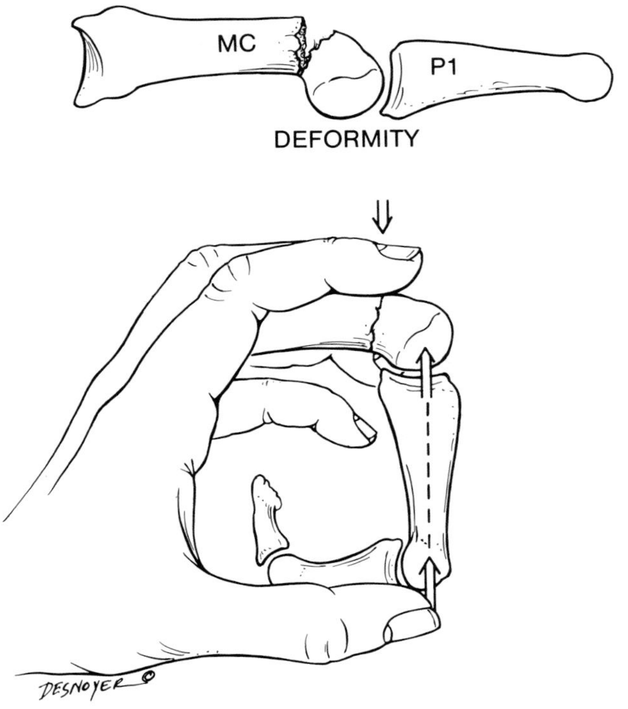

Figure 7–9 The Jahss maneuver for reducing metacarpal neck fractures. Volar to dorsal force is applied through the proximal phalanx to the head of the metacarpal with dorsal to volar force applied directly over the apex of the fracture.

When early return to play is essential, the K-wires should be cut subcutaneously to lessen the likelihood of infection and facilitate application of a protective splint. When splinting is not possible and unrestricted use of the hand is required, closed reduction is performed and the fracture supported by multiple K-wires for intermedullary fixation. Internal fixation is accomplished by creation of a small cortical window at the proximal metaphysis of the fractured metacarpal, reduction of the fracture through a

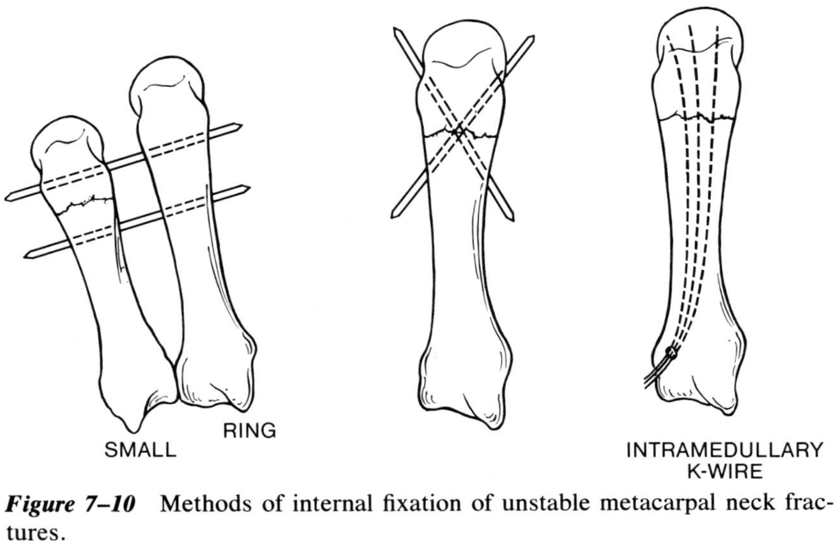

Figure 7–10 Methods of internal fixation of unstable metacarpal neck fractures.

Jahss maneuver, and insertion of multiple 0.035 K-wires down the shaft and across the fracture (Fig. 7–11*A* to *E*). Single intramedullary pin fixation (Fig. 7–12) and external fixation (Fig. 7–13) are seldom used. The fracture is opened only in cases of extensor tendon entrapment or unreducible fracture displacement. In such instances, fixation is best applied through an oblique K-wire and dorsally positioned tension band wire, or a 2.0 mm miniblade plate.[4, 7, 15]

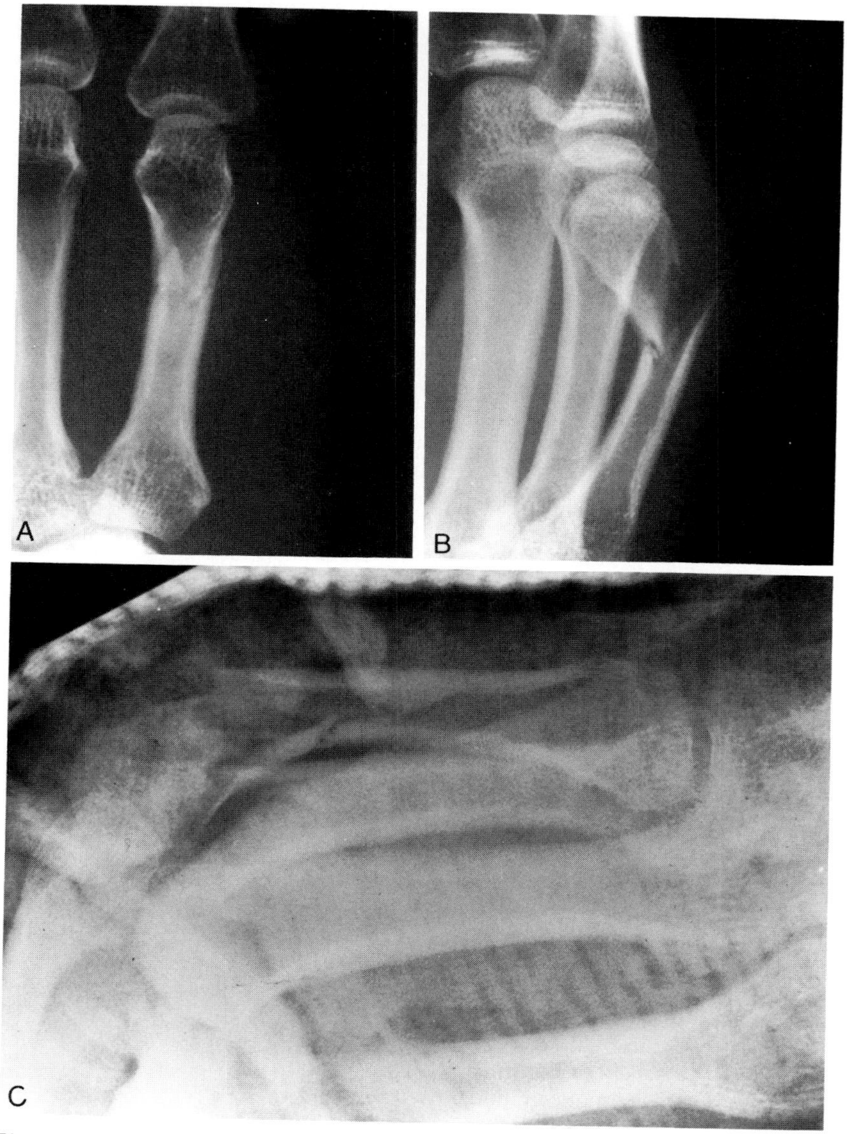

Figure 7–11 Anteroposterior (*A*) and lateral (*B*) views of metacarpal fracture with marked dorsal angulation and protruding dorsal bony spike. Partial reduction of fracture with cast immobilization (*C*).

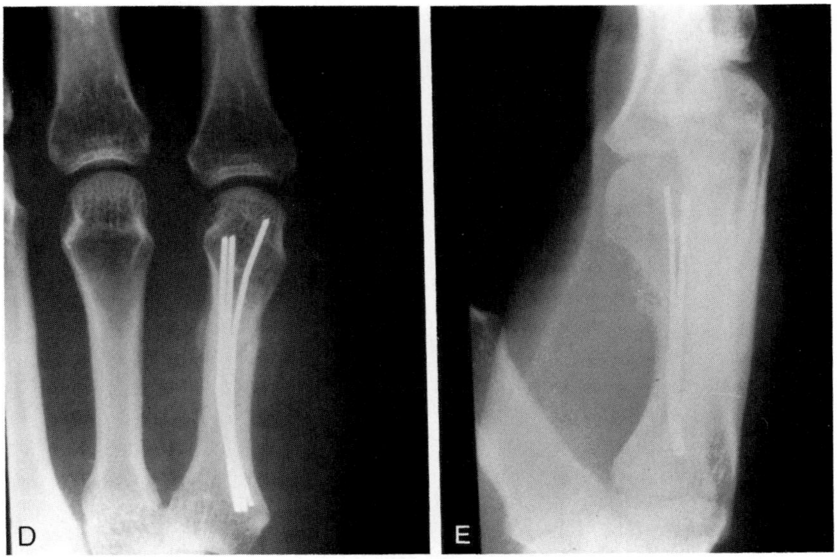

Figure 7–11 Continued Anteroposterior (*D*) and lateral (*E*) views of fracture after closed reduction and fixation with intramedullary K-wires inserted through cortical window at metaphyseal base of metacarpal.

METACARPAL SHAFT FRACTURES

Treatment of metacarpal shaft fractures depends upon (1) the fracture location and configuration, (2) the degree of fracture displacement, and (3) the number of metacarpal fractures.

Transverse Fractures

Dorsal angulation is not tolerated for the index and middle metacarpals. Index and middle metacarpal fractures without angulation or malrotation and ring and small metacarpal fractures without rotational displace-

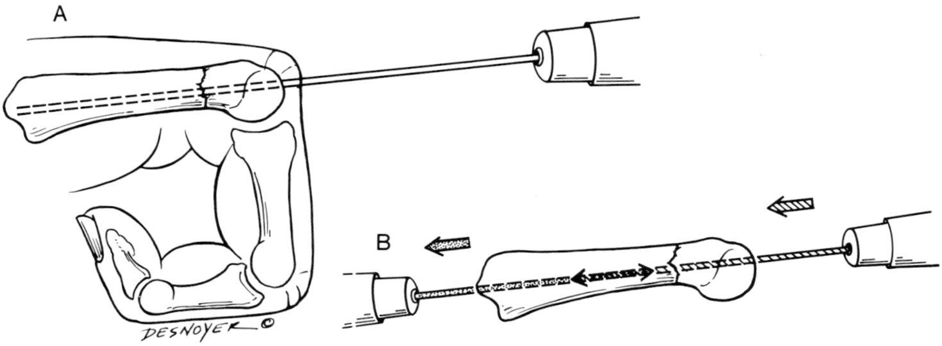

Figure 7–12 Intramedullary Steinmann pin fixation of metacarpal fracture. The MCP joint is flexed, and the fracture is reduced by the Jahss maneuver. *A*, A Steinmann pin is placed through the metacarpal head and down the metacarpal, the wrist palmar flexed, and the K-wire withdrawn from the dorsal wrist area. *B*, The pin is withdrawn such that the distal part lies within the metacarpal head, allowing active range of motion of the MCP joint. Maintenance and protection of wrist palmar flexion are required to avoid irritation of the pin in the dorsal wrist area.

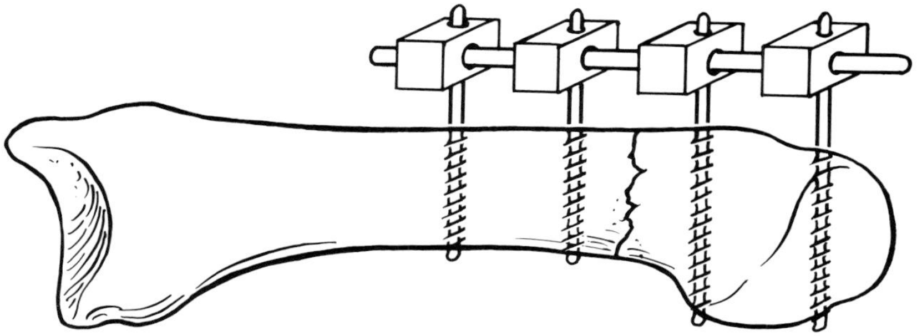

Figure 7–13 Example of external fixation principle of metacarpal fracture. This is best applied in a dorsolateral plane.

ment and with minimal dorsal angulation can be treated in a short arm cast. Dorsal and volar splints that hold the wrist in dorsiflexion, the MCP joints in flexion, and the IP joints in relative extension, are an alternative for these fractures. Immobilization must include an adjacent unfractured digit. When displacement is rotational, closed reduction is performed. The wrist is immobilized in dorsiflexion and the MCP joints in flexion. The injured digit is buddy taped to an adjacent digit and active motion is encouraged. Maintenance of full digital flexion will encourage proper rotational alignment of the fractured digit.[8, 9] When angular and rotational displacement requires reduction, casting or splinting may not be reliable in maintaining the reduction. If the fracture is closed and can be anatomically reduced, the simplest way of maintaining reduction is through placement of transverse K-wires between the fractured metacarpal[21] and an adjacent unfractured metacarpal. Active range of motion may be allowed, but in between exercise periods, supplemental immobilization is required for 6 weeks. The K-wires should be cut underneath the skin to avoid interference with the postoperative orthosis.

Open reduction and internal fixation are reserved for multiple closed metacarpal fractures and most open fractures. Cross K-wires alone have long been recommended for controlling rotation but are inefficient in counteracting dorsal angular forces. They should be supplemented by a single dorsally placed tension band wire (Fig. 7–14). An alternative method is to use a dorsal tension band compression plate (see Fig. 7–14), which provides strength equal to or greater than that of the strongest interosseous wiring techniques.[4, 24] Either a four-hole 2.7 mm 1/4 tubular plate or a 2.0 mm dynamic compression plate is advised.[16, 17] Active range of motion of the hand is encouraged postoperatively. A small orthoplast splint is utilized between exercises for 6 weeks, including wrist and MCP joints of the injured and adjacent normal metacarpal. The IP joints are left free for motion. A similar soft athletic orthosis is fabricated for play, again allowing full PIP and DIP motion.

Oblique Fractures

Oblique fractures cause metacarpal shortening more frequently than transverse fractures. Shortening does not necessarily lead to malrotation, as the distal metacarpals are rotationally supported by the deep inter-

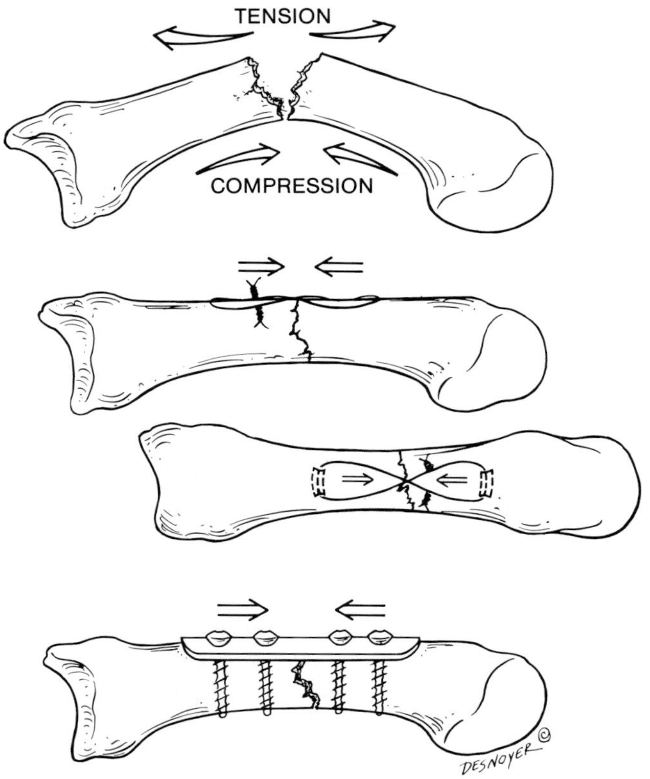

Figure 7–14 Principle of tension band fixation of transverse metacarpal fractures. As transverse fractures of metacarpals angulate dorsally, either a plate or a wire will function as a dorsal tension band, preventing separation of the dorsal cortex. Cortex-to-cortex apposition is required on the palmar side.

metacarpal ligaments. Displacement and shortening are more common on the border index and small digits, which are supported by a deep intermetacarpal ligament on one side. Treatment depends upon the amount of shortening and the presence or absence of rotational displacement. At least 3 mm of shortening can be accepted without significant impairment.[5]

Fractures with acceptable rotational alignment and length are treated with a short arm cast holding the wrist in dorsiflexion and the MCP joints in flexion and assuring immediate full active motion of the IP joints. Shortening beyond 3 mm can lead to extensive weakening of the intrinsic muscles and disruption of the distal transverse metacarpal arch. When shortening is excessive or rotational malalignment is present, open reduction and internal fixation are required. If the fracture surface length is greater than twice the diameter of the metacarpal, several interfragmentary 2.0 mm compression screws are used. Fractures with an angle of greater than 45° or with a fracture surface less than twice the metacarpal diameter are treated with K-wires supplemented by a dorsal tension band wire or an interfragmentary compression screw supplemented by a dorsal neutralization plate.[4, 15–17, 22]

Spiral Fractures

Spiral fractures are more apt to rotate than oblique fractures, particularly when involving the index or small digits (see Fig. 7–6). Reduction can be maintained only by reduction and internal fixation, either through several percutaneous K-wires or through open reduction and internal fixation. If shortening and malrotation are minimal, a short arm cast that includes the MCP joint in flexion is applied and active range of motion is prescribed. Functional use will encourage rotational realignment. If immediate return to play is needed and an orthosis can be utilized, closed reduction and percutaneous K-wires across the fracture is the safest choice. If a protective orthosis is contraindicated (e.g., diving, swimming), open reduction and internal fixation are warranted.

Comminuted Fractures

With injuries caused by projectiles or similar severe force, transverse, oblique, or spiral fractures may be comminuted and thus rendered additionally unstable. The same criteria in choice of treatment apply as discussed previously. Frequently, nondisplaced comminuted fractures occur from a direct blow, and AP splints in a safe position are utilized. When the fracture is displaced, rigid internal fixation with or without distal radius cancellous bone grafting is advised to render fracture stability. This will offset the delay in expected union and allow early mobilization of the hand for prevention of arthrofibrosis and peritendinous adhesions.

FRACTURES OF THE METACARPAL PROXIMAL METAPHYSIS

Because of the stabilizing intermetacarpal ligaments, intrinsic muscles, and fascia, fractures through the base of the metacarpal are minimally displaced or nondisplaced. Careful physical examination is required to rule out rotational problems. Radiographs must be evaluated for intra-articular involvement, which when displaced can lead to carpometacarpal posttraumatic arthrosis. When displacement is minimal, early return to athletics is allowed with a short arm orthosis that holds the wrist in mild dorsiflexion, the injured and adjacent MCP joints in flexion, and the IP joints free. In most instances, closed reduction and percutaneous K-wire fixation suffices, but when comminution is extensive, a 2.7 mm 1/4 tubular T-plate or a 2.0 mm condylar plate is utilized as a strut plate and the defect bone grafted.[14, 7, 16]

THUMB METACARPAL FRACTURES

The thumb is susceptible to the same type of metacarpal fractures as the index through small digits. Most thumb metacarpal extra-articular fractures occur at the proximal base and are either transverse or oblique. When the fracture is significantly displaced and associated with marked swelling, reduction may be difficult to maintain by splint or cast. Oblique fractures often require percutaneous K-wire fixation. The majority of thumb metacarpal fractures are amenable to thumb spica immobilization. Because of the multiple planes of thumb motion, up to 30° of angulation and/or rotation is acceptable.

Phalangeal Fractures

Proximal Phalangeal Fractures

Fractures of the proximal phalanx occur when rotational or angular forces that do not result in injury to the PIP joint are transmitted proximally. In childhood, fractures commonly occur through the distal neck of the proximal phalanx, while in teenagers, the phalanx is weakest, resulting in physeal fractures of the base of the proximal phalanx. In adult athletes, fracture results are through the shaft or into the condylar area of the proximal phalanx.

Extra-articular Fractures of Base of Proximal Phalanx

The most common fracture in childhood is a Salter-Harris II fracture of the base of the proximal phalanx involving the small digit (Fig. 7–15*A* and *B*).[1, 20] Force applied in an ulnar and dorsal direction results in a radial fracture and volar angulation. Fracture occurs through the physis exiting through the metaphysis. When displacement is significant, the digit will rest in abduction. Clinicians are taught to place a pencil between the fourth and fifth digits, against which the small finger can be reduced. However, because of the distal position of the web with respect to the base of the proximal phalanx, the position of the pencil falls too far distal, and rather than assist in reduction, its use can lead to injurious compression of the epiphyseal plate (Fig. 7–16).

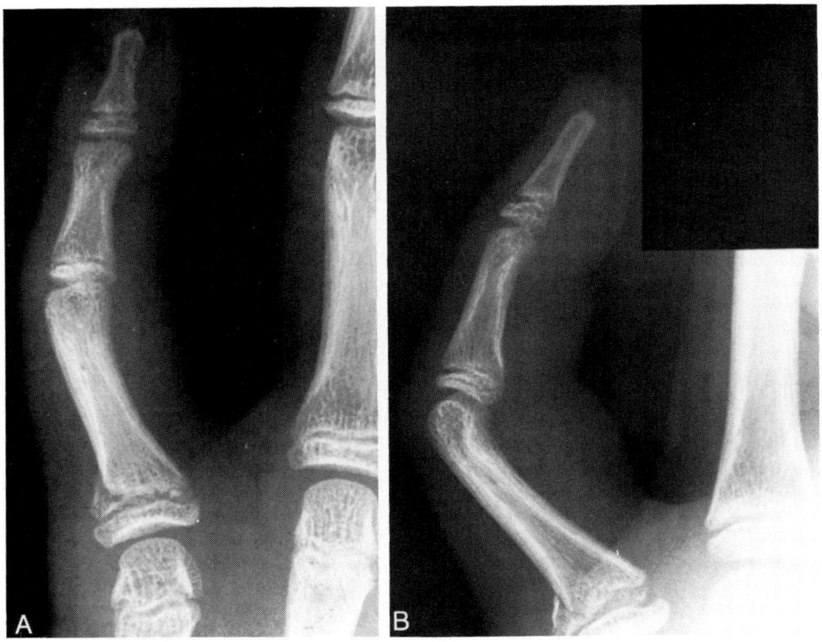

Figure 7–15 Palmar (*A*) and radial (*B*) angulation of a typical Salter-Harris II fracture at the base of the proximal phalanx.

that of the normal unfractured bone, allowing immediate resumption of activity with minimal protection and early functional return. The exact treatment plan and length of impairment will vary according to fracture location, pattern, and displacement.

REFERENCES

1. Aitken, A.P.: Fractures of the epiphyses. Clin. Orthop. 41:19, 1965.
2. Alms, M.: Fracture mechanics. J. Bone Joint Surg. 43B:162, 1961.
3. Belsky, R., Eaton, R.G., Lane, L.B.: Closed reduction and internal fixation of proximal phalangeal fractures. J. Hand Surg. 9A:725, 1984.
4. Belsole, R.J., Greene, T.L.: Comparative strengths of internal fixation techniques. J. Hand Surg. 10A:315, 1985.
5. Bloem, J.J.: The treatment and prognosis of uncomplicated dislocated fractures of the metacarpals and phalanges. Arch. Chir. Neerl. 23:55, 1971.
6. Brooks, D.B., Burstein, A.H., Frankel, V.H.: The biomechanics of torsional fractures. J. Bone Joint Surg. 52A:507, 1970.
7. Buchler, U., Fischer, T.: Use of a minicondylar plate for metacarpal and phalangeal periarticular injuries. Clin. Orthop. 214:53, 1987.
8. Burkhalter, W.E.: Closed treatment of hand fractures. J. Hand Surg. 14A:390, 1989.
9. Burkhalter, W.E., Reyes, F.A.: Closed treatment of fractures of the hand. Bull. Hosp. Joint Dis. Orthop. Inst. 44(2):145, 1984.
10. Carr, D., Johnson, R.J., Pope, M.H.: Upper extremity injuries in skiing. Am. J. Sports Med. 9:378, 1981.
11. DeMuth, W.E., Smith, J.M.: High-velocity bullet wounds of muscle and bone: the basis of rational early treatment. J. Trauma 6:744, 1966.
12. Dimond, F.C., Rich, N.M.: M-16 rifle wounds in Vietnam. J. Trauma 7:619, 1967.
13. Dixon, G.L., Moon, N.F.: Rotational supracondylar fractures of the proximal phalanx in children. Clin. Orthop. 83:151, 1972.
14. Frankel, V.H., Burstein, A.H.: Orthopaedic Biomechanics. Philadelphia, Lea & Febiger, 1970.
15. Greene, T.L., Noellert, R.C., Belsole, R.J.: Treatment of unstable metacarpal and phalangeal fractures with tension band wiring techniques. Clin. Orthop. 214:78, 1987.
16. Hastings, H., II: Unstable metacarpal and phalangeal fracture treatment with screws and plates. Clin. Orthop. 214:37, 1987.
17. Hastings, H., II: Point/counterpoint. Orthopedics 12:911, 1989.
18. Jahss, S.A.: Fractures of the metacarpals. A new method of reduction and immobilization. J. Bone Joint Surg. 20:178, 1938.
19. Lane, C.S.: Detecting occult fractures of the metacarpal head: The Brewerton view. J. Hand Surg. 2:131, 1977.
20. Salter, R.B., Harris, W.R.: Injuries involving the epiphyseal plate. J. Bone Joint Surg. 45A:587, 1963.
21. Saypol, G.M., Slattery, L.R.: Observations on displaced fractures of the hand. Surg. Gynecol. Obstet. 79:522, 1944.
22. Segmuller, G.: Surgical Stabilization of the Skeleton of the Hand. Baltimore, Williams & Wilkins, 1977.
23. Spinner, M.: Kaplan's Functional and Surgical Anatomy of the Hand, 3rd ed. Philadelphia, J.B. Lippincott, 1984.
24. Vanik, R.K., Weber, R.C., Matloub, H.S., et al.: The comparative strengths of internal fixation techniques. J. Hand Surg. 9A:216, 1984.

CHAPTER

8

Carpal Fractures

Norman P. Zemel, M.D.

Most injuries to athletes, whether they occur in adolescents or adults, are minor sprains, strains, or contusions that readily heal with conservative treatment and appropriate rehabilitation. Compressive loading of the wrist from an uncontrolled fall onto the dorsiflexed wrist is a frequent occurrence during athletic activities and can cause injury of the distal radius, carpal bones, and ligaments or a fracture-dislocation of the carpus. Mayfield and co-workers described a sequence of injuries to the carpus from a fall on the outstretched extremity with the wrist in dorsiflexion, ulnar deviation, and intercarpal supination.[28] Other injuries can occur with the wrist in dorsiflexion and radial deviation.

If seemingly minor injuries to the wrist do not improve with conservative treatment and a nagging ache or pain persists, additional evaluation is indicated. The individual should not be summarily dismissed as a "crybaby." Misdiagnosis of serious wrist injury such as a scaphoid fracture or ligament tear as a simple sprain can have a significant impact on the length of time an athlete must be out of action. In addition, a delay in treatment often reduces the therapeutic options available.

Fractures of the scaphoid are the most prevalent and well known of the carpal bone fractures.[6, 7, 10] Hook of the hamate fractures occur most commonly in golf, tennis, baseball, racquetball, and squash. Injuries to the other carpal bones, including the body of the hamate, are much less common but must be included in the differential diagnosis of an acutely injured wrist or an injury that has not responded to treatment.

Scaphoid Fractures

The scaphoid, which is almost completely covered by articular cartilage, articulates with the radius and lunate proximally, the capitate on its ulnar border, and distally forms the scaphotrapezialtrapezoidal joint. It spans the proximal and distal carpal rows. Mechanically it serves as a link between the two rows of carpal bones.[16] In normal wrists, a strong volar ligament acts as a sling and maintains the bone in 30° to 60° of flexion in relationship to the lunate.[25]

Gelberman and colleagues studied the extraosseous and intraosseous vascularity of the human carpus.[21] The extraosseous blood supply comes from an anastomotic network of three dorsal and palmar arches from the radial and ulnar arteries; additional anastomoses are supplied by the anterior interosseous artery. Between 70 and 80 percent of the intraosseous blood supply, including the entire proximal pole, is from branches of the radial artery that enter the dorsal ridge of the bone near the waist. Branches from the volar radial artery supply 20 to 30 percent of the scaphoid in the region of the distal tuberosity. Gelberman and Menon concluded that a volar operative approach to the scaphoid would be the least harmful to the blood supply of the proximal pole.[19] However, the scaphoid is at great risk for avascular necrosis following a fracture because it has large intraosseous areas that are dependent upon one vessel.[35] It has been estimated that 30 percent of middle third fractures and almost 100 percent of proximal fifth fractures of the scaphoid will develop avascular necrosis of the proximal pole.[32]

Because of its anatomic position in the wrist, the scaphoid is highly susceptible to injury when the wrist is loaded in an extended position. Weber and Chao were able to produce fractures through the waist of cadaver scaphoids when the wrists were in 95° to 100° of dorsiflexion and the load was primarily on the radial aspect of the palm.[46] The load on the articular surface between the radius and scaphoid was four times that on the palm. The proximal pole of the scaphoid was trapped between the radius and capitate, and the fracture occurred at the unsupported waist of the scaphoid. Experimentally, and probably in clinical cases as well, the scaphoid waist fracture originates on the volar ulnar surface of the bone (tension side) and extends to the dorsal lateral surface (compression side). In a study on fractures of the distal radius, Frykman was also able to consistently produce fractures of the waist of the scaphoid when the wrist was dorsiflexed greater than 90° and radially deviated.[17] If a lesser degree of dorsiflexion were present, the fracture would occur in the distal radius.

Tenderness over the dorsoradial aspect of the wrist and in the anatomic snuffbox is a common finding in patients with scaphoid fractures. Associated swelling of the wrist, particularly in the snuffbox, should alert the physician to the possibility of such a fracture. A six-view series of roentgenograms (scaphoid series) should consist of a posteroanterior (PA), lateral, right, and left oblique as well as PA view of the wrist in radial and ulnar deviation with the fingers flexed. The ulnar deviation view profiles the scaphoid (Fig. 8–1). If no fracture is seen, the wrist should be immobilized in a splint and the roentgenogram repeated in 10 to 14 days. Resorption at the fracture site may render it visible radiologically at that time.

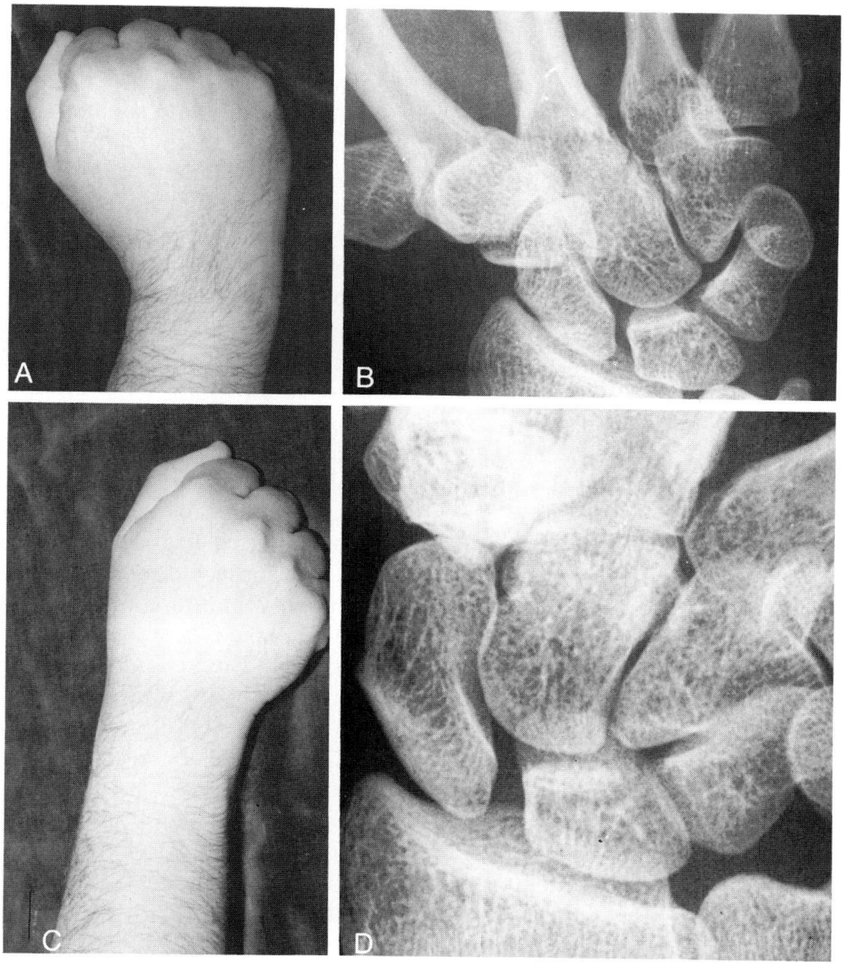

Figure 8–1 *A*, The wrist in radial deviation. *B*, A PA roentgenogram of the wrist in radial deviation with the scaphoid palmar flexed. *C*, The wrist in ulnar deviation. *D*, A PA roentgenogram of the wrist in ulnar deviation and fingers flexed shows a profile view of the scaphoid.

MIDDLE THIRD FRACTURES

Fractures of the scaphoid occur most commonly through the middle third or waist of the bone (70%), followed by the proximal third (20%), and least commonly in the distal third (10%). Russe classified the fractures into three groups, depending on the relationship of the fracture line to the longitudinal axis of the scaphoid.[37] The horizontal oblique (35%) and the transverse (60%) fractures were reasonably stable and tended to heal with less than 3 months of immobilization. The less common vertical oblique fracture (5%) was inherently unstable and required a longer period of cast immobilization. If diagnosed within a few days from injury and properly immobilized, 95 percent of undisplaced or minimally displaced fractures of the scaphoid will unite within 3 months.[10, 37, 41, 45] Our preference is to immobilize the hand and wrist in a well-molded, below-elbow cast with the wrist in slight radial deviation and in neutral position with regard to flexion. The thumb should be included in the cast. The cast is changed every 3 to 4 weeks to insure effective immobilization of the wrist. Others have advocated an above-elbow cast to prevent forearm rotation and eliminate pull of the volar radioscaphoid ligament on the fractured scaphoid.[44]

The displaced or unstable scaphoid fracture cannot be treated by cast immobilization alone, as the union rate is significantly lower than that for undisplaced fractures.[10, 45] Cooney and associates hold that there is a displaced unstable fracture of the scaphoid when there is greater than 1 mm of offset on the anteroposterior or oblique roentgenographic views (Fig. 8–2).[10] Other criteria used were a lunocapitate angle of greater than 15° or a scapholunate angle of greater than 45° on the lateral roentgenogram. The authors stressed the position of the lunate as an indication of carpal instability secondary to the fracture of the scaphoid. Dorsal angulation at the fracture site of the scaphoid causes the lunate to rotate dorsally and produce a dorsal intercalated segment instability (DISI collapse deformity). The displaced or unstable scaphoid fracture must be treated by open reduction and internal fixation in order to realign the articular surfaces of the bone, prevent malunion of the scaphoid, place the lunate in proper alignment, and prevent future arthrosis of the wrist.

An open reduction of the scaphoid is best done through a volar-radial approach as advocated by Russe.[37] The volar capsule of the radiocarpal joint is incised and the fracture site identified. By gently manipulating the bone fragments, the fracture is reduced and immobilized with two fine Kirschner wires (Fig. 8–3). These wires are cut off beneath the skin and removed later under general anesthesia when the fracture has united. Unless there is comminution at the fracture site, a bone graft is not necessary. When the scaphoid fracture is reduced and stabilized, the malalignment of the lunate is also corrected. A posteroanterior and lateral roentgenogram in the operating room is useful to determine if a proper reduction of the bones has been obtained.

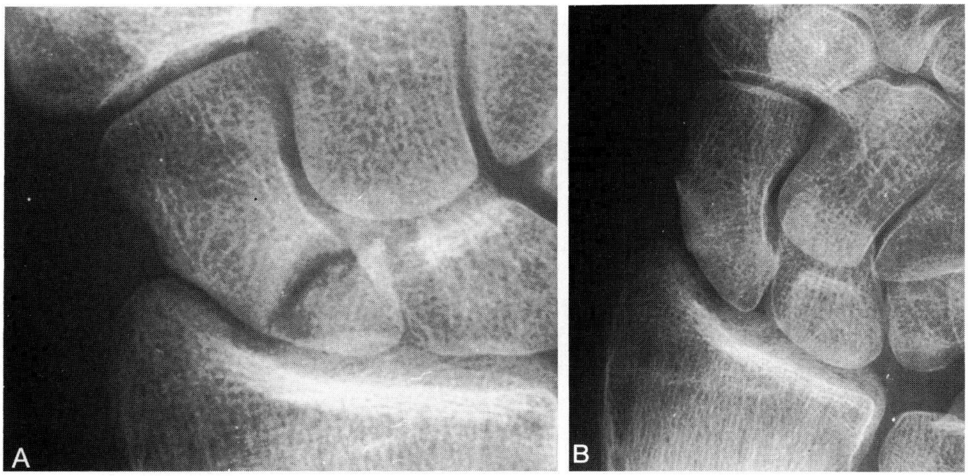

Figure 8–2 *A*, An acute fracture of the scaphoid with a 3-mm offset of the articular surface. *B*, Four months after operation the fracture is healed.

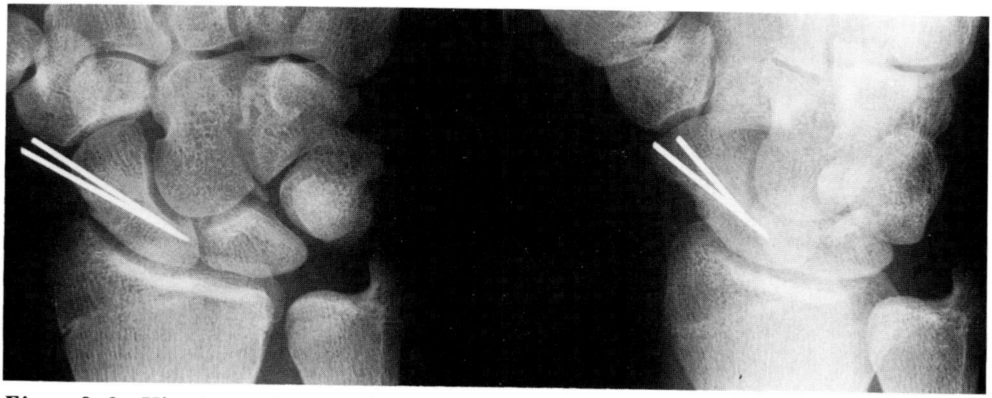

Figure 8–3 Kirschner wires provide excellent fixation of an acute fracture of the scaphoid.

The hand and wrist are immobilized in an above-elbow thumb spica cast for 8 weeks followed by a below-elbow thumb spica cast until the fracture has united. Avascular necrosis, which sometimes occurs in the proximal pole, does not affect the rate of fracture healing. However, healing can be prolonged. Herbert advocates the use of a threaded bone screw to provide rigid internal fixation of a scaphoid fracture.[23] He discontinues plaster immobilization after 6 weeks in order to begin active wrist motion. If the fracture is not united in an additional 2 to 3 weeks, he recommends an additional operation. This is an exceedingly aggressive approach. There has been no increase in morbidity in those patients treated with Kirschner wire fixation and a longer period of plaster immobilization. In our view it is better to continue plaster immobilization for an additional 1 to 3 months than to proceed with a second operation 8 to 10 weeks after the initial procedure.

If there is a persistent radiolucent line at the fracture site after adequate cast immobilization alone or open reduction, internal fixation, and cast immobilization, then a delay in bony union (3 to 4 months) or a nonunion (6 months) of the fracture must be considered. Additional roentgenographic studies are imperative to evaluate the status of fracture healing. Planar or trispiral tomography is useful in evaluating bony union (Fig. 8–4),[10] and computed tomography (CT) even more reliably shows the presence or absence of bone across the fracture site. Even with a cast, multiplanar cuts of the fracture site can be obtained with the CT scan, and one can accurately determine whether the fracture is healed, partially healed, or ununited (Fig. 8–5). If a delayed union is present (i.e., there is partial bone healing), then additional cast immobilization is indicated. Electrical stimulation in a delayed union of the scaphoid is probably not indicated. If after 6 months of continuous immobilization, the scaphoid fails to heal, it is best to do a bone grafting procedure. Some have recommended continued cast immobilization in conjunction with electrical stimulation of the bone.[4, 18, 33]

Nonunion of the scaphoid has been attributed to inadequate immobilization, fracture displacement, instability of the fracture fragments, carpal instability, and inadequate blood supply to the proximal fragment. Bone

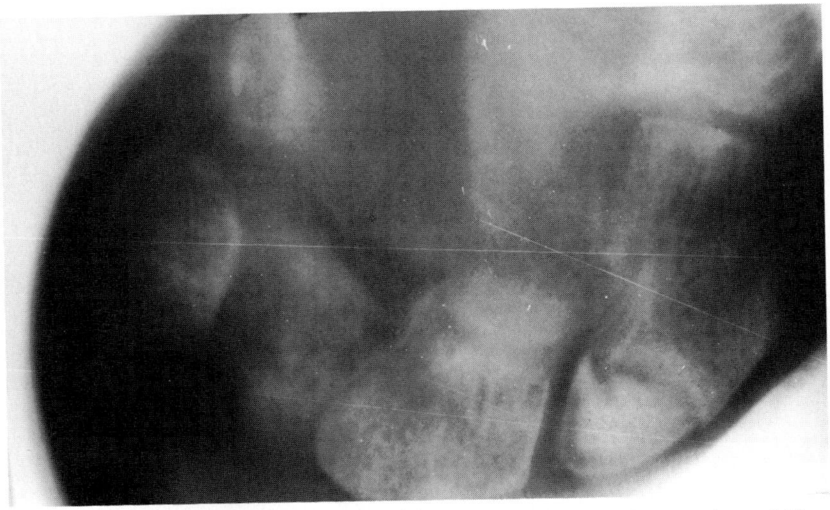

Figure 8–4 Three months after an acute fracture treated by cast immobilization, a tomogram shows delayed union of the scaphoid.

grafting in conjunction with internal fixation has proven to be an excellent method of obtaining union of the scaphoid. Between 86 and 97 percent of ununited scaphoid fractures have healed with bone grafting procedures.[11, 37, 38, 47]

Our preference is the volar radial approach as described by Russe.[37] Once the nonunion site is identified, a cavity is made on the volar aspect of both fragments and the dead bone is removed. The humpback deformity of the bone is corrected by realigning the dorsal and lateral cortices of both fragments and immobilizing them with two small Kirschner wires. The wires can be inserted into the bone under direct vision prior to inserting the bone graft. The DISI collapse deformity can often be corrected by realigning and internally fixing the scaphoid. Cortical cancellous bone taken from the iliac crest is then inserted into the cavities, the joint capsule is repaired, and the hand and wrist are immobilized in an above-elbow thumb spica cast for 2 months and then a below-elbow thumb spica cast until the nonunion has healed (Fig. 8–6), usually within 3 to 4 months. Slight radiocarpal arthritis as noted on roentgenograms, cystic changes in the bone, and avascular necrosis of the proximal segment of the bone are not considered contraindications to bone grafting a nonunited scaphoid. Athletes can return to competitive sports after the bone has united.

PROXIMAL THIRD FRACTURES

Twenty percent of scaphoid fractures occur through the proximal third of the bone. The studies of the vascular supply of the bone by Gelberman and Menon[19] and Taleisnik and Kelly[42] show that this end of the bone is particularly at risk for avascular necrosis and that healing takes longer than for middle third fractures. This has been corroborated by clinical studies.[11, 37] An acute, undisplaced fracture of the proximal third of

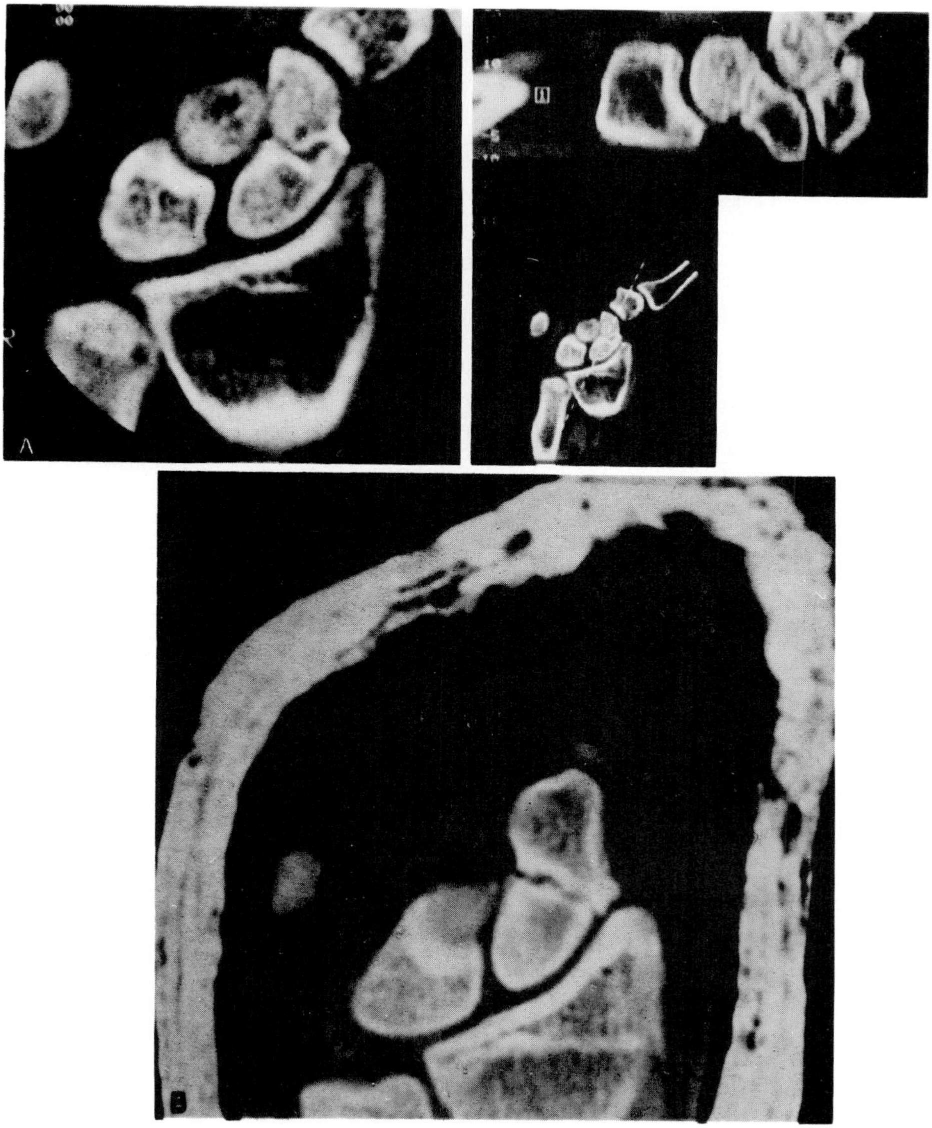

Figure 8–5 *A*, Multiplanar CT views of an ununited scaphoid. *B*, A nonunion of the scaphoid is identified even though the wrist is immobilized in plaster.

Illustration continued on following page

the scaphoid should be treated by cast immobilization. If the fracture is displaced, it should be treated by open reduction and internal fixation. The bone will probably unite in 3 to 4 months. If a nonunion develops, then the treatment depends in part upon the size of the proximal fragment. If the proximal fragment is large enough and has sufficient bone (i.e., it is not a cartilage shell), then a bone grafting procedure in conjunction with internal fixation should be done. When the proximal fragment is very small, sclerotic, deformed, or fragmented, it can be excised and a carved Silastic spacer inserted (Fig. 8–7).[25] Although these wrists will have some loss of motion and some weakness of grip, patients can return to recreational

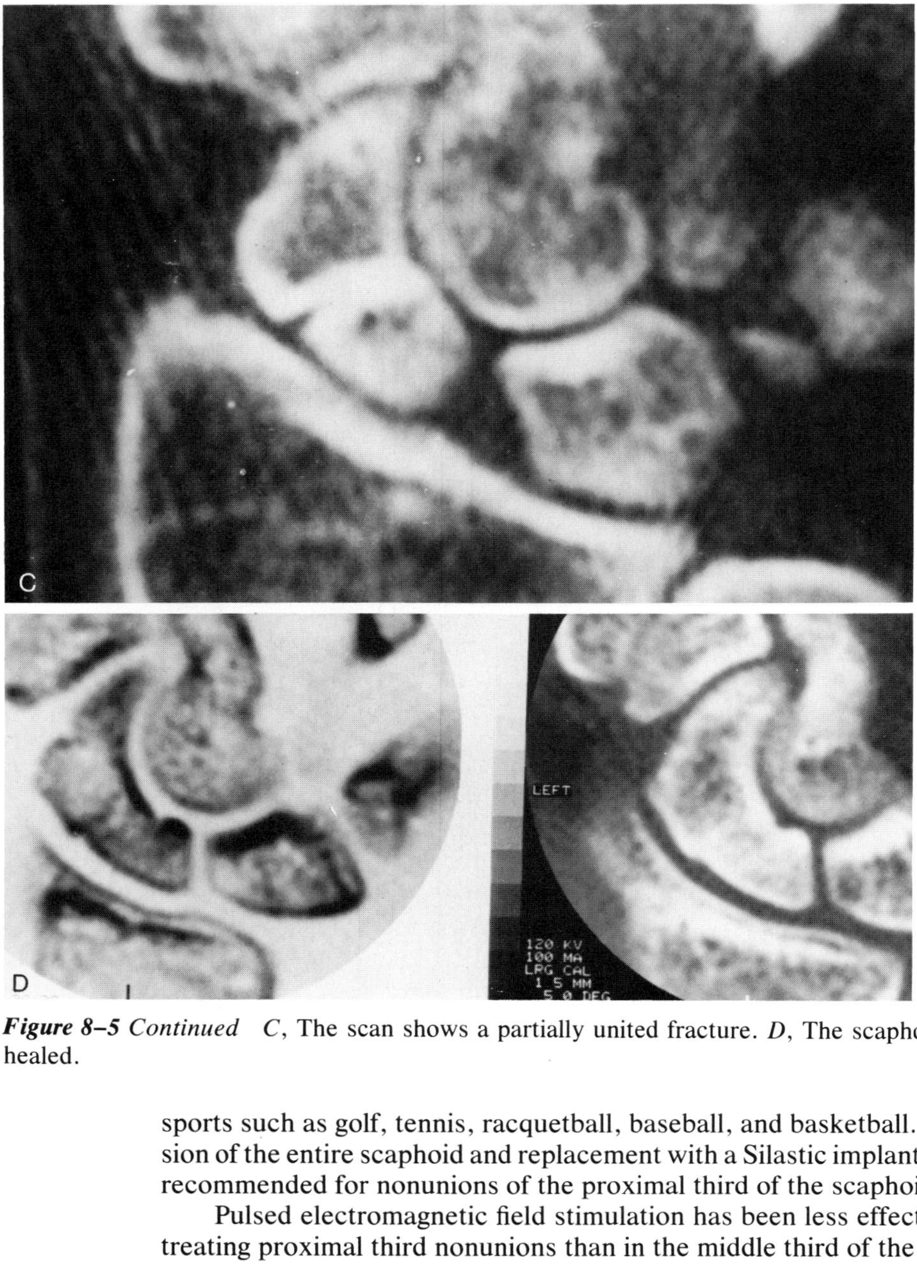

Figure 8–5 *Continued* C, The scan shows a partially united fracture. *D*, The scaphoid has healed.

sports such as golf, tennis, racquetball, baseball, and basketball. Excision of the entire scaphoid and replacement with a Silastic implant is not recommended for nonunions of the proximal third of the scaphoid.

Pulsed electromagnetic field stimulation has been less effective in treating proximal third nonunions than in the middle third of the bone. Frykman and associates found that 62.5 percent of proximal third nonunions healed compared with 83 percent in the middle and distal thirds.[18]

DISTAL THIRD FRACTURES

Fewer than 10 percent of all scaphoid fractures occur in the distal third. These readily heal in 6 to 8 weeks with plaster immobilization. When the rare nonunion occurs, it should be treated by bone grafting and internal fixation (Fig. 8–8).

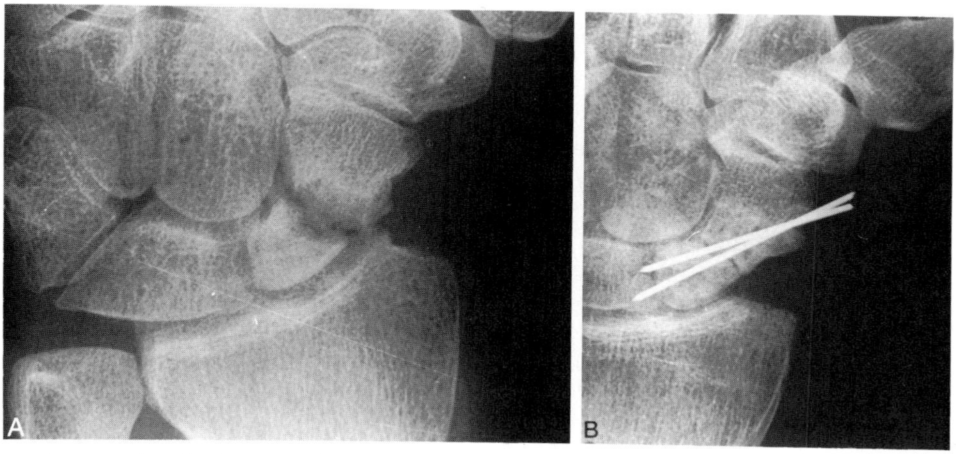

Figure 8–6 *A*, A failed bone graft to the scaphoid using the radial styloid as the graft donor site. *B*, Three months after an open reduction with bone grafting using the iliac crest and internal fixation with Kirschner wires.

NONUNIONS

Scaphoid nonunion can occur in both treated and untreated individuals. If the nonunion is left untreated, for whatever reason, the end result seems to be degenerative arthritis of the wrist. Mack and colleagues[26] and Ruby and co-workers[36] described the natural history of scaphoid nonunion

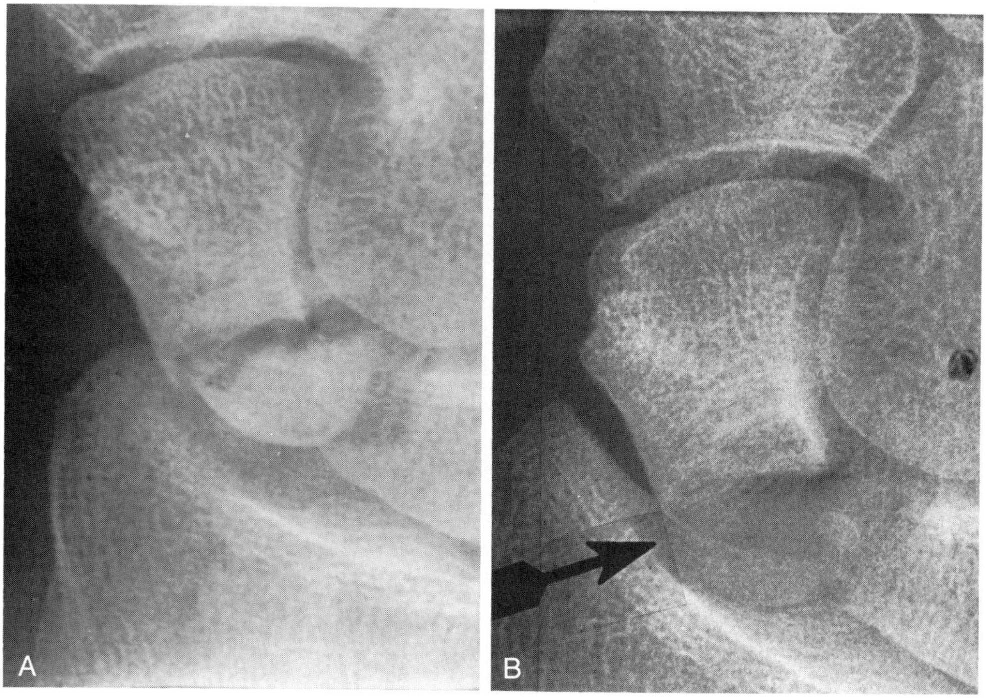

Figure 8–7 *A*, At operation, the proximal fragment of the scaphoid was small and comminuted. *B*, A hand-carved Silastic spacer (*arrow*) was used to replace the proximal pole of the scaphoid. This individual was able to resume playing golf.

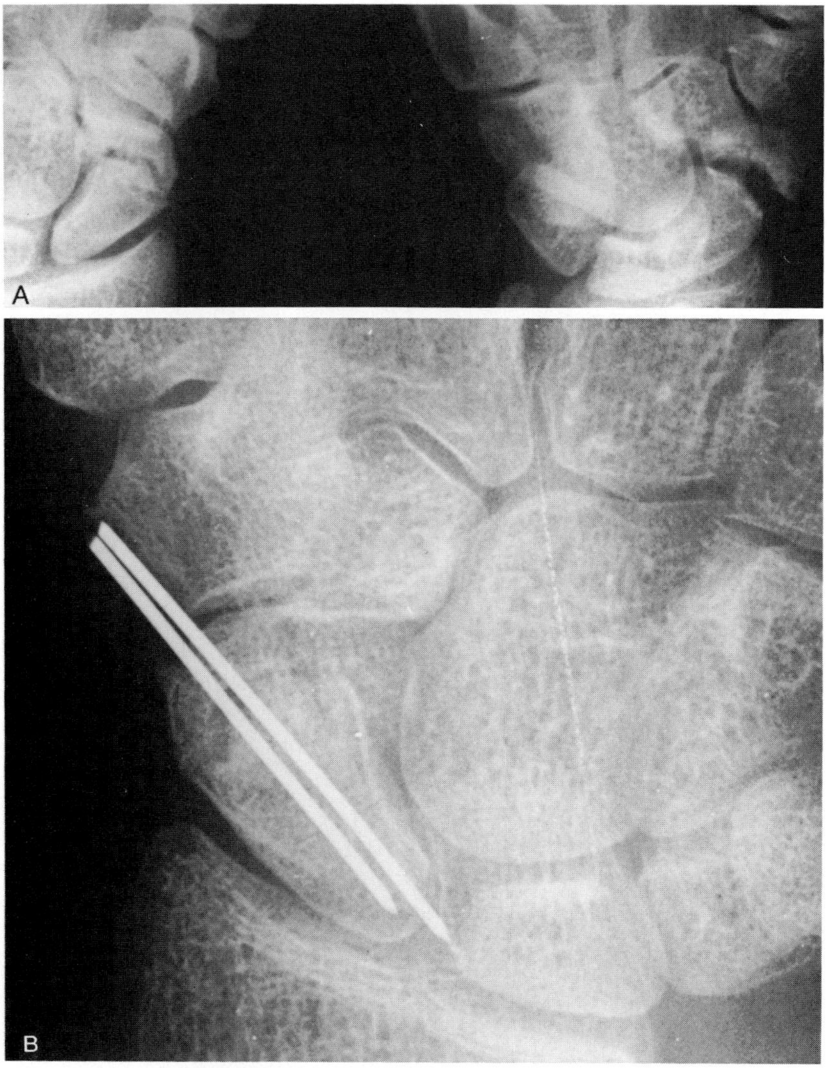

Figure 8–8 *A*, A nonunited distal third fracture of the scaphoid in a 17-year-old football player. *B*, Two months after operation.

and concluded that a significant percent of patients with untreated scaphoid nonunions will develop varying degrees of degenerative arthritis of the wrist within 5 to 10 years. The severity of the arthritis in the wrist increases with time.

Fracture of the Hamate

A fracture of the hook of the hamate frequently occurs during athletic competition, especially in golf, tennis, baseball, squash, and racquetball. Located in the proximal row, the body of the hamate is on the dorsal ulnar aspect of the wrist. The hook extends into the base of the hypothenar eminence and can be easily palpated in the palm. Attached to this bony process are the pisohamate ligaments, the short flexor and opponens muscles of the little finger, and the transverse carpal ligament. When the hook is fractured, usually at its base where it joins the body of the bone, these structures exert intermittent tension on the broken bone and prevent it from healing. The motor branch of the ulnar nerve lies ulnar to the hook and adjacent to its base. The sensory branch of the nerve is near the apex of the hook. The flexor tendons to the ring and little fingers are adjacent to the radial side of the hook in the carpal tunnel.

In a sports-related injury, the hook of the hamate most probably fractures as a result of direct trauma. The bone is usually broken when an individual is playing a racquet-type sport, golf, or baseball.[9, 30, 39] The racquet, golf club, or baseball bat rests against the distal end of the hook in the hypothenar eminence (Fig. 8–9), and the fracture is thought to occur during a swing when the end of the racquet, club, or bat strikes the hook. In baseball the fracture occurs during a forceful or checked swing. A fracture of the hook of the hamate can also occur when a tennis player loses control of the racquet or from a routine swing or a ''dubbed'' shot in golf.[39]

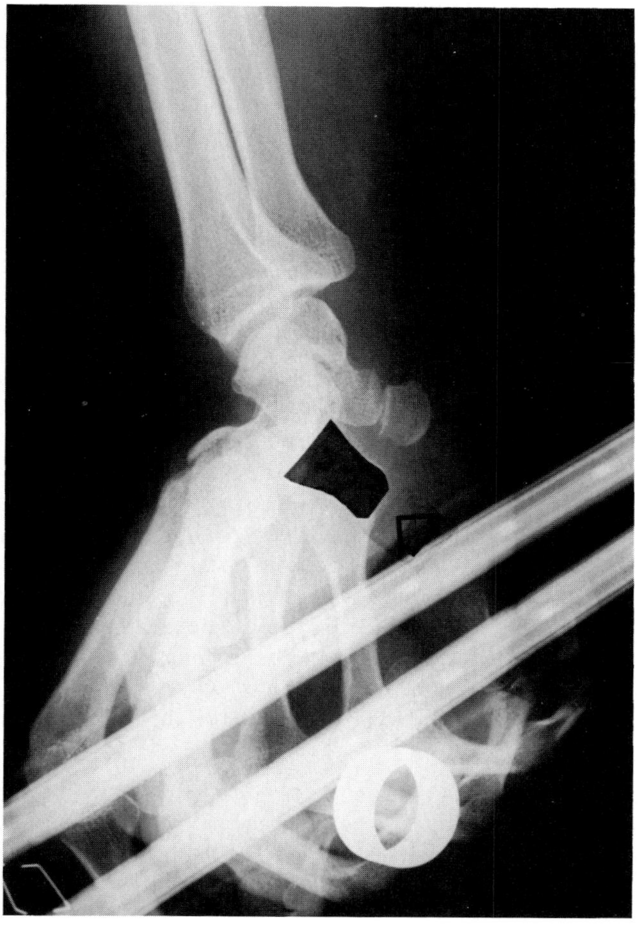

Figure 8–9 The impact from the handle of a tennis racquet in the hypothenar eminence can fracture the tip of the hook of the hamate.

This diagnosis must be strongly considered in athletes participating in racquet sports, golf, or baseball who complain of persistent pain on the ulnar side of the wrist and proximal palm. This is especially true if their complaints are unrelieved by conservative treatment. This fracture is frequently misdiagnosed as a wrist sprain or tendinitis. While activities of daily living will produce few complaints, attempts to play a sport that requires forceful grip of a club, bat, or racquet will produce significant pain and cause the individual to play poorly or cease playing altogether. Occasionally there will be irritability of the ulnar nerve. There is often tenderness with direct pressure over the end of the hook in the hypothenar eminence; occasionally, it is restricted to the dorsal ulnar aspect of the wrist. Ruptured flexor tendons have been reported in patients with undiagnosed fractures of the hook of the hamate.[13, 39]

Roentgenographic examination must be used to prove the diagnosis. Although several roentgenographic signs have been described,[31] it is extremely difficult to identify a broken hook of the hamate on routine roentgenographic views. A carpal tunnel view as described by Hart and Gaynor[22] frequently shows the fracture line (Fig. 8–10). The lateral profile of the hook can be shown by an oblique roentgenogram of the wrist with the forearm supinated and the wrist dorsiflexed (Fig. 8–11). If these special views do not show the fracture, then tomograms or preferably a CT scan should be done. The CT scan is particularly useful when the diagnosis is suggested but not clearly demonstrated by the other roentgenographic techniques (Fig. 8–12).[14, 47]

The best treatment for a fracture of the hook of the hamate is to excise the bony process.[39] The hook is exposed through a curved incision in the hypothenar eminence. The ulnar nerve, ulnar artery, and their branches are identified and protected. After incising the periosteum over the tip, the hook of the hamate is exposed by subperiosteal dissection. The loose bone fragment (hook) is removed and the base of the bone smoothed with a rongeur. The periosteum and adjacent fascial structures are repaired, and the hand and wrist are immobilized in a plaster splint for 3 weeks. Athletic activity can usually be resumed in 4 to 6 weeks.

Fractures of the body of the hamate are much less common in athletic activities, and frequently occur in conjunction with dislocations and fractures of the bases of the fourth and fifth metacarpals (Fig. 8–13). An intra-articular fracture of the hamate at the carpometacarpal joint usually displaces proximally and dorsally. This injury frequently follows a direct blow on the hand such as when striking a football helmet.

The fracture is best seen on an oblique view of the hand and wrist. If displaced, it should be treated by open reduction and internal fixation, and the associated dislocations of the metacarpals reduced. After operation, the hand and wrist are immobilized for 4 to 6 weeks in plaster followed by an appropriate therapy program.

Fractures of the Other Carpal Bones

Fractures of the other six carpal bones occur less frequently as a result of athletic injuries than those of the scaphoid or hook of the hamate. Nevertheless, they must be considered when examining a painful wrist following a sports injury.

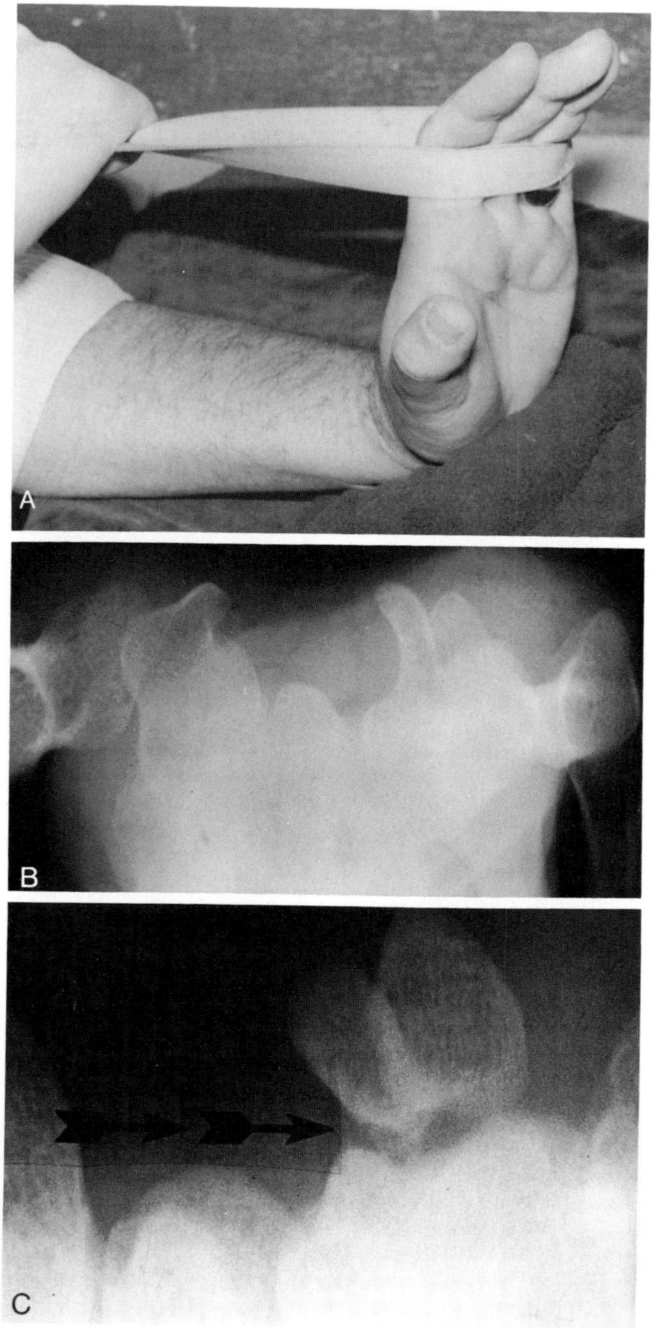

Figure 8–10 *A*, Wrist position for a carpal tunnel view. The tube is angled 20 to 25° and the beam is directed toward the base of the hypothenar eminence. *B*, A normal hook of the hamate is seen on the ulnar side, and the trapezial ridge is on the radial side. *C*, An ununited fracture of the hook of the hamate in a baseball player.

FRACTURES OF THE CAPITATE

In a review of fractures of the capitate, Adler and Shaftan[1] found the injuries to be of three types: isolated fractures of the capitate, navicular-capitate syndrome, and capitate fractures in combination with a variety of other carpal injuries. Although a direct blow to the

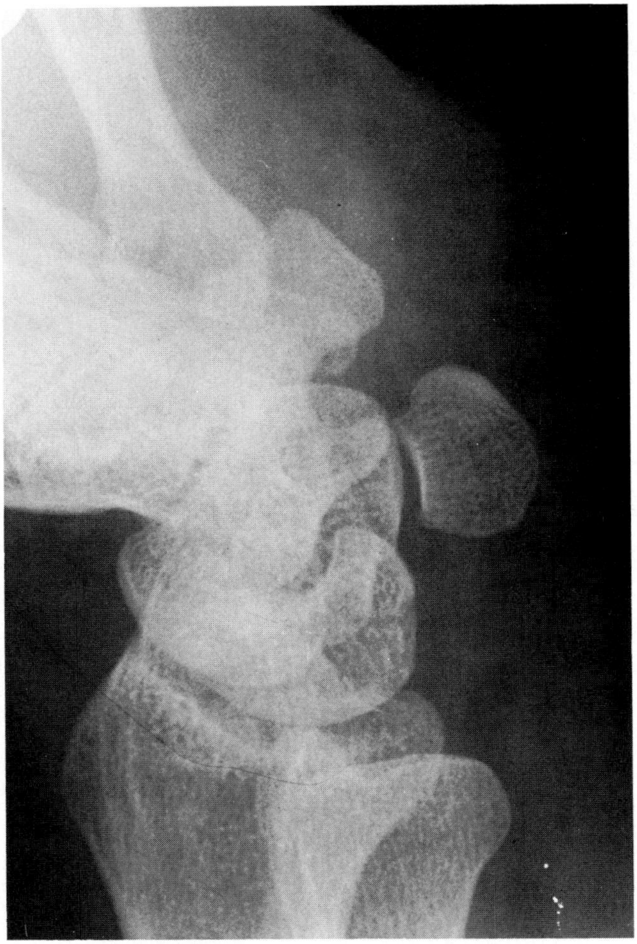

Figure 8–11 A supinated oblique view of the wrist shows the hook of the hamate in lateral profile.

wrist can cause a fracture of the capitate, the more common mechanism of injury is a fall on the dorsiflexed wrist. During a fall, with the wrist in dorsiflexion and radial deviation, the radial styloid can impinge on the scaphoid and fracture it. If the force is sufficiently strong, the capitate will also fracture, and the fracture will be in line with that of the scaphoid. The fractured head of the capitate can rotate 180°. Fenton described this condition as the naviculocapitate syndrome.[15] Using cadavers, Stein and Siegel[40] noted that the scaphoid fractures under tension when the wrist is dorsiflexed. Increased extension of the wrist forces the capitate under the lip of the radius, causing the capitate to fracture. The head of the capitate rotates as the wrist returns to a neutral position.

An acute fracture, in which the head of the capitate is rotated 90° or 180°, usually cannot be reduced by closed manipulation. Open reduction and internal fixation are needed to reduce the fracture of both the capitate and the scaphoid. The scaphoid is exposed through a volar incision and the capitate through a dorsal incision. The displaced frac-

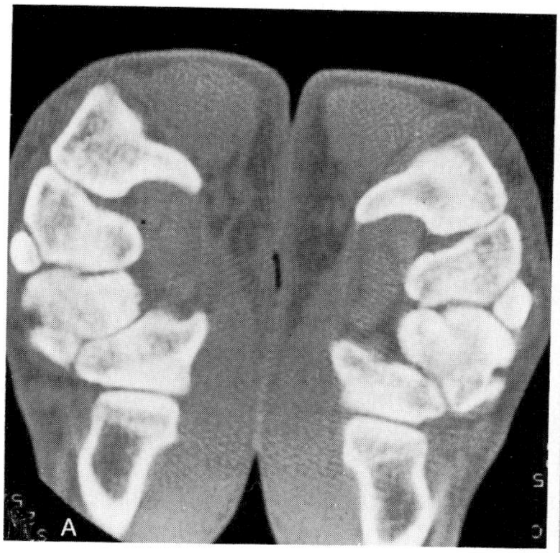

Figure 8–12 *A*, A normal hook of the hamate as shown on the CT scan. *B*, A fracture of the hook of the hamate was found in a golfer with a 6-month history of pain in the wrist.

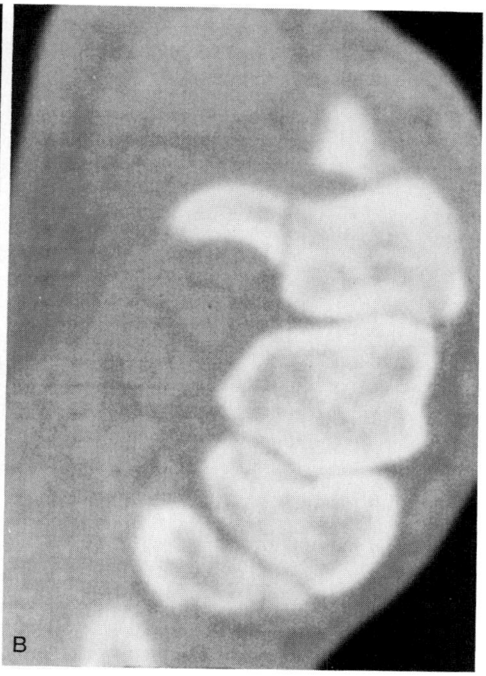

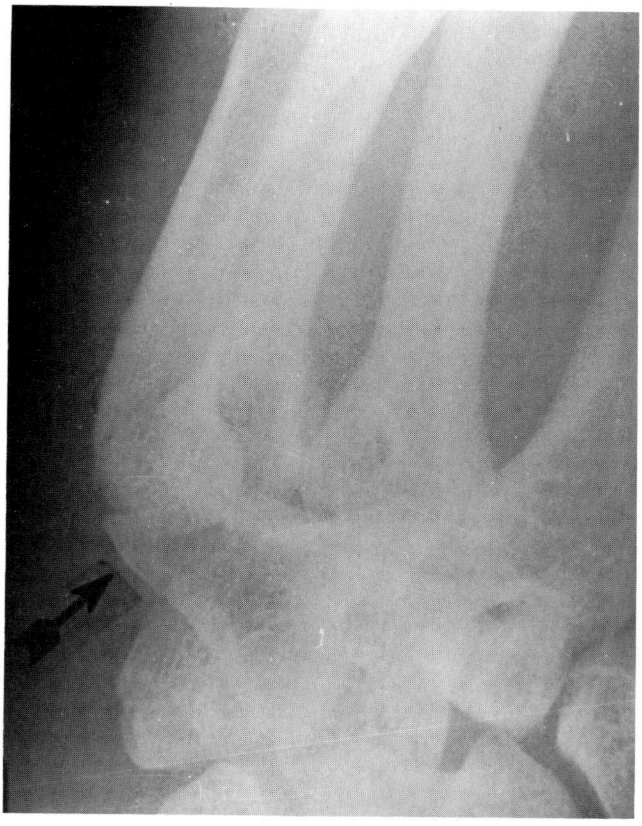

Figure 8–13 A 17-year-old linebacker sustained this fracture of the hamate in conjunction with a dislocation of the fourth and fifth metacarpals.

tures are reduced and immobilized with Kirschner wires. The hand and wrist are immobilized in plaster until the fractures have united. Following a fracture, the head of the capitate is prone to develop avascular necrosis because the proximal segment is supplied by a single intraosseous vessel.[21] Injuries that are neglected may develop painful midcarpal arthritis. This is best treated by a midcarpal fusion.

FRACTURES OF THE LUNATE

Although there is still significant controversy as to the cause of Kienböck's disease, recent reports implicate a stress or compression fracture of the lunate.[2, 5, 20] The avascular process is secondary to the loss of blood supply to the fractured segments. Repetitive minor injuries probably account for a significant number of cases of Kienböck's disease. Athletes are often seen with stiff, painful wrists but without a history of significant injury.

Trispiral tomography,[5] computerized tomography, and magnetic resonance imaging are newer techniques currently used to detect fractures of the lunate, which are difficult to identify on plain roentgenograms. If an acute fracture of the lunate is diagnosed, the wrist should be immobilized in plaster for about 8 weeks. If avascular necrosis of the lunate develops there are two basic principles of treatment. Prior to collapse of the bone, a procedure should be done to decrease the compressive forces on the lunate and allow it to revascularize or to somehow augment the blood supply to the lunate. After the bone has collapsed and/or fragmented, either the lunate should be replaced with a prosthesis or autogenous material or an intercarpal fusion should be done.

FRACTURES OF THE PISIFORM

The pisiform is a sesamoid bone in the flexor carpi ulnaris tendon that articulates with the triquetrum to form the pisotriquetral joint. The pisiform is attached to the fifth metacarpal, triquetrum, and hamate by ligaments. Fractures are usually the result of direct trauma on the hypothenar eminence. Fractures of the pisiform may be linear, comminuted, or of the avulsion type.[43] These fractures are best seen on a supinated oblique or carpal tunnel view of the wrist. Acute isolated fractures of the pisiform can be treated by 4 to 6 weeks of plaster immobilization. Arthritis at the pisotriquetral joint, whether from a fracture or previous repetitive injury, is best treated by excision of the pisiform. Athletes can resume competitive activities, including racquet sports, 8 weeks after operation.

FRACTURES OF THE TRAPEZIUM

Fractures of the trapezium account for fewer than 5 percent of all carpal fractures. They are either vertical fractures,[12] often associated with dislocation of the base of the thumb metacarpal, or avulsion fractures of the trapezial ridge.[29, 34] The trapezial ridge fractures are best seen on a carpal tunnel view (Fig. 8–10*B*).

Undisplaced vertical fractures of the trapezium or avulsion fractures of the trapezial ridge are treated by plaster immobilization of the wrist. Small, widely displaced bony fragments should be excised, while larger fragments should be reduced and stabilized with Kirschner wires.

FRACTURES OF THE TRIQUETRUM

Fractures of the triquetrum are seldom a significant problem to athletes, even though they are the second[3] or third[8] most common carpal fracture.

DISLOCATIONS OR FRACTURE-DISLOCATIONS OF THE CARPUS

A wide variety of fractures and ligament disruptions can occur in the wrist. Although these injuries are described by their initial roentgenographic appearance (e.g., perilunate dislocation), every wrist injury is a specific stage of a progressive disorder. The particular stage in a specific patient is determined by (1) the degree of force loading; (2) the duration and magnitude of the force; (3) the position of the hand at the time of impact; and (4) the biomechanical properties of the bones and ligaments of the individual.

The mechanism of carpal dislocation is ulnar deviation and supination of the wrist.[27] Fracture of the carpal bones about the lunate in conjunction with a dislocation is called a greater arc injury; dislocation of the perilunar carpal bones without fracture is known as a lesser arc injury.[24] Dorsal trans-scaphoid perilunate dislocations, dorsal perilunate dislocations, and volar lunate dislocations are sometimes seen following athletic injuries.

REFERENCES

1. Adler, J.B., and Shaftan, G.: Fractures of the capitate. J. Bone Joint Surg. 44A:1537, 1962.
2. Almquist, E.A.: Kienbock's disease. Clin. Orthop. 202:68, 1986.
3. Bartone, N.F., Grieco, R.V.: Fractures of the triquetrum. J. Bone Joint Surg. 38A:353, 1956.
4. Beckenbaugh, R.D.: Noninvasive pulsed electromagnetic stimulation in the treatment of scaphoid nonunion. Orthop. Trans. 9:444, 1985.
5. Beckenbaugh, R.D., Shives, T.C., Dobyns, J.H., et al.: Kienbock's disease: the natural history of Kienbock's disease and consideration of lunate fractures. Clin. Orthop. 149:98, 1980.
6. Borgeskov, S., Christiansen, B., Kjaer, A., et al.: Fracture of the carpal bones. Acta Orthop. Scand. 37:276, 1986.
7. Boyes, J.H.: Bunnell's Surgery of the Hand, 5th ed. Philadelphia, J.B. Lippincott, 1970.
8. Bryan, R.S., Dobyns, J.H.: Fractures of the carpal bones other than lunate or navicular. Clin. Orthop. 149:107, 1980.
9. Carter, P.R., Eaton, R.G., Littler, J.W.: Ununited fracture of the hook of the hamate. J. Bone Joint Surg. 59A:583, 1977.

10. Cooney, W.P., Dobyns, J.H., Linscheid, R.L.: Fractures of the scaphoid: a rational approach to management. Clin. Orthop. 149:90, 1980.
11. Cooney, W.P., Dobyns, J.H., Linscheid, R.L.: Nonunion of the scaphoid: analysis of the results from bone grafting. J. Hand Surg. 5:343, 1980.
12. Cordrey, L.J., Ferrer-Torells, M.: Management of fractures of the greater multangular. J. Bone Joint Surg. 42A:1111, 1960.
13. Crosby, E.B., Linscheid, R.L.: Rupture of the flexor profundus tendon of the ring finger secondary to ancient fracture of the hook of the hamate. Review of the literature and report of 2 cases. J. Bone Joint Surg. 56A:1076, 1974.
14. Egawa, M., Asai, T.: Fracture of the hook of the hamate: report of six cases and the suitability of computerized tomography. J. Hand Surg. 8:393, 1983.
15. Fenton, R.L.: The naviculo-capitate syndrome. J. Bone Joint Surg. 38A:681, 1956.
16. Fisk, G.R.: Carpal instability and the fractured scaphoid (Hunterian Lecture, 1968). Ann. R. Coll. Surg. Engl. 46:63, 1970.
17. Frykman, G.: Fractures of the distal radius including sequelae—shoulder hand-finger syndrome, disturbance in the distal radio-ulnar joint, and impairment of nerve function: a clinical and experimental study. Acta Orthop. Scand. (Suppl.) 108:1, 1967.
18. Frykman, G.K., Taleisnik, J., Peters, G., et al.: Treatment of nonunited scaphoid fractures by pulsed electro-magnetic field and cast. J. Hand Surg. 11A:344, 1986.
19. Gelberman, R.H., Menon, J.: The vascularity of the scaphoid bone. J. Hand Surg. 5:508, 1980.
20. Gelberman, R.H., Bauman, T.D., Menon, J., et al.: The vascularity of the lunate bone and Kienböck's disease. J. Hand Surg. 5:272, 1980.
21. Gelberman, R.H., Panagis, J.S., Taleisnik, J., et al.: The arterial anatomy of the human carpus. I. The extraosseous vascularity. J. Hand Surg. 8:367, 1983.
22. Hart, V.L., Gaynor, V.: Roentgenographic study of the carpal canal. J. Bone Joint Surg. 23:382, 1941.
23. Herbert, T.J.: Use of the Herbert bone screw in surgery of the wrist. Clin. Orthop. 202:79, 1986.
24. Johnson, R.P.: The acutely injured wrist and its residuals. Clin. Orthop. 149:33, 1980.
25. Linscheid, R.L., Dobyns, J.H., Beabout, J.W., et al.: Traumatic instability of the wrist: diagnosis, classification and pathomechanics. J. Bone Joint Surg. 54A:1612, 1972.
26. Mack, G.R., Bosse, M.J., Gelberman, R.H., et al.: The natural history of scaphoid non-union. J. Bone Joint Surg. 66A:504, 1984.
27. Mayfield, J.K.: Mechanism of carpal injuries. Clin. Orthop. 149:45, 1980.
28. Mayfield, J.K., Johnson, R.P., Kilcoyne, R.K.: Carpal dislocations: pathomechanics and progressive perilunar instability. J. Hand Surg. 5:226, 1980.
29. McClain, E.J., Boyes, J.H.: Missed fractures of the greater multangular. J. Bone Joint Surg. 48A:1525, 1966.
30. Nisenfield, F.G., Neviaser, R.J.: Fracture of the hook of the hamate: a diagnosis easily missed. J. Trauma 14:612, 1974.
31. Norman, A., Nelson, J.R., Green, S.: Fractures of the hook of the hamate: radiographic signs. Radiology 154:49, 1985.
32. Obletz, B.E., Halberstein, B.M.: Nonunions of fractures of the carpal navicular. J. Bone Joint Surg. 20:424, 1938.
33. Osterman, A.L., Bora, F.W.: Electrical stimulation applied to bone and nerve injuries in the upper extremity. Orthop. Clin. North Am. 17:353, 1986.
34. Palmer, A.K.: Trapezial ridge fracture. J. Hand Surg. 6:561, 1981.
35. Panagis, J.S., Gelberman, R.H., Taleisnik, J., et al.: The arterial anatomy of the human carpus. II. The intraosseous vascularity. J. Hand Surg. 8:375, 1983.
36. Ruby, L.K., Stinson, J.R., Belsky, M.R.: The natural history of scaphoid non-union. J. Bone Joint Surg. 67A:428, 1985.
37. Russe, O.: Fracture of the carpal navicular: diagnosis, non-operative treatment and operative treatment. J. Bone Joint Surg. 42A:759, 1960.
38. Stark, H.H.: Unpublished data.
39. Stark, H.H., Jobe, F.W., Boyes, J.H., et al.: Fracture of the hook of the hamate in athletes. J. Bone Joint Surg. 59A:575, 1977.
40. Stein, F., Siegel, M.W.: Naviculo-capitate fracture syndrome. J. Bone Joint Surg. 51A:391, 1969.

41. Stewart, M.J.: Fractures of the carpal navicular (scaphoid). A report of 436 cases. J. Bone Joint Surg, 51A:391, 1969.
42. Taleisnik, J., Kelly, P.J.: Extraosseous and intraosseous blood supply of the scaphoid bone. J. Bone Joint Surg. 48A:1125, 1966.
43. Vasilas, A., Grieco, R.V., Bartone, N.F.: Roentgen aspects of injuries to the pisiform bone and pisotriquetral joint. J. Bone Joint Surg. 42A:1317, 1960.
44. Verdan, C., Narakas, A.: Fractures and pseudarthrosis of the scaphoid. Surg. Clin. North Am. 48:1083, 1968.
45. Weber, E.R.: Biomechanical implications of scaphoid waist fractures. Clin. Orthop. 149:83, 1980.
46. Weber, E.R., Chao, E.Y.: An experimental approach to the mechanism of scaphoid wrist fractures. J. Hand Surg. 3:142, 1978.
47. Zemel, N.P., Stark, H.H.: Fractures and dislocations of the carpal bones. Clin. Sports Med. 5:709, 1986.
48. Zemel, N.P., Stark, H.H., Ashworth, C.R., et al.: Treatment of selected patients with an ununited fracture of the proximal part of the scaphoid by excision of the fragment and insertion of a carved silicone-rubber spacer. J. Bone Joint Surg. 66A:510, 1984.

CHAPTER

9

Tendon Injuries

Joseph P. Leddy, M.D.
Thomas R. Dennis, M.D.

Hand and upper extremity injuries are common during sporting activities. Much attention has been paid to athletic injuries of the knee, ankle, and shoulder, but relatively little has been written about the athlete's hand. These injuries are common and when diagnosed early and treated properly, a successful result is often possible. Unfortunately, however, a serious injury is often misdiagnosed as a sprained or jammed finger and little or no treatment is given; a permanent disabling deformity may be the end result.[88] This chapter discusses closed tendon injuries to the athlete's hand including mallet finger deformity, boutonnière deformity, boxer's knuckle, dislocation of the extensor tendons at the metacarpophalangeal joint level, and avulsion of the flexor digitorum profundus tendon.

Anatomy

It is essential to have a basic understanding of the functional anatomy of the extensor and flexor mechanisms in the hand in order to properly diagnose and treat these injuries.[44] Extension of the finger is accomplished by action of the intrinsic and extrinsic musculotendinous units working in harmony with the digital flexor tendons.[35] Landsmere[49] has shown that any disruption along this pathway may affect another part of the mechanism, causing dysfunction or deformity at a different level. The extrinsic extensor system is innervated by the radial nerve, while the intrinsic system is innervated by the median and ulnar nerves.[18] The extensor indicis proprius, extensor digiti quinti proprius, extensor pollicis longus, and extensor pollicis brevis have a comparatively independent origin. In contrast, the extensor digitorum communis contains four distinct tendons that arise from a common muscle and have a limited ability to function independently.[44] Extensor tendons enter the hand through six fibro-osseous tunnels at the wrist level.[16] Proximal to the metacarpophalangeal (MCP) joint, the communis tendons are interconnected by the juncturae tendinum.[44, 107] At the MCP joint level, the extensor tendon is centrally located over the metacarpal head, held in place by the extensor hood mechanism.[44] The extensor indicis proprius and the extensor digiti quinti proprius are located on the ulnar side of their respective communis tendons.[16, 44, 107] The sagittal bands arise from the transverse metacarpal ligaments and terminate on the sides of the extensor tendon, forming the proximal portion of the extensor hood.[18, 44] The proximal margin of each sagittal band is free while the distal border is intimately associated with the dorsal hood fibers from the intrinsic tendons.[118] The principal function of the sagittal bands is to extend the proximal phalanx on the metacarpal head through the hood mechanism.[107] As the extensor tendon pulls proximally, the sagittal bands, through their attachment to the transverse metacarpal ligament and volar plate, lift the base of the proximal phalanx and extend the MCP joint. Some investigators have found a connection between the undersurface of the extensor tendon and the dorsal capsule of the MCP joint and have postulated that this also contributes to active extension at this joint.[44, 118] The sagittal bands also serve to stabilize the extensor communis tendon over the MCP joints, limit excursion of the extensor tendons, prevent dorsal bowstringing at this level, and provide a tunnel for the passage of the interosseous tendons (Fig. 9–1).[118, 127]

The main function of the extrinsic extensor tendons is to extend the MCP joint. The intrinsic system prevents hyperextension of this joint and thus allows the extrinsics to secondarily extend the PIP joint.[44] The central extensor tendon trifurcates over the proximal phalanx into one central and two lateral slips, which coalesce with the expansions from the intrinsic tendons.[35, 118] The central slip inserts into the base of the middle phalanx. The triangular ligament is located just distal to the insertion of the central slip and maintains the lateral bands dorsal to the axis of rotation at the PIP joint.[35, 119] Disruption of this mechanism at the PIP joint level may result in a boutonnière deformity.

The concept of differential loading of the lateral bands and central slip at the level of the PIP joint has been discussed by several authors.[49, 77, 101] Studies have shown that the extensor mechanism at the trifurcation level is composed of a layered, criss-cross fiber pattern that alters its geometric arrangement during flexion and extension of the PIP joint.[103] The most central fibers are tensed in flexion and the lateral fibers are tighter in extension.[77]

The lateral bands are formed by a combination of fibers from the lateral portion of the central slip and the intrinsic tendons that coalesce over the dorsum of the middle phalanx to form the terminal extensor tendon. This tendon is responsible for DIP joint extension.[111] The central slip and the terminal extensor tendon are adherent to the joint capsules of the PIP and DIP joints, respectively.[69]

The intrinsic system in the hand is composed of the lumbricals and the dorsal and volar interossei. The lumbricals originate in the palm on the

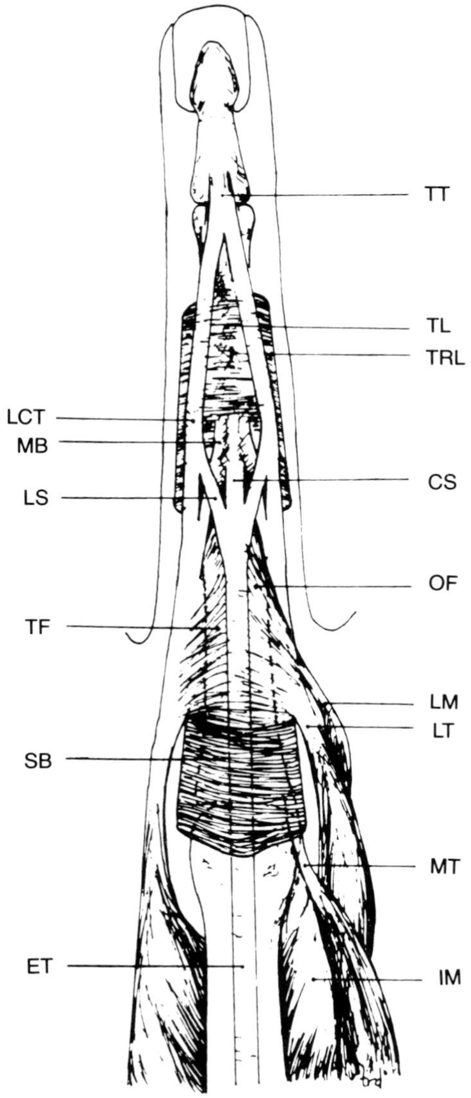

Figure 9–1 Extensor mechanism of the middle finger. ET, common extensor tendon; IM, interosseous muscle, deep head of the second dorsal; MT, medial tendon, superficial head of the second dorsal interosseous; SB, sagittal bands; LT, lateral tendon of the deep head of the second dorsal interosseous; LM, lumbrical muscle; TF, transverse fibers of the interossei; OF, oblique fibers of the interossei; LS, lateral slip of the common extensor; CS, central slip of the common extensor; MB, medial interosseous band; LCT, lateral conjoined tendon; TRL, transverse retinacular ligament; TL, triangular ligament; TT, terminal tendon.

flexor digitorum profundus tendon and travel palmar to the axis of the transverse metacarpal ligament. They form the radial border of the dorsal aponeurosis and terminate on the radial lateral bands of the extensor tendons.[22, 44, 107, 118, 119] This unique arrangement allows the lumbricals to act as extensors of the PIP and DIP joints during MCP joint flexion and extension.[22, 119] Contraction of the lumbricals facilitates DIP extension by advancing the flexor profundus tendon.[22, 56, 107, 111] Normally there are three volar interosseous muscles whose tendons insert into the dorsal aponeurosis. One inserts on the ulnar side of the index finger, the second into the radial side of the ring finger, and the third into the radial side of the little finger. The dorsal interossei have two separate components. There is a deeper portion that inserts primarily into bone at the base of the proximal phalanx and a more superficial portion that blends with the volar interossei to become the dorsal aponeurosis.[22, 107] The percentage that inserts into bone versus into the aponeurosis varies from one finger to another.[22]

The retinacular system has two parts. The transverse retinacular ligament encircles the finger at the PIP joint level.[49] It arises from the flexor sheath and envelops both lateral bands and the central slip. This ligament limits dorsal migration of the lateral bands during extension and assists lateral band descent during flexion.[107, 118, 119] The oblique retinacular ligament arises from the palmar aspect of the proximal phalanx and the flexor sheath, then passes dorsally and distally to join the lateral bands and terminal extensor tendon. It is palmar to the axis of PIP joint rotation and dorsal to the axis of DIP joint rotation.[107, 111, 118, 119] This retinacular or "link" ligament may contribute to synchronized flexion and extension at the PIP and DIP joints.[107, 111]

The flexor tendons enter the hand through the carpal canal. Distal to this, the lumbrical muscles originate on the flexor digitorum profundus tendons. The superficialis and profundus tendons then enter the synovial sheaths starting at the level of the distal palmar skin crease. The sheaths provide low friction gliding and supply the tendons with synovial fluid for nutritional purposes. The annular and cruciform pulleys are thickened areas within the sheath (Fig. 9–2). The very thick annular pulleys prevent

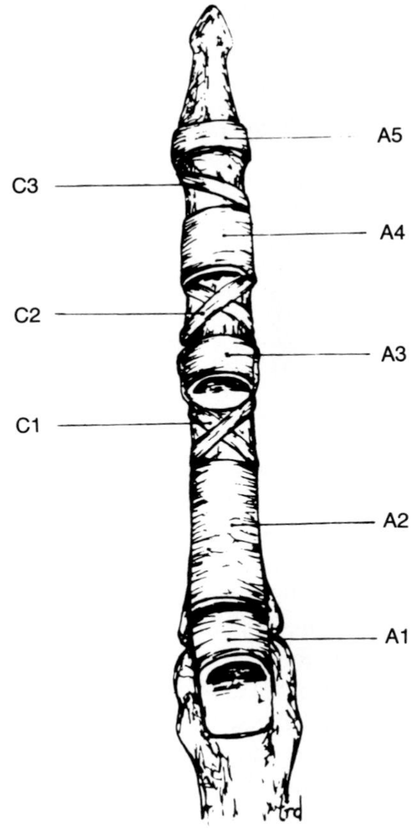

Figure 9–2 Pulley mechanism of flexor tendon. A, annular pulleys; C, cruciform pulleys.

tendon bowstringing during finger flexion, while the thinner cruciate pulleys give the sheath the ability to conform to the position of flexion by collapsing and allowing the annular pulleys to approximate each other.[52] The superficialis tendon inserts into the midportion of the middle phalanx. Distal to this level, the profundus lies in the sheath beneath the A4, C3, and A5 pulleys as it proceeds to its broad fan-shaped insertion into the distal phalanx.[52] In the thumb, there are three constant pulleys on the top of the sheath and closely applied to it. The A1 and oblique pulleys are the most important.[52] The flexor pollicis longus has a broad insertion into the base of the distal phalanx.

There has been some disagreement regarding nutrition of the flexor tendons. Leffert and associates[55] in 1974 and Ochiai and associates[82] in 1979 described in detail the vincular system of blood supply to the flexor tendons (Fig. 9–3). The distal portion of the profundus tendon in the finger receives its blood supply from the short vinculum. Proximal to this, the profundus tendon receives its blood supply from the long vinculum near the level of the PIP joint. Following avulsion of the tendon insertion, the damage to the vincular system may help determine the level to which the tendon retracts.[51, 52, 54] An intact long vinculum can prevent the avulsed tendon from retracting proximally into the palm. The flexor tendons within the digital sheath have a dual nutritional source: they receive vascular perfusion from the vincular system and also diffusion of nutrients from the synovial fluid. Manske[60, 61, 63–68] and others[58, 59, 86] have demonstrated the relative importance of diffusion from the synovial fluid to the flexor tendons. It is now believed that diffusion is more important than perfusion in the nutrition of the flexor tendons within the digital sheath.

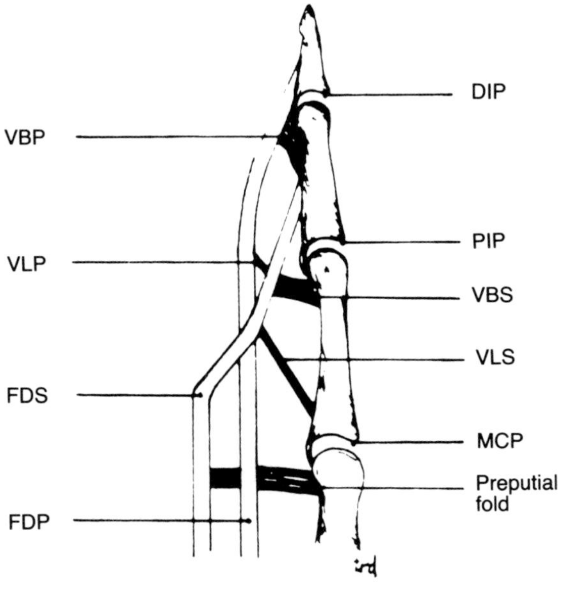

Figure 9–3 The vincular system. FDP, flexor digitorum profundus; FDS, flexor digitorum superficialis; VLP, vinculum longum profundus; VBP, vinculum breve profundus; MCP, metacarpal phalangeal joint; VLS, vinculum longum superficialis; VBS, vinculum breve superficialis; PIP, proximal interphalangeal joint; DIP, distal interphalangeal joint.

Mallet Finger

The terms "mallet finger," "drop finger," and "baseball finger" are used interchangeably.[1, 88] The injury results from a blow to the tip of the extended finger that forces the distal phalanx into flexion, disrupting the extensor mechanism over the dorsum of the DIP joint.[5, 69] The characteristic deformity results, with the DIP joint held in the flexed position (Fig. 9–4). If there is generalized joint laxity, there may be hyperextension at the PIP joint with an early swan neck deformity visible immediately following the injury.[16, 30, 98, 117] There is tenderness and swelling over the dorsum of the finger distally and inability to actively extend the DIP joint. If the disruption of the terminal extensor mechanism takes place entirely through the substance of the tendon, radiographs will be normal except for a flexion deformity at the DIP joint. Often, however, the terminal extensor tendon avulses a portion of bone from the base of the distal phalanx at the time of injury.[1, 33, 98, 113, 123] In this instance, three different clinical roentgenographic presentations may be seen (Fig. 9–5): (1) a small fleck of bone may be avulsed from the base of the distal phalanx; (2) a large portion of bone may be avulsed comprising up to a third or more of the articular surface; or (3) a large portion of bone may be avulsed with a palmar subluxation of the remaining portion of the distal phalanx.[123] It has been postulated that the degree of flexion present during disruption of the extensor tendon will determine whether or not there is an associated bony avulsion. In cadaver studies, Zancolli[127] has shown that bony avulsion occurs when the distal phalanx is forcibly flexed beyond 90° while the PIP joint remains extended. The mallet finger deformity has been reported to occur from trivial trauma.[1, 33, 69, 113] This happens more frequently in the older population with degenerative joint disease; in the younger athletic population significant force is often required. Obviously the injury can occur in any sport and is the most common closed tendon injury of the hand seen in the athletic population.[88] On rare occasions, these injuries may be compound and open into the DIP joint. In young children, there

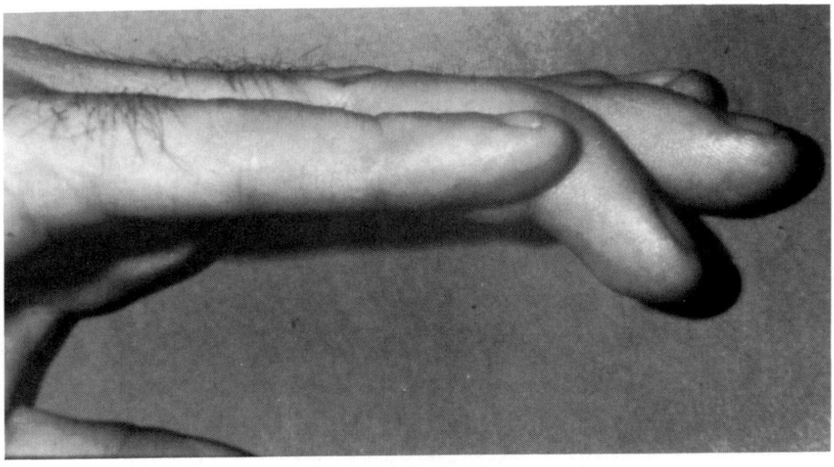

Figure 9–4 Mallet finger deformity.

visualize and perform the open reduction and internal fixation.[12, 34] The tendon is then repaired prior to skin closure. We prefer to use the technique advocated by Stark and colleagues.[112, 113] One collateral ligament, usually the ulnar, is divided and the hematoma at the fracture site is removed. Joint subluxation can be corrected if necessary by reduction and intramedullary pinning. The fragment can then be reduced into its bed anatomically and held in place either by small smooth K-wires or by a pull-out wire and button technique. After 6 weeks of splinting in extension, gentle motion exercises are begun and the finger is splinted in the extended position for 2 to 4 more weeks at night. Satisfactory results can be achieved by this method but rarely does the patient regain a full range of motion following this type of surgical procedure.

A mallet injury is rare in the thumb and we have treated only three cases in athletes (Fig. 9–11). Din and Meggitt[15] have recommended surgical treatment while others state that conservative treatment is preferable.[1, 78, 84, 94] We have utilized the same principles in treating the mallet thumb that we have in the mallet finger. We use conservative treatment unless there is palmar subluxation of the distal phalanx, and we have not encountered this in the thumb. Splinting of the interphalangeal joint in extension for 6 weeks and then at night for 2 to 4 more weeks has produced satisfactory results.

Compound mallet injuries are open joint injuries. We treat these with thorough debridement and irrigation of the wound and repair of the extensor mechanism. The joint is then treated in as outlined above. Epiphyseal injuries to the base of the distal phalanx in children should be treated with closed reduction and splinting for 3 to 4 weeks. Occasionally, a markedly displaced epiphyseal fracture will require open reduction and internal fixation with a smooth K-wire.[123]

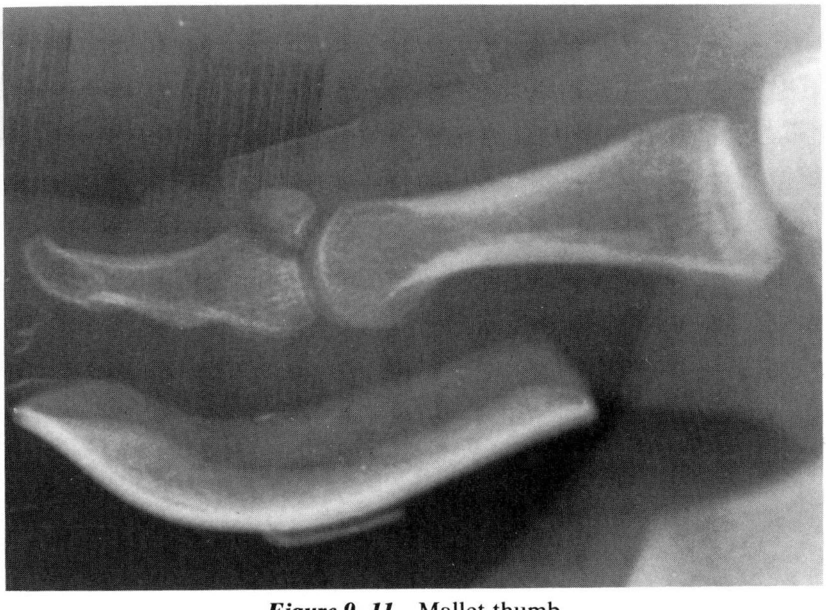

Figure 9–11 Mallet thumb.

Boutonnière Deformity

The boutonnière, or button hole, deformity results from an injury to the central slip near or at its insertion into the base of the middle phalanx. The characteristic deformity consists of flexion at the PIP joint and hyperextension at the DIP joint (Fig. 9–12). The head of the proximal phalanx can "button hole" through the defect in the extensor mechanism, hence the term "boutonnière." In athletes, the injury may result from a blow to the dorsum of the middle phalanx that forces the PIP joint into flexion while the athlete is attempting to extend his finger. This causes a disruption in the central slip at or near its insertion into the base of the middle phalanx. However, the injury is probably more commonly caused by an unrecognized palmar dislocation of the PIP joint that reduces spontaneously or is pulled back into place on the athletic field by the athlete or the trainer.[53] The typical deformity is rarely seen immediately following the closed injury. There is swelling and tenderness at the base of the middle phalanx near the central slip insertion. Weakness of active extension at the PIP joint is seen, particularly when the MCP joint is flexed. Immediately following the injury, the lateral bands are still in their proper position and can extend the PIP joint weakly. If the injury is not recognized and treated properly, the central extensor mechanism begins to retract, the triangular ligament stretches out, and the lateral bands fall palmar to the axis of rotation at the PIP joint. The lateral bands thus become flexors of the PIP joint and, as they retract proximally, hyperextend the DIP joint. The characteristic deformity is thus produced. In the early stages there is full passive motion of the PIP and DIP joints, but contractures may soon develop without proper splinting.

A thorough understanding of the anatomy and a high index of suspicion are necessary to diagnose these lesions and treat them properly to prevent this disabling deformity. This injury must always be kept in mind when an athlete has "jammed" a finger or has pulled a finger back into place after an injury.[72, 73] If there are swelling and tenderness dorsally at

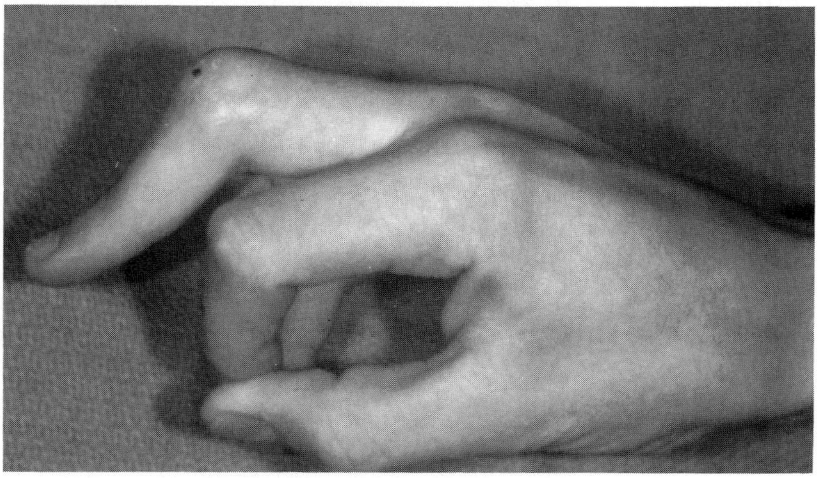

Figure 9–12 Boutonnière deformity.

the base of the middle phalanx and weakness on extension of the PIP joint with the MCP joint flexed, then radiographs should be taken and the finger splinted in the appropriate position until the damaged structures have healed.

In athletes, most of these are closed injuries caused by blunt trauma. We think that many are secondary to palmar lateral dislocations of the PIP joint that are pulled back into place on the athletic field, with the true extent of the injury going unrecognized. Leddy and Coyle[53] reported on a series of 27 acute palmar PIP dislocations, mostly in athletes. There were three distinct types: Type I were straight palmar dislocations, with the mechanism of injury being blunt trauma with straight downward pressure over the base of the middle phalanx. These patients presented with an obvious deformity of the PIP joint, and radiographs showed the base of the middle phalanx sitting directly beneath the head of the proximal phalanx with no lateral deviation or rotational deformity (Fig. 9–13). Four of six patients avulsed a small fleck of bone from the base of the middle phalanx at the insertion of the central slip. In each instance, closed reduction was easily achieved by traction and manipulation under digital block anesthesia, but each patient was left with a profound extensor lag at the PIP joint indicative of the disruption of the central slip insertion. Type II were

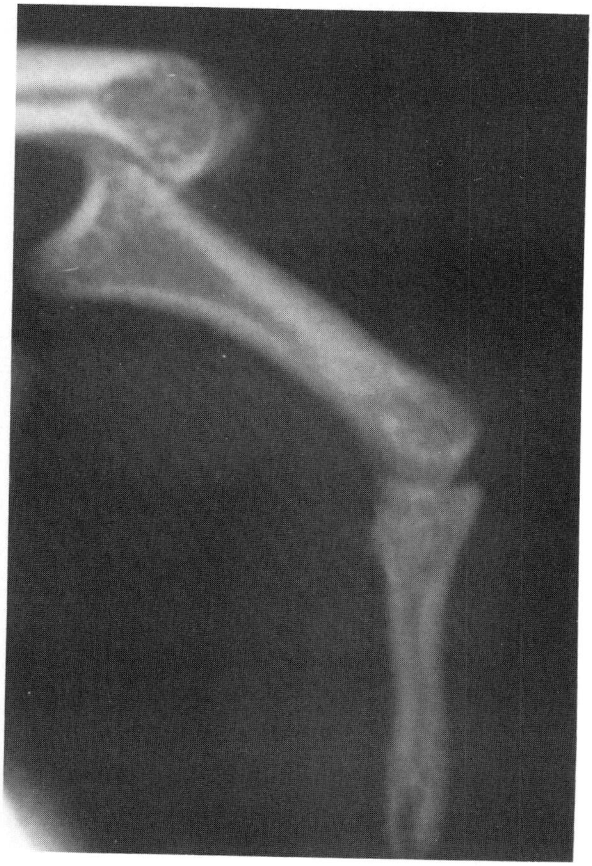

Figure 9–13 Straight palmar dislocation with no lateral or rotational component.

palmar lateral dislocations, and there were sixteen of these. These injuries were caused by a palmar and laterally directed force on the middle phalanx. The PIP joint was flexed and laterally deviated, usually to the ulnar side, with a tear of the radial collateral ligament. Roentgenograms showed the palmar and lateral displacement of the base of the middle phalanx on the head of the proximal phalanx (Fig. 9–14). Six of the sixteen patients avulsed a fleck of bone from the base of the middle phalanx, indicating a disruption of the central slip insertion. Closed reduction was easily accomplished by traction and manipulation. After reduction, there was tenderness over the insertion of the central slip into the base of the middle phalanx and over one collateral ligament complex (usually the radial side). Most of these patients had an immediate extensor lag at the PIP joint and others had demonstrable weakness of extension. All had laxity of the involved collateral ligament. It was postulated that these patients had rupture of one collateral ligament and partial to complete tears of the central slip and volar plate. Type III injuries were irreducible dislocations. There were five of these cases, and as far as could be determined there was a rotational component along with the palmar and lateral force causing the dislocation (Fig. 9–15). The deformity was less obvious than in the pre-

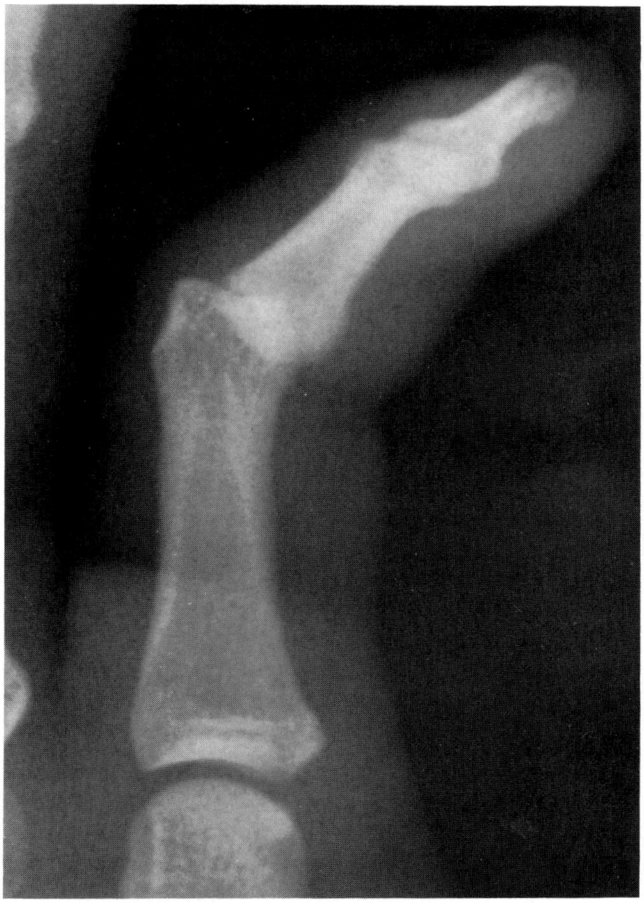

Figure 9–14 Palmar lateral dislocation.

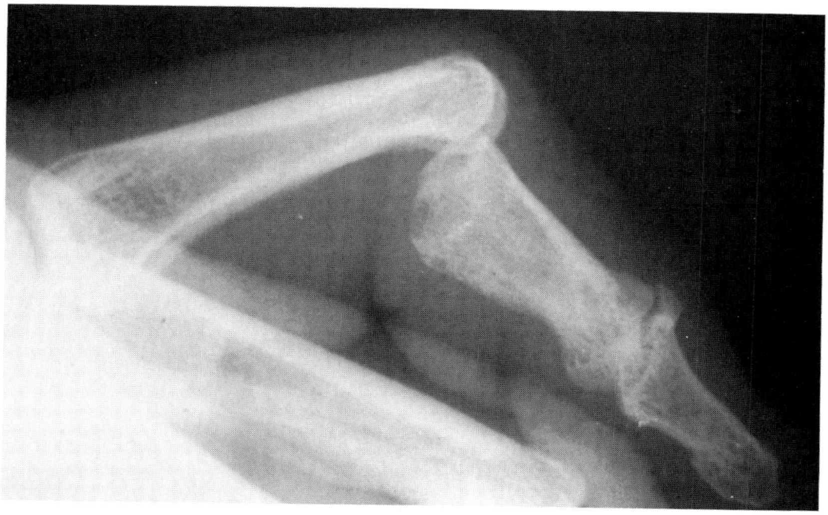

Figure 9–15 Irreducible palmar dislocation with rotational component.

vious two types. Multiple attempts at closed reduction under anesthesia with the MCP and PIP joints in various positions were unsuccessful due to soft tissue interposition (Fig. 9–16). Open reduction, removal of the interposed tissues, and repair of the damaged structures were performed. The type and duration of postoperative splinting depended on whether or not the central slip was damaged. Three of these five patients had an intact central slip and were splinted only long enough to allow soft tissue healing.

Surgical intervention is the treatment of choice in chronic unrecognized palmar PIP dislocation.[85, 90] However, many different forms of treatment have been proposed for the acute boutonnière deformity and for the acute palmar dislocation of the PIP joint with damage to the central slip.[17, 85, 110, 115] Some have recommended operative repair of the torn central slip, while others have advocated percutaneous pinning of the PIP joint in extension and still others splinting. We prefer to treat all of these injuries in a closed fashion with a safety pin splint as soon as possible following injury. The only exception would be a large displaced intra-articular fragment at the PIP joint or soft tissue interposition preventing a congruent reduction in a palmar PIP dislocation.*

A small bony fragment avulsed from the base of the middle phalanx by the central slip insertion is not an indication for surgical intervention in our opinion. The safety pin splint holds the MCP and PIP joints in extension and allows active and passive flexion at the DIP joint, which should be encouraged (Fig. 9–17). This active and passive flexion at the DIP joint permits the lateral bands to assume and maintain their normal position at the PIP joint, thereby preventing them from displacing palmar to the axis of motion and causing an increase in the flexion moment. It also prevents the lateral bands from retracting proximally and causing hyperextension at the DIP joint. Holding the PIP joint in extension allows the damaged

---

* See refs. 14, 27, 43, 47, 79, 80, 83, 91, 104.

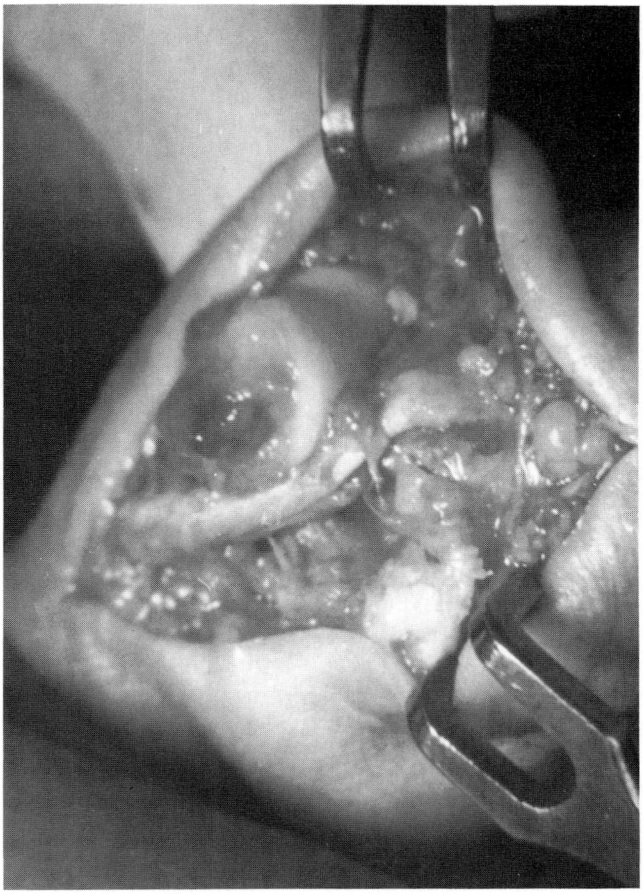

Figure 9–16 Irreducible palmar dislocation with collateral ligament rupture and extensor mechanism interposition.

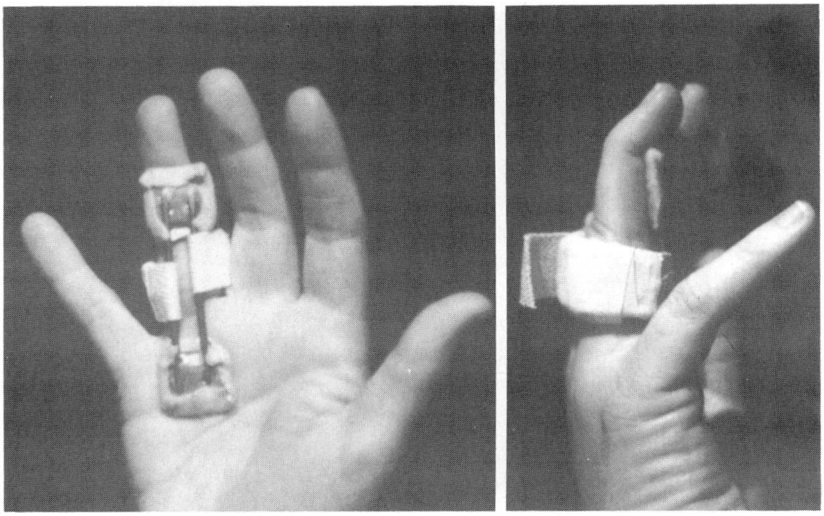

Figure 9–17 Safety Pin Splint, allowing active and passive flexion at the DIP joint.

central slip to heal. These splints are worn for a total of 6 weeks. During this period, great care is taken to prevent accidental flexion of the PIP joints (and disruption of early healing) when the splint is removed to cleanse the finger. Splinting is discontinued at 6 weeks, and gentle active and passive flexion exercises are begun at the PIP joint. Occasionally, the splint may be worn at night for another 2 weeks. This regimen has proven to be successful for the treatment of complete disruption of the central slip insertion in a great majority of our patients (including several with a small bony fleck avulsed from the base of the middle phalanx).

In our hands, results of closed treatment have been greatly superior to those obtained with operative treatment. Many athletes can participate in their sport while wearing this splint, which can be wrapped and padded if necessary. In our opinion, the only indications for surgical treatment of a closed injury to the central slip insertion are (1) an irreducible palmar PIP dislocation due to soft tissue interposition and (2) a large displaced intra-articular PIP joint fracture at the base of the middle phalanx.

In the series cited above,[53] the palmar lateral dislocations were the most common. These easily reducible injuries may occur more often than we realize. Many are pulled back into place immediately after injury and the true extent of soft tissue damage is not appreciated. These patients will develop a boutonnière deformity with a painful unstable collateral ligament. We have seen several of these, particularly in the small fingers of athletes, such as basketball players, with unstable radial collateral ligaments. Awareness of this injury and a high index of suspicion are mandatory, and these athletes should be carefully examined following any significant injury to their fingers.

Prior to surgical reconstruction of an established boutonnière deformity, a full passive range of motion of the PIP joint must be obtained either by splinting or by surgical release.[19, 20, 108, 109] We prefer to use the method described by Elliot[19] because it reconstructs the extensor mechanism in an anatomic fashion. The central slip is shortened appropriately and the lateral bands are brought back to their proper position. Postoperatively, we immobilize the PIP joint in the extended position with a K-wire. This is removed 3 weeks later and a safety pin splint is applied for another 3 weeks. During this entire period, active and passive flexion of the DIP joint is encouraged. At 6 weeks after surgery, active and passive range of motion exercises are begun at the PIP joint and night splinting may be continued for another 2 weeks. Although a full range of motion is rarely, if ever, obtained, satisfactory results can be achieved by this method (Fig. 9–18).

The true boutonnière deformity must be distinguished from the pseudo-boutonnière deformity since they resemble each other in appearance, but their causes and treatments are vastly different. In a typical pseudo-boutonniere deformity, the flexion contracture at the PIP joint is fixed and passive extension is not possible. This normally results from a hyperextension injury to the PIP joint where the volar plate and one collateral ligament have been damaged.[72, 73] As these structures heal and then contract, a fixed flexion deformity is produced at the PIP joint with a secondary mild hyperextension deformity at the DIP joint. In a normal boutonnière deformity, following disruption of

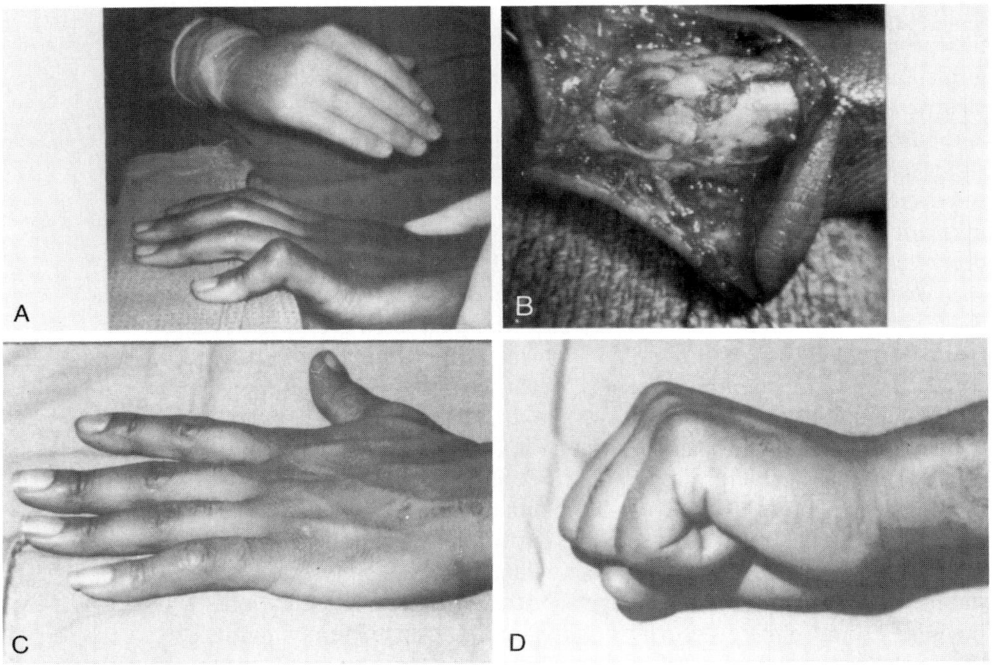

Figure 9–18 *A*, Boutonnière deformity. *B*, Operative reconstruction. *C, D,* Postoperative result.

the central slip, there is full passive extension of the PIP joint unless a later contracture develops due to inadequate treatment. In a pseudo-boutonnière deformity, roentgenograms may show calcification along the volar lateral aspect of the proximal phalanx on the side of the collateral ligament injury (Fig. 9–19). If these deformities are seen before the fixed flexion contracture is greater than 45°, treatment with a safety pin splint or joint jack may be successful in gradually restoring full extension to the PIP joint. However, if the flexion contracture is greater than 45° when first seen, then surgical release may be necessary to restore extension to the affected joint.[73] In these cases, the central slip was not damaged at the time of the injury and loss of extension is due to scarring and contracture on the palmar aspect of the joint.

Extensor Tendon Injuries at the Metacarpophalangeal Joint Level

The soft tissues overlying the MCP joint are prone to repetitive injury from direct impact during sports activities.[88, 89] A sudden flexion and/or ulnar deviation force to the finger may cause damage to the extensor hood mechanism over the MCP joint. The problems at this level that warrant discussion are (1) the "boxer's knuckle" or "soft knuckle" and (2) dislocation or subluxation of the extensor tendon mechanism.

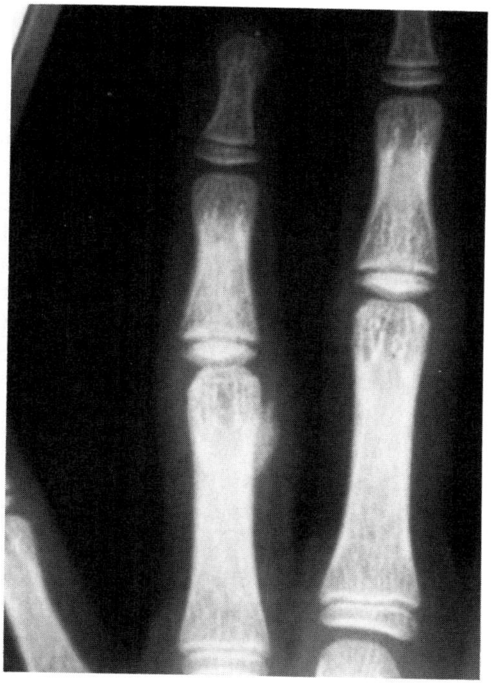

Figure 9–19 Pseudo-boutonnière deformity with calcification on the radial aspect of the proximal phalanx.

BOXER'S KNUCKLE

In 1957, Gladden[28] used the term "boxer's knuckle" to describe an injury to the dorsal soft tissue structures at the MCP joint level. The boxer usually gave a history of a specific event that caused the injury and then subsequent repetitive trauma causing pain and swelling over the dorsum of the MCP joint. The surgical findings included thickening of the soft tissue over the MCP joint with a tear in the tendon, sagittal fibers, or dorsal capsule itself.

Koniuch and colleagues[48] described a similar injury secondary to direct blows over the dorsum of the MCP joint in nine patients. All had chronic pain and swelling over the MCP joint without extensor tendon subluxation. Each had a partial arcuate tear of the sagittal fibers on the ulnar side with scarring of the dorsal capsule. Surgical repair of these tears produced satisfactory results.

In a recent article, Posner and Ambrose[89] reported on six patients with closed injuries who sustained tears in the dorsal capsule of the MCP joint. The injuries occurred in the index or middle finger MCP joint, usually in the dominant hand of professional boxers. Surgical repair of the defect in the dorsal capsule and sagittal fibers of the extensor hood produced excellent results.

The training process in karate is designed to develop bursae and fibrotic tissue over the metacarpal heads to enable them to perform the required wood breaking techniques during competition.[75] Gardner[26] presented a case of a karate athlete who developed a painful restriction of extension at the MCP joint from hypertrophic infiltrative tendinitis as a result of his training program. Schultz[102] has described a similar post-traumatic entrapment of the extensor digiti minimi proprius tendon.

The diagnosis of "boxer's knuckle" is not usually difficult. There is a history of a closed injury followed by multiple repetitive episodes of trauma and chronic painful swelling of the MCP joint (Fig. 9–20).[89] Radiographs are usually within normal limits and there is no subluxation of the extensor tendon. Normally the condition is chronic before the athlete seeks medical help. Conservative treatment, consisting of rest and splinting, may be of little or no benefit in these cases.[48, 89] At the time of surgery, the joint should be inspected for loose bodies and arthritic changes. The dorsal capsule, sagittal fibers, and extensor tendon should be carefully inspected for tears, which should be repaired. Postoperatively, these joints should be immobilized in a moderately flexed position for approximately 4 weeks, after which range of motion and strengthening exercises should be instituted. Contact should be avoided for 6 months following repair of these injuries.[89]

DISLOCATION-SUBLUXATION OF THE EXTENSOR TENDONS AT THE METACARPOPHALANGEAL JOINT LEVEL

Traumatic subluxation or dislocation of the extensor tendons at the MCP joint is a rare occurrence in athletes. It can result from a direct blow forcing the finger into flexion or with forced flexion and ulnar deviation of the finger.[5, 125] The middle finger is most commonly involved, with ulnar subluxation of the extensor digitorum communis tendon.[45, 125] Radial subluxation or dislocation is extremely rare.[48] Kettlekamp and co-workers[45] presented an excellent clinical, anatomic,

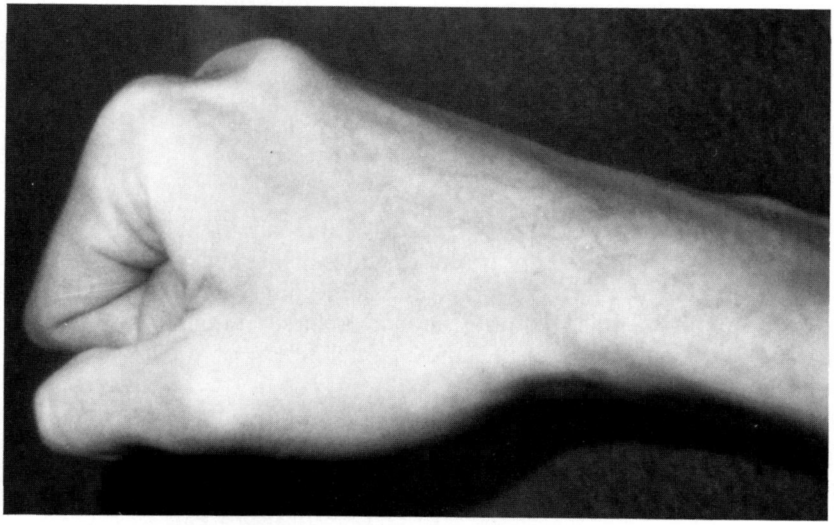

Figure 9–20 Boxer's knuckle.

and biomechanical study of traumatic dislocations of the long finger extensor tendon. They showed that the extensor tendon of the middle finger is more round than the other extensors and, therefore, more prominent and that the attachment to the underlying transverse lamina is weaker in this finger, especially on the radial side. This may explain why the majority of traumatic extensor tendon dislocations occur in the long finger to the ulnar side. In addition, the line of pull of the extensor and flexor tendons in the index and middle fingers is in an ulnar direction. Fresh cadaver dissections performed on 44 MCP joints showed that neither partial nor complete division of the ulnar sagittal fibers allowed radial dislocation of the extensor tendon. However, transection of just two thirds or more of the radial fibers did produce ulnar dislocation of this tendon.[48]

Ritts and associates[97] recommend immobilizing an acute extensor tendon dislocation with the MCP joint in extension for 4 to 6 weeks. However, there are no reports of a large series of these cases being treated successfully in this manner. A number of operative techniques have been proposed to treat these injuries if conservative treatment fails or if the condition is chronic and recurrent when first seen by the treating physician.* Primary repair of the sagittal fibers has been recommended by Kettlekamp and colleagues.[45] If the tissue is attenuated and there is difficulty relocating the extensor tendon centrally, then release of the ulnar sagittal fibers is performed and the radial side is then reefed to hold the extensor tendon in place.[16, 40, 45] Wheeldon[125] used the junctura tendinum to reinforce the repair, while Bunnell[5] advocated using the palmaris longus tendon for this purpose. Others have recommended using a part of the extensor tendon looped around the lumbrical or the radial collateral ligament to reinforce the repair on the radial side of the extensor hood.[7, 8, 21, 46, 71]

In an acute case, in which the tendon is relocated by extending the MCP joint, we would recommend splinting the MCP joint in extension for a total of 4 to 6 weeks. It is rare to see this injury acutely and we have treated only one case successfully in this manner. It is much more common to see the injury after multiple repetitive episodes of pain and swelling associated with a snapping sensation in the finger. Usually with the fingers in the extended position, the tendon is centrally located, but as the finger is slowly flexed, the extensor tendon will subluxate or dislocate to the ulnar side of the MCP joint (Fig. 9–21). If the condition is chronic and painful, surgical correction should be considered.

We prefer to expose the area through a slightly curved longitudinal incision. If the extensor tendon can be easily relocated without undue tension and the radial sagittal fibers can be freshened and repaired, then a direct repair is performed. If, however, there is difficulty in relocating the extensor tendon, the ulnar sagittal fibers are divided and a tendon loop reconstruction as advocated by Carroll and associates is performed.[8] Postoperatively, the MCP joints are immobilized in extension for 3 to 4 weeks, but active and passive motion of the PIP joints is

---

* See refs. 5, 7, 8, 16, 21, 36, 40, 45, 46, 71, 100, 125.

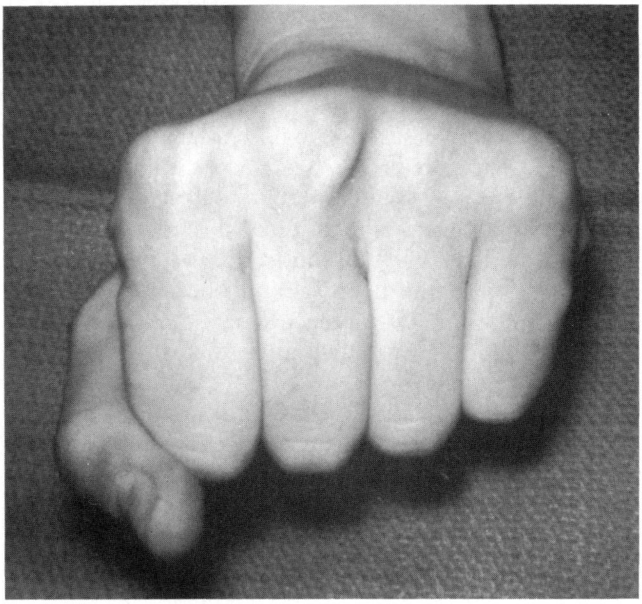

Figure 9–21 Ulnar dislocation of the extensor tendon of the MP joint of the middle finger.

encouraged. During the next 2 to 3 weeks, active motion is instituted at the MCP joint in a dynamic extension splint. Six weeks after surgery, splinting is discontinued. The patient is not allowed to return to competition until there is a full active range of motion and grip strength has been restored.

Avulsion of the Profundus Tendon Insertion

Avulsion of the profundus tendon insertion occurs with relative frequency in athletes. In 1891, Von Zander[122] described a rupture of the flexor pollicis longus tendon and since then, several reports have been published.* McMaster,[76] in a classic paper in 1933, showed that the tendon was the strongest link in the musculotendinous chain and that rupture rarely occurred in the substance of a normal tendon. He proved experimentally that rupture usually occurred at the bony insertion and less often at the musculotendinous junction. When there is rupture of a flexor tendon within the tendon substance, usually there is a pathologic process responsible such as rheumatoid arthritis, tenosynovitis, or fracture of the hook of the hamate.[6]

Avulsion of the profundus tendon insertion occurs most frequently in young adult males. The ring finger is affected in more than 75 percent of the cases, but the injury has been reported in all fingers and the thumb and can occur at any age in either sex. Gunter[32] believes that the common flexor muscle belly of the profundus to the middle, ring, and

* See refs. 3, 6, 9, 11, 23, 32, 38, 50–52, 54, 87, 99, 106, 124.

little fingers makes the ring finger more susceptible to this injury. The anatomic arrangement of the extensor tendons may also play a role. Manske and Lesker[62] showed in a cadaver study that the breaking strength of the flexor digitorum profundus insertion of the ring finger is significantly less than that of the middle finger. Each of these factors may play a role in the increased susceptibility of the ring finger to this injury.

Avulsion of the tendon insertion occurs when the finger is forcibly extended during a maximum contraction of the profundus muscle. Many of these injuries occur in football, flag football, and rugby, when, in a desperate effort to make a tackle, the shorter little finger of the player slips away from the opposing player's pants or jersey. The little finger continues to flex and as the opponent pulls away, the ring finger, caught in the pants or jersey, is forcibly extended while the profundus is contracting and the insertion gives way.[51, 52, 54] The diagnosis is often missed initially, particularly if the physician or trainer is not aware of this entity. Unless one specifically tests for the presence of active flexion at the DIP joint the injury will not be recognized. Radiographs are often negative. Pain, swelling, and ecchymosis are not always present. The pathognomonic feature of this diagnosis is inability to actively flex the DIP joint of the affected finger (Fig. 9–22).

Factors that influence the prognosis and treatment of this injury include the level to which the tendon retracts and, therefore, the remaining blood supply to the tendon, the length of time between injury and treatment, and the presence and size of a bony fragment on the radiograph. This injury has been classified into three main types and the mechanism of injury is presumed to be the same for each.[51, 52, 54]

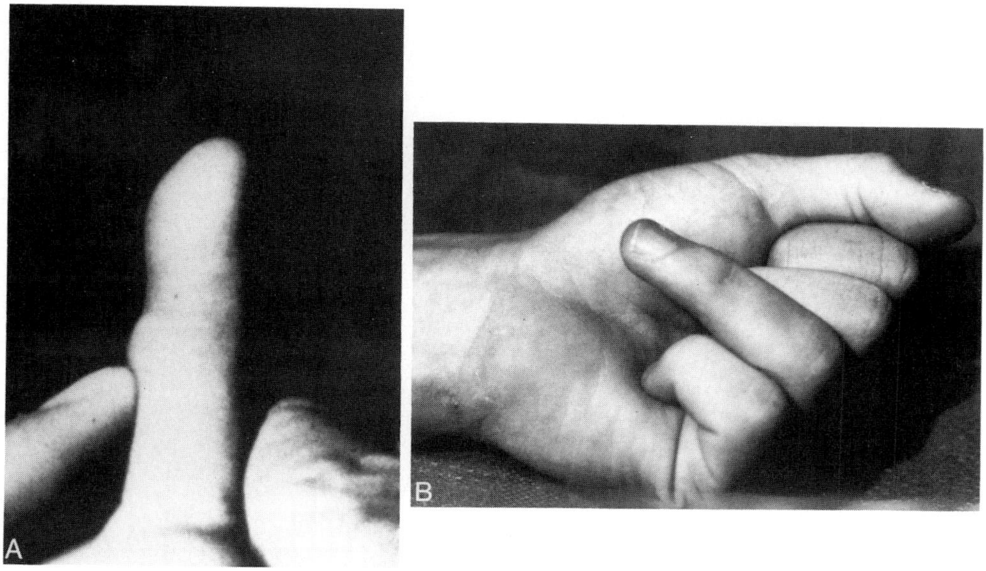

Figure 9–22 The absence of active flexion at the DIP joint is diagnostic of avulsion of the profundus tendon insertion.

TYPE I

In this type, the tendon retracts all the way into the palm. Both vinculae have been ruptured, and therefore a substantial portion of the blood supply to the tendon is lost. There is also loss of diffusion of nutrients into the tendon from the synovial fluid. There may be some tenderness over the area of the insertion into the distal phalanx and there may also be some swelling and tenderness in the palm at the level of the retracted tendon near the lumbrical origin. This tendon should be reinserted into the distal phalanx within 7 to 10 days of injury before the tendon becomes shriveled and contracted, making advancement and reinsertion impossible (Fig. 9–23). A midlateral or palmar zigzag incision is made on the finger, exposing the flexor sheath from the area of the insertion of the profundus tendon to just proximal to the PIP joint. An opening in the sheath is made just distal to the A2 pulley. If the tendon is not found at this level, it has retracted into the palm, and a slightly curved incision is made just proximal to the distal palmar crease, exposing the flexor sheath proximal to the A1 metacarpal pulley. There is some hemorrhage found within the sheath. An incision is made and the distal end of the profundus tendon is located. A small pliable catheter is passed retrograde from distal to proximal beneath the sheath and pulleys to the level of the proximal end of the A1 pulley. The flexor tendon is attached to the catheter with nonabsorbable sutures and the catheter is pulled distally, threading the profundus tendon back

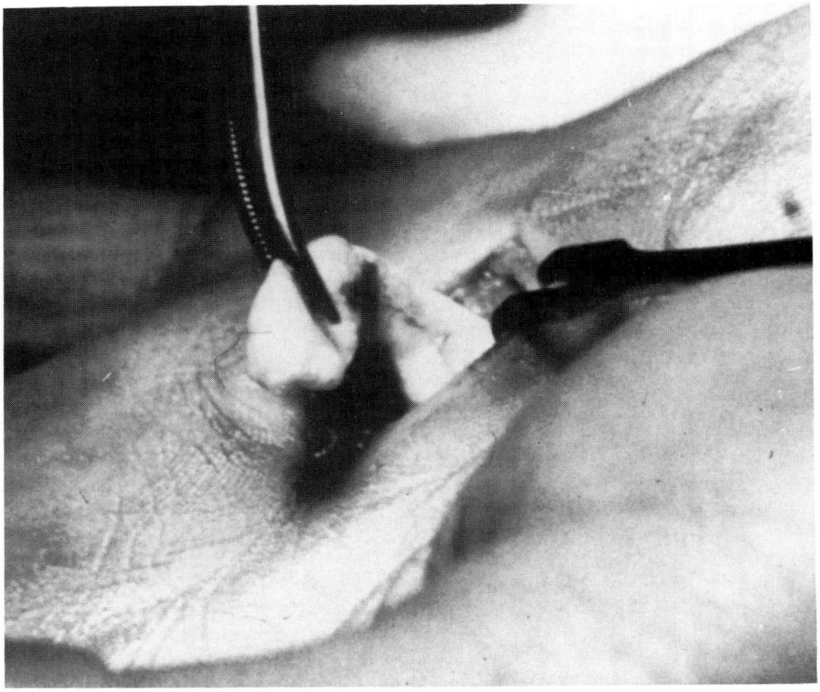

Figure 9–23 Shriveled, contracted profundus tendon that cannot be reinserted into the distal phalanx.

beneath the pulleys and through the superficialis to the level of the distal phalanx. Passing the tendon beneath the A4 pulley may be difficult. We reinsert the tendon into the base of the distal phalanx through a raised osteoperiosteal flap with a standard pull-out wire and button technique using either No. 34 monofilament stainless steel wire or a synthetic monofilament suture such as 4-0 Prolene. No pull-out wire is necessary if the synthetic monofilament suture is used (Fig. 9–24). When it is time to remove the button, one slip of the suture can be divided beneath the button and the remainder can be pulled out through the tendon and bone. Suturing the tendon to the surrounding periosteum and soft tissues following avulsion of the insertion is not an acceptable method of anchoring the tendon into the distal phalanx. The volar plate at the DIP joint should not be injured while reinserting the tendon. A dorsal plaster splint is used to hold the wrist in slight flexion, the MCP joints in 75° of flexion, and the PIP and DIP joints in relative extension. Passive flexion exercises can be instituted very early on. The splint is removed at 3 weeks and active exercises are begun. The pull-out wire and button may be removed at 3 to 4 weeks postoperatively. The remaining care is similar to that for other flexor tendon injuries.

TYPE II

In this instance, the tendon retracts to the level of the PIP joint, leaving the long vinculum intact and thereby preserving more of the blood supply to the tendon and retaining more of its length. Some nutrition from synovial fluid diffusion is also preserved. Anteroposterior and lateral radiographs of the finger should be taken because occasionally a small bony fleck is avulsed with the tendon and can be seen on the lateral radiograph at the level of the PIP joint (Fig. 9–25). There is no active flexion at the DIP joint and there is pain, swelling, tenderness, and some loss of motion at the PIP joint. This type is also best treated by early reinsertion of the tendon into the distal phalanx. However, because a greater length of the tendon is preserved and there is better blood supply and synovial fluid diffusion, these tendons can be reinserted at a later date if the injury was not recognized initially. The tendon does not become shriveled and contracted as in type I injuries.

A midlateral or zigzag incision is made on the affected finger to expose the flexor tendon mechanism. An incision is made in the sheath just distal to the A2 pulley and the tendon is found at this level, held in

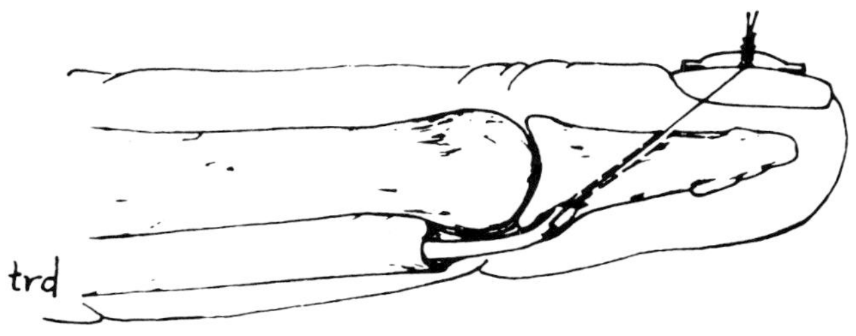

Figure 9–24 Profundus reinsertion through an osteoperiosteal flap in the distal phalanx using synthetic monofilament suture.

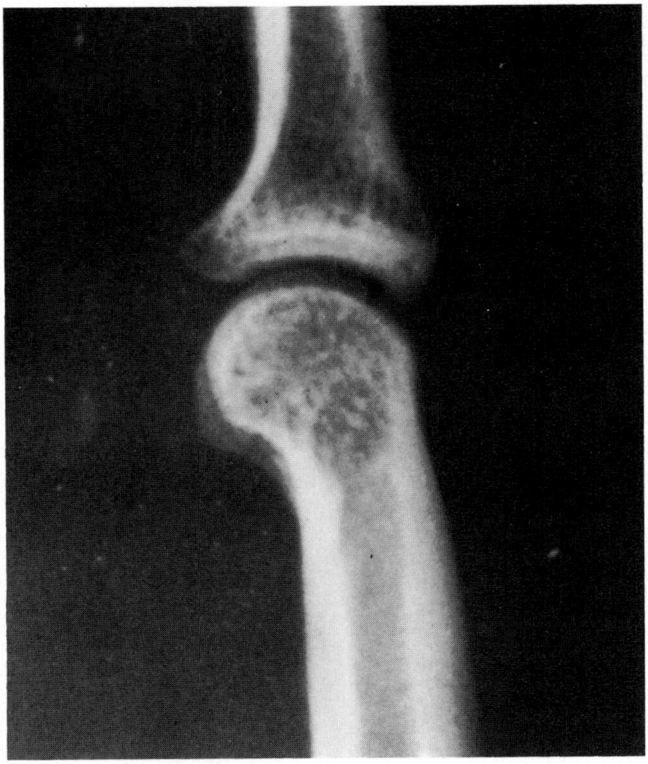

Figure 9–25 Small bony fleck adjacent to PIP joint.

place by the long vinculum. If the injury is more than a few weeks old, any granulation tissue at this level should be excised and a full passive range of motion restored prior to reinserting the tendon. The tendon is then passed beneath the sheath and pulleys to the level of the distal phalanx and reinserted as described previously. Postoperative care is the same. Successful treatment may be possible a few months postinjury. A type II injury may also convert to a type I injury when the tendon slips away from the level of the PIP joint into the palm, thus rupturing the long vinculum. It is then treated as a type I injury.

TYPE III

In this instance, there is usually a large bony fragment that is held in place by the A4 pulley. There may be some comminution of the fragment, a comminuted intra-articular fracture of the DIP joint, or both. Both vinculae are intact and tendon length is preserved as is the nutrition from synovial fluid diffusion. There are marked swelling, ecchymosis, and tenderness over the distal end of the middle phalanx just proximal to the DIP joint and no active flexion at the DIP joint. A large bony fragment can be seen on the lateral radiograph just proximal to the DIP joint (Fig. 9–26). Open reduction and internal fixation of the fragment will normally give a satisfactory result. Postoperative care is the same as for the other two types. Active motion is instituted as soon as bony healing permits.

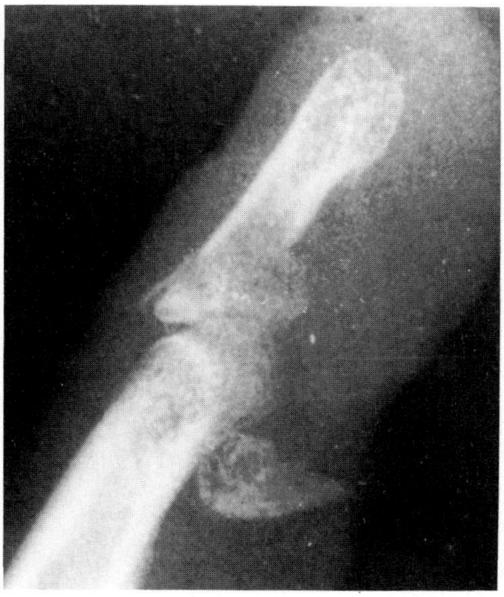

Figure 9–26 Type III avulsion with large bony fragment.

There have been a few reports[50, 99, 106] of type III fractures with simultaneous avulsion of the profundus tendon from the fracture fragment. This is an unusual injury and we have treated only two (Fig. 9–27). In this instance, bony continuity should be restored by open reduction and internal fixation if possible and then the avulsed profundus tendon should be treated as a type I or II injury depending on the level of retraction.

Not all authors agree on the management of old, untreated cases that are too late for operative reinsertion. In our opinion, those that are asymptomatic should be left alone. Limitation of motion at the PIP joint is rare 6 months postinjury. If there is no instability at the DIP joint and no special requirement for active flexion at this joint, then no surgical treatment is indicated. If there is instability of the DIP joint with weakness of pinch or recurrent dorsal dislocations, joint fusion or tenodesis should be considered. We prefer fusion, which provides joint stability and will not interfere with the function of the superficialis tendon (Fig. 9–28). If there is a tender lump in the palm, the retracted tendon can be excised at the time of the DIP joint fusion. Tenodesis at this level can be a difficult procedure since the tendon has to be inserted into both the distal and the middle phalanges because there is no remaining tendon on the distal phalanx. It may also stretch out with the passage of time.

Use of a flexor tendon graft in the presence of an intact functioning superficialis tendon has been reported by several authors.* While it may be a worthwhile procedure, particularly in the index and middle fingers of young people, it must be recognized that there are significant complications whether the procedure is done in one or two stages. Since more than 75 percent of these injuries occur in the ring finger, it may be that the potential risks of a flexor tendon graft outweigh the possible advantages in most individuals. Some people, such as musicians or skilled

* See refs. 9, 11, 25, 29, 32, 38, 39, 42, 70, 95, 114, 121, 126.

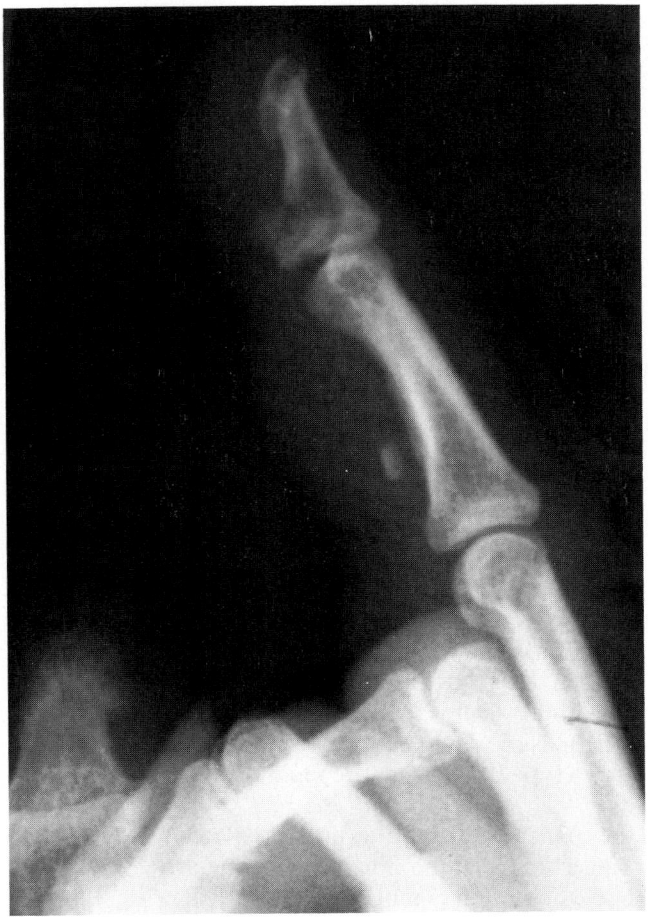

Figure 9–27 Avulsion of a large fragment from the base of the distal phalanx with simultaneous avulsion of a small bony fleck by the profundus tendon.

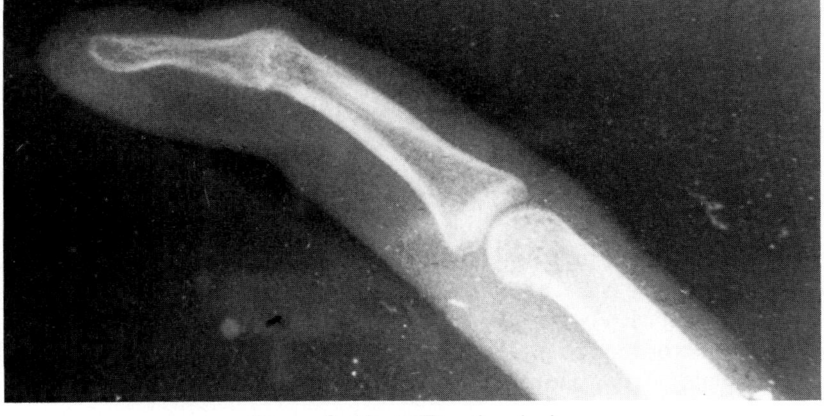

Figure 9–28 DIP arthrodesis.

technicians, may require active flexion at the DIP joint of the ring finger, and in these instances the procedure may be indicated.

In those patients who are diagnosed and treated early with reinsertion of the tendon, a satisfactory result is usually obtained. although there may be a small 10 to 15° loss of extension at the DIP joint, grip strength approaches normal, and patients who undergo fusion or tenodesis will have grip strength equivalent to that of the late untreated group. A successful tendon graft can stabilize the DIP joint and increase grip strength.[51, 52, 54]

REFERENCES

1. Abouna, J.M., Brown, H.: The treatment of mallet finger. Brit. J. Surg. 55:653, 1968.
2. Albertoni, W.M.: The Brooks-Graner procedure for correction of mallet finger. In Tubiana, R. (ed.): The Hand, Vol. 3. Philadelphia, W.B. Saunders, 1988, pp. 97–100.
3. Blazina, M.E., Lane, C.: Rupture of the insertion of the flexor digitorum profundus tendon in student athletes. J. Am. Coll. Health Assn. 14:248, 1966.
4. Bowers, W.H., Hurst, L.C.: Chronic mallet finger: the use of Fowler's central slip release. J. Hand Surg. 3:373, 1978.
5. Boyes, J.H.: Bunnell's Surgery of the Hand, 5th ed. Philadelphia, J.B. Lippincott, 1970.
6. Boyes, J.H., Wilson, J.N., Smith, J.W.: Flexor tendon ruptures in the forearm and hand. J. Bone Joint Surg. 42A:637, 1960.
7. Bracey, D.J., Jeffreys, T.E.: Habitual extensor tendon dislocation. Hand 2:284, 1979.
8. Carroll, C., IV, Moore, J.R., Weiland, A.J.: Posttraumatic ulnar subluxation of the extensor tendons: a reconstructive technique. J. Hand Surg. 12A:227, 1987.
9. Carroll, R.E., Match, R.M.: Avulsion of the profundus tendon insertion. J. Trauma 10:1109, 1970.
10. Casscells, S.W., Strange, T.B.: Intramedullary wire fixation of mallet-finger. J. Bone Joint Surg. 39A:521, 1957.
11. Chang, W.H., Thoms, O.J., White, W.L.: Avulsion injury of the long flexor tendons. Plast. Reconstr. Surg. 50:260, 1972.
12. Cohn, B.T., Froimson, A.I.: Case report of a rare mallet finger injury. Orthopedics 9:529, 1986.
13. Crawford, G.P.: The molded polythene splint for mallet finger deformities. J. Hand Surg. 9A:231, 1984.
14. DeSmet, L., Vercauteren, M.: Palmar dislocation of the proximal interphalangeal joint requiring open reduction: a case report. J. Hand Surg., 9A:717, 1984.
15. Din, K.M., Meggitt, B.F.: Mallet thumb. J. Bone Joint Surg. 65B:606, 1983.
16. Doyle, J.R.: Extensor tendons—acute injuries. In Green, D.P. (ed.): Operative Hand Surgery, Vol. 3, 2nd ed. New York, Churchill Livingstone, 1988, pp. 2045–2072.
17. Dray, G.J., Eaton, R.G.: Dislocations and ligament injuries in the digits. In Green, D.P. (ed.): Operative hand surgery, Vol. 1, 2nd ed. New York, Churchill Livingstone, 1988, pp. 785–786.
18. Eaton, R.G.: The extensor mechanism of the fingers. Bull. Hosp. Joint Dis. 30:39, 1969.
19. Elliott, R.A., Jr.: Injuries to the extensor mechanism of the hand. Orthop. Clin. North Am. 1:335, 1970.
20. Elliott, R.A., Jr.: Splints for mallet and boutonniere deformities. Plast. Reconstr. Surg. 52:282, 1973.
21. Elson, R.A.: Dislocation of the extensor tendons of the hand. Report of a case. J. Bone Joint Surg. 49B:324, 1967.
22. Eyler, D.L., Markee, J.E.: The anatomy and function of the intrinsic musculature of the fingers. J. Bone Joint Surg. 36A:1, 1954.

23. Folmar, R.C., Nelson, C.L., Phalen, G.S.: Ruptures of the flexor tendons in hands of non-rheumatoid patients. J. Bone Joint Surg. 54A:579, 1972.
24. Fowler, S.B.: Extensor apparatus of the digits. Proceedings of the British Orthopaedic Association. J. Bone Joint Surg. 31B:477, 1949.
25. Gaisford, J.C., Hanna, D.C., Richardson, G.S.: Tendon grafting: a suggested technique. Plast. Reconstr. Surg. 38:302, 1966.
26. Gardner, R.C.: Hypertrophic infiltrative tendinitis (HIT syndrome) of the long extensor. J.A.M.A., 211:1009, 1970.
27. Garroway, R.Y., Hurst, L.C., Leppard, J., et al.: Complex dislocations of the proximal interphalangeal joint. Orthop. Rev. 13:21, 1984.
28. Gladden, R.J.: Boxer's knuckle. Am. J. Surg. 93:388, 1957.
29. Goldner, J.L., Coonrad, R.W.: Tendon grafting of the flexor profundus in the presence of a completely or partially intact flexor sublimis. J. Bone Joint Surg. 51A:527, 1969.
30. Green, D.P., Rowland, S.A.: Fractures and dislocations in the hand. In Rockwood, C., Green, D. (eds.): Fractures in Adults. Vol. 1, 2nd ed. Philadelphia, J.B. Lippincott, 1984, pp. 313–409.
31. Grundberg, A.B., Reagan, D.S.: Central slip tenotomy for chronic mallet finger deformity. J. Hand Surg. 12A:545, 1987.
32. Gunter, G.S.: Traumatic avulsion of the insertion of flexor digitorum profundus. Aust. N.Z. J. Surg. 30:1, 1960.
33. Hallberg, D., Lindholm, A.: Subcutaneous rupture of the extensor tendon of the distal phalanx of the finger: "mallet finger." Acta Chir. Scand. 119:260, 1960.
34. Hamas, R.S., Horrell, E.D., Pierret, G.P.: Treatment of mallet finger due to intra-articular fracture of the distal phalanx. J. Hand Surg. 3:361, 1978.
35. Harris, C., Rutledge, G.L.: The functional anatomy of the extensor mechanism of the finger. J. Bone Joint Surg. 54A:713, 1972.
36. Harvey, F.J., Hume, K.F.: Spontaneous recurrent ulnar dislocation of the long extensor tendons of the fingers. J. Hand Surg. 5:492, 1980.
37. Hillman, F.E.: New technique for treatment of mallet fingers and fractures of distal phalanx. J.A.M.A., 161:1135, 1956.
38. Honner, R.: The late management of the isolated lesion of the flexor digitorum profundus tendon. Hand 7:171, 1975.
39. Honner, R., Meares, A.: A review of 100 flexor tendon reconstructions with prosthesis. Hand 9:226, 1977.
40. Iftikhar, T.B., Hallman, B.W., Kaminski, R.S., et al.: Spontaneous rupture of the extensor mechanism causing ulnar dislocation of the long extensor tendon of the long finger. J. Bone Joint Surg. 66A:1108, 1984.
41. Iselin, F., Levame, J., Godoy, J.: A simplified technique for treating mallet fingers: tenodermodesis. J. Hand Surg. 2:118, 1977.
42. Jaffe, S., Weckesser, E.: Profundus tendon grafting with the sublimis intact. J. Bone Joint Surg. 49A:1298, 1967.
43. Johnson, F.G., Greene, M.H.: Another cause of irreducible dislocation of the proximal interphalangeal joint of a finger. J. Bone Joint Surg. 48A:542, 1966.
44. Kaplan, E.B.: Anatomy, injuries and treatment of the extensor apparatus of the hand and the digits. Clin. Orthop. 13:24, 1959.
45. Kettlekamp, D.B., Flatt, A.E., Moulds, R.: Traumatic dislocation of the long-finger extensor tendon. J. Bone Joint Surg. 53A:229, 1971.
46. Kilgore, E.S., Graham, W.P., Newmeyer, W.L., et al.: Correction of ulnar subluxation of the extensor communis. Hand 7:272, 1975.
47. Kilgore, E.S., Newmeyer, W.L., Brown, L.G.: Post-traumatic trapped dislocations of the proximal interphalangeal joint. J. Trauma 16:481, 1976.
48. Koniuch, M.P., Peimer, C.A., VanGorder, T., et al.: Closed crush injury of the metacarpophalangeal joint. J. Hand Surg. 12A:750, 1987.
49. Landsmeer, J.M.F.: The anatomy of the dorsal aponeurosis of the human finger and its functional significance. Anat. Rec. 104:31, 1949.
50. Langa, V., Posner, M.A.: Unusual rupture of a flexor profundus tendon. J. Hand Surg. 11A:227, 1986.
51. Leddy, J.P.: Avulsions of the flexor digitorum profundus. In Strickland, J.W. (ed.):

elbow flexion between 120° and 135° either Struther's ligament or lacertus fibrosus level of compression should be suspected.[38, 39] Pain produced by resistance of long finger flexion, however, indicates compression of the nerve at the sublimis arch (Fig. 10–9). There is usually a Tinel's sign (sensitivity to tapping or percussion at the site of compression giving rise to tingling or "electric" sensations) in the forearm at the site of compression, but Tinel's and Phalen's signs (maximum wrist flexion for about 1 minute resulting in reproduction of symptoms) are absent at the level of the wrist. The most sensitive clinical test is reproduction of the patient's symptoms with direct, firm, deep pressure over the area of nerve compression for 60 seconds. Electrodiagnostic studies should be obtained but seldom aid in confirmation of this diagnosis (less than 10 percent in the Mayo Clinic series).[17] Conservative treatment consisting of rest and splinting for 4 to 6 weeks should initially be tried. Weight training has frequently been implicated in this syndrome and often will need to be discontinued or modified before any improvement is noted. Exploratory surgery should be reserved for refractory cases and must include complete decompression from above the elbow to the flexor digitorum sublimis arch.

Anterior Interosseous Nerve Syndrome This is also clinically manifested by vague activity-aggravated myalgia in the proximal forearm but without sensory complaints in the hand.[37] Occasionally, this clinical picture follows the onset of sudden, severe forearm pain terminating in a few hours. Clinical examination of a "junk ball" pitcher or a tennis player who attempts to impart a great deal of topspin will reveal weakness of the index profundus, flexor pollicis longus, and pronator quadratus (Fig. 10–10). This syndrome is usually caused by repetitive trauma to the forearm or by constricting tendinous bands that can arise from either the deep head of the pronator teres or the muscle origins of the sublimis, palmaris, profundus, or flexor carpi radialis. Accessory muscles, aberrant vessels, an enlarged bicipital bursa, and trauma are other etiologic factors. Electrodiagnostic

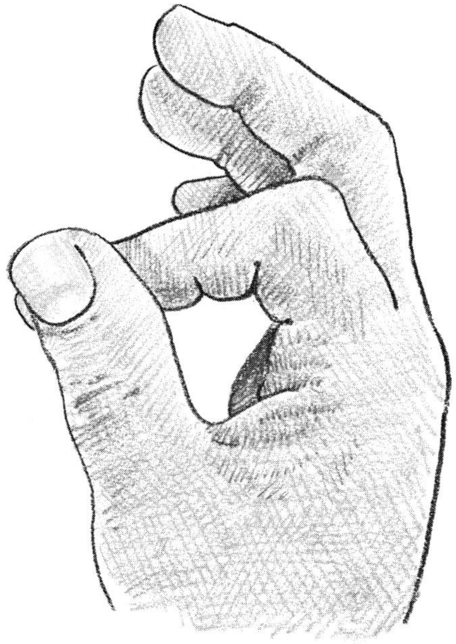

Figure 10–10. Anterior osseous nerve paralysis, demonstrating the characteristic pinch of this paralysis. (From Spinner, M.:Injuries to the Major Branches of the Forearm, 2nd ed. Philadelphia, W. B. Saunders, 1978.)

studies are occasionally helpful, especially if the involved muscles are specifically tested. Treatment is similar to that outlined for the pronator syndrome.

Carpal Tunnel Syndrome This is the most common compressive neuropathy in the upper extremity.[9] Closed wrist trauma with or without a fracture is the most common cause of this problem. Patients with this syndrome complain of activity-aggravated weakness or clumsiness of the hand along with paresthesias in the lateral three and one-half digits. Frequently, nightpain and paresthesias will awaken the patient, presumably secondary to acute wrist flexion during sleep. Clinical examination reveals a Tinel's sign at the wrist with a Phalen's sign as well. There may be thenar weakness or atrophy along with hypohidrosis and demonstrable sensory deficits on examination. These findings, however, usually indicate a chronic entrapment neuropathy. There is no identifiable weakness of flexor pollicis longus or index profundus strength on examination, and there is normal sensation in the proximal palm. Electromyography (EMG) and nerve conduction studies establish the diagnosis and differentiate it from more proximal nerve compressions. Further diagnostic work-up may be indicated depending on the clinical situation, including routine wrist roentgenograms with carpal tunnel views and pertinent laboratory data (erythrocyte sedimentation rate, glucose, uric acid, thyroid panel, and rheumatoid factor).

Treatment depends on the severity of the disease. If thenar atrophy is absent and sensory complaints are minimal, a cock-up splint and anti-inflammatory medication should be tried for 3 to 4 weeks. A steroid injection[13] into the carpal tunnel along with various diuretics may be tried. Surgical decompression should be reserved for patients who fail conservative treatment or those with established sensory and/or motor deficits.

Palmar Cutaneous Nerve Compression This syndrome is manifested clinically by dysethetic pain over the thenar eminence and proximal palm[41] A positive Tinel's sign is present in this area but the remaining clinical signs of carpal tunnel entrapment are absent.[36] Conservative measures such as padding the area, various physical therapeutic modalities, and local steroid injection may be tried initially. Rarely is surgery indicated, as the majority of these injuries are secondary to blunt trauma and hence result in only transient neuropraxic conduction blockage.

Bowler's Thumb In this disorder, a traumatic neuroma of the ulnar digital nerve to the thumb develops due to repeated friction between the thumb and the ball during bowling (Fig. 10–11). The nerve lies superficial to the sesamoid bone and can be trapped during the repeated insertion and withdrawal of the thumb. This condition is also seen in racquet sports where it is caused by similar repetitive pressure on this ulnar digital nerve. Clinically, these patients complain of sensitivity over the nerve and hyperesthesia in the area of irritation. Atrophy of the overlying skin or callus formation is usually present, and palpable induration of the nerve is invariably identifiable, which allows the examiner to "roll" the nerve over the metacarpophalangeal joint prominence and reproduce the patient's complaints. Early recognition and treatment are imperative as this condition may cause permanent disability if unrecognized. Conservative measures should include adjustment of size and spacing along with the fit and slope of the hole in the bowling ball. The racquet player must discontinue

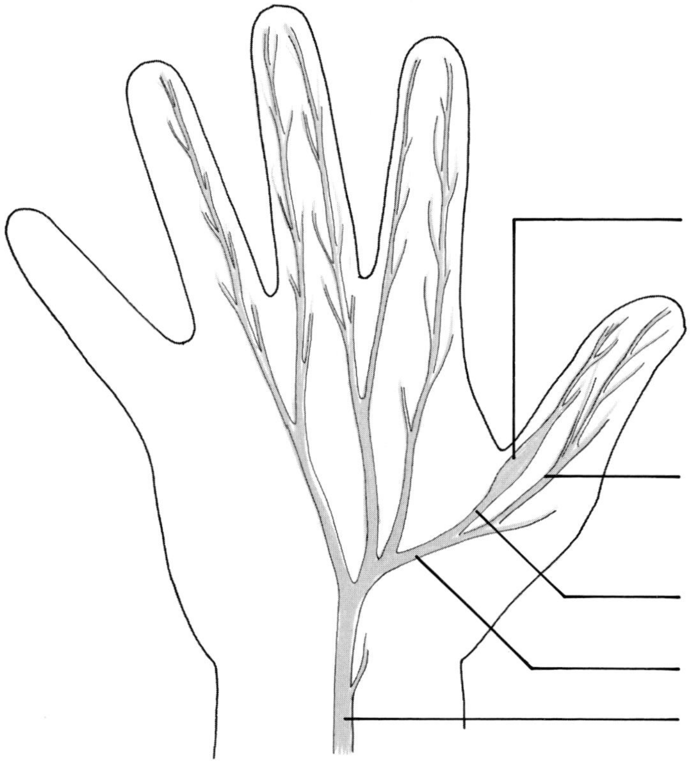

Figure 10–11. Bowler's thumb. Distal sensory branches of the median nerve in the hand and location of perineurial fibrosis of the proper ulnar digital nerve of the thumb. (From Minkow, F. V., Bassett, F. H., III: Clin. Orthop. 83:115, 1972.)

playing for a period of time and shift his or her grip and adjust the thumb position to eliminate repetitive trauma. Protective guards may be tried but patient compliance is poor because of their bulk. Surgery in the form of a neurolysis[7] may be beneficial if symptoms are severe and intractable. Transposition of the nerve posterior to the adductor pollicis tendon has been proposed[22] and seems a practical approach to this repetitive pressure problem. However, surgical treatment will probably never restore the thumb to normal in chronic cases, as nerve damage is usually permanent.

Repetitive trauma to other digital neurovascular bundles can create a similar picture in adjacent digits of the hand. Handball players are frequently affected. Diagnosis and treatment is similar to that for bowler's thumb, with early recognition and conservative treatment being important principles.

Compression Neuropathies of the Ulnar Nerve

Ulnar neuropathy is usually caused by compression or stretching of the nerve at the elbow, proximal forearm, or wrist. The nerve is particularly vulnerable at the elbow, where it passes subcutaneously under a thick band of fascia around the medial epicondyle and is then tethered by the flexor carpi ulnaris as it passes deep to the thick fascial confluence of their two heads. Neuropathy can occur at the elbow by direct trauma, stretching due to cubitus valgus, or repetitive subluxation of the nerve over the epicondyle following rupture of the transverse ligament. The latter has been described in baseball pitchers and is presumably related to microtears in the ligament caused by the throwing mechanism. Compression secondary to hypertrophy of the confluence of the flexor carpi ulnaris heads can also occur in pitchers.[14] An unusual case has been reported in a cross-country skier, apparently related to forceful poling. Extension and pronation of the elbow with simultaneous contraction of the flexor carpi ulnaris and triceps narrows the cubital tunnel, causing nerve irritation.[11]

Patients with ulnar neuropathy will present with elbow pain and paresthesias, frequently radiating to the ring and little fingers. The diagnosis can be made by reproducing the symptoms; if the patient cannot do this by performing the inciting activity, the examiner can usually elicit pain and/or paresthesias by hyperflexing the elbow or percussing the nerve in the groove. In addition, a subluxing nerve can be readily palpated with elbow motion. Motor involvement or objective sensory loss is infrequent and usually indicates prolonged compression. Motor loss is manifested by weakness of wrist flexion (flexor carpi ulnaris) and ring and fifth finger flexion (profundi flexors). Hypothenar and interossei weakness may also be present with weakness of thumb adduction. Clawing of the ring and little fingers can occur, although this sign is usually more pronounced with wrist lesions.

Treatment of early compression consists of rest and avoidance of the causative activity. Nighttime use of an elbow splint for 4 to 6 weeks should be tried as well. Recurrence of symptoms following a rest period may be treated surgically in patients who wish to continue the causative activity or sport. Electrodiagnostic confirmation should be obtained prior to exploration. The presence of motor weakness or intrinsic atrophy indicates more severe nerve damage and is a more definite indication for surgery. The nerve should first be identified proximal to the medial epicondyle and decompressed from the ligament of Struther to the point where it courses between the two heads of the flexor carpi ulnaris. Indications for transposition include failure to find a compressed area, a positive elbow flexion test preoperatively (paresthesias in the ulnar nerve distribution following hyperflexion of the elbow for at least 30 seconds), and the presence of cubitus valgus.[12]

Ulnar neuropathy at the wrist is much less common than median neuropathy, as the nerve passes outside the confines of the carpal canal. Compressive ulnar neuropathies are almost always traumatic because there are no tendons in Guyon's canal to initiate swelling through inflammation. Occasionally, ganglions or lipomas can produce this condition. In patients with a history and symptoms suggestive of a distal ulnar nerve injury, a logical and thorough examination can easily distinguish this from a more proximal lesion. The presence of sensation on the dorsal medial side of the hand suggests that compression is distal to the origin of the dorsal sensory branch; conversely, weakness of the flexor carpi ulnaris or ulnar profundi flexors indicates a more proximal injury. Electromyography and nerve conduction studies help confirm the diagnosis. Roentgenograms, including a carpal tunnel view, should be obtained to diagnose fractures of the hamate and pisiform (Fig. 10–12). Calcific tendinitis of the flexor carpi ulnaris, arthropathy of the pisotriquetral joint, and ligamentous wrist injuries are other causes of pain in this region but are seldom associated with neuropathy.

There are three variations in the motor and sensory loss of the ulnar nerve at the wrist, depending on the point of compression. Type I injuries cause motor weakness of all ulnar intrinsics plus a sensory deficit to the hypothenar palm and ulnar two fingers. This localizes the lesion within or proximal to the canal. Again, normal sensation on the dorsomedial side of the hand excludes forearm or elbow compression. Type II lesions are characterized by normal sensation with weakness of the ulnar innervated intrinsics. The nerve is compressed where it exits from the canal of Guyon next to the hook of the hamate (Fig. 10–12) or

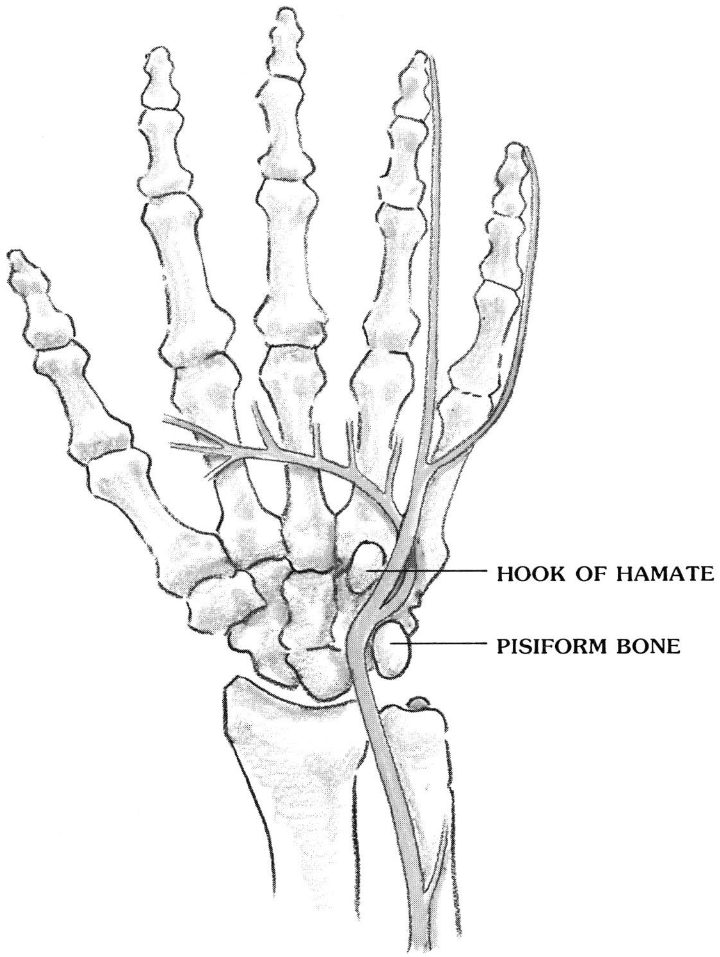

Figure 10–12. Ulnar nerve at Guyon's canal.

more distal in intrinsic musculature. In type III injuries there is a sensory deficit on the palmar medial side of the hand and fingers with no motor deficit. Injury is at the end of or distal to the canal.[34]

Ulnar neuropathy can occur with fractures of the pisiform, hook of the hamate, triquetrum, or base of the fourth or fifth metacarpal.[1] Most fractures can be treated by closed reduction and casting. Type II lesions predominate and complete return of motor function may take up to 6 months or more. Exploration may be indicated in the presence of a large compressive hematoma or if no clinical or EMG evidence of return is observed by 3 months.[27]

Ulnar neuropathy occurs frequently in bicycle riders and has been termed "cyclist's palsy." The condition typically develops following a prolonged road trip or a period of heavy training. Nerve compression is probably caused by direct pressure over the hypothenar eminence as the rider supports the weight of the trunk on the handlebars. Hyperextension of the wrist may also be contributory. The neuropathy almost always presents as a type I lesion with both motor and sensory involvement, although pure motor lesions have been reported. Weakness and atrophy of the dorsal interossei, the abductor digiti minimi, and the adductor pollicis, with or without numbness in the ring and little fingers, are the usual clinical findings. EMG and nerve conduction studies in these patients have confirmed both sensory and motor involvement, with evidence of major axonal destruction in severe cases. The lesion may occur in both hands but usually affects only the dominant extremity, suggesting stronger physical involvement of this hand during cycling.[28] Early diagnosis and interruption of longer cycling tours are the best means of avoiding more severe lesions; wearing gloves and padding the handlebars are good preventive measures. The patient should also be asked about the position of the handlebars, as deeply mounted handlebars for faster cycling have been implicated as a contributing factor. Avoiding a hyperextended hand position and frequent changing of the hand position are also helpful. In patients with objective clinical findings, cycling should be avoided or at least limited to occasional noncompetitive short sessions. Cyclist's palsy tends to resolve spontaneously but can seriously limit the normal use of the hand and ability to work for months. If there is evidence of progressive deterioration or persistence of denervation beyond 3 months, exploration of the nerve should be considered.[10]

Compression Neuropathies of the Radial Nerve

Neuropathies related to radial nerve compression from the elbow to the hand are unusual in their presentation and frequently misdiagnosed. Because motor involvement of the radial nerve is usually the exception rather than the rule, physical findings and symptoms are seldom specific enough to support a diagnosis. The clinical complaints following a radial nerve injury in this area are of weakness and pain. Pain rather than a motor deficit is the cause of this weakness and often involves structures innervated deep within the forearm and wrist.

Compression of the Radial Nerve in the Forearm

Radial tunnel syndrome has been called resistant tennis elbow because the patient has often been treated unsuccessfully for lateral epicondylitis by various conservative measures before the diagnosis of this much rarer condition is made. Indeed, early clinical findings typically mimic those of tennis elbow with pain and tenderness over the lateral epicondyle. Careful examination, however, will also reveal tenderness over the radial tunnel with digital compression of the nerve in the radial tunnel four finger breadths distal to the lateral epicondyle. In addition, there is usually pain with resisted supination of the extended forearm and a positive middle finger sign (resisted extension of the middle finger elicits pain in the proximal forearm by compressing the fibrous edge of the extensor carpi radialis brevis against the nerve). These findings, combined with localized tenderness along the radial tunnel (when compared with the opposite side), are considered a relative indication for surgical decompression. The EMG is very helpful when positive, showing significant delay in motor latencies when measured from the spiral groove to the extensor digitorum communis.[31] Conservative measures should be tried initially and include rest, splinting the extremity with the forearm in a neutral or most comfortable position, and anti-inflammatory medication. The differential diagnosis should include wrist extensor tendinitis, stenosis of the orbicular ligament, fibrillation of the radial head, and cervical spine disorders.[19] Surgery is reserved for refractory cases and should include a complete radial nerve decompression. The nerve is exposed just above the elbow flexor crease where it lies between the brachioradialis and brachialis. It is then followed through the radial tunnel and supinator muscle to the point where the nerve arborizes. All impinging structures in the radial tunnel are released and refractory lateral epicondylitis surgery carried out where appropriate.

An unusual radial neuropathy called *runner's radial palsy* should not be confused with radial tunnel neuritis. It is manifested by numbness in the sensory distribution of the left forearm and hand in runners who keep their arms acutely flexed at the elbow. This is thought to be caused by compression of the radial nerve between the humerus and the triceps. Symptoms will resolve by simply having the patient run with the elbows in a more extended posture.[30]

Distal Posterior Interosseous Nerve Syndrome

Dorsal wrist pain in athletes is almost always related to repetitive, forceful hyperextension. The more frequent causes include the scaphoid or radial impaction syndrome, tears of the scapholunate ligament, occult ganglia, and carpometacarpal sprains. These injuries are seen most commonly in gymnasts.[16]

Distal posterior interosseous nerve impingement should be considered a diagnosis of exclusion after these more common causes have been ruled out. Such a work-up should include radiographs, including a motion series (ulnar deviation, radial deviation, flexion and extension, and a clenched fist view), to rule out carpal instability patterns. Also, one should look carefully at the dorsal radioscaphoid joint for osteophytes or loose bone fragments, which could cause this dorsal wrist pain.

On clinical examination, no masses are identified, there is absence of painful clicking or snapping in the wrist, and the motor and sensory findings are normal. Pain is elicited by forced wrist extension or digital compression over the dorsal wrist in flexion. If rest, splinting, and anti-inflammatory drugs fail to resolve the symptoms, the nerve should be injected with 0.5% bupivacaine just proximal to the wrist joint. If there is immediate relief of symptoms with recurrence later, then surgical transection of the nerve should be considered.[2]

Superficial Radial Nerve Compression

Cheiralgia paresthetica, or Wartenberg's disease, is not usually related to any specific sports activity but may be seen in athletes who wear a tight wristwatch or other wristband, such as those worn by weight lifters. It is mentioned because it is the second most common mononeuropathy, after meralgia paresthetica (irritation of the lateral femoral cutaneous nerve in the lower extremity).[35] It also can be confused with other problems, including DeQuervain's tenosynovitis, sprain or arthropathy of the thumb carpometacarpal joint, and gamekeeper's thumb.

Patients usually present with numbness or decreased sensation over the dorsoradial hand and the dorsum of the thumb and index finger. The clinical findings include a false-positive Finkelstein sign (forced thumb flexion with ulnar deviation provoking first dorsal compartment pain). However, there will be a Tinel's sign over the superficial branch of the radial nerve in the midforearm and decreased sensation over the dorsoradial hand and thumb when compared with the opposite side. In addition, thumb extension or abduction should not elicit pain in the absence of coexisting first dorsal extensor tenosynovitis. Symptoms usually resolve after removing the constricting band. Occasionally, this neuritis will occur in the absence of a constricting band, and these patients usually report direct trauma to the radial forearm or a twisting injury to the wrist or forearm. Treatment in these groups should be rest and splinting.

Electrodiagnostic studies are not helpful, and in resistant cases, a diagnostic block should be performed prior to surgically exploring the nerve. It is recommended to first block the lateral antebrachial cutaneous nerve to rule out an associated injury of this nerve.[6]

Compartment Syndrome

Any condition in which the circulation and function of tissue within a closed space is compromised by increased pressure within that space can be referred to as a compartment syndrome. This condition is well recognized in the upper extremity but unfortunately has been given various names, such as Volkmann's ischemia[34] and crush syndrome.[32] A useful clinical approach is to thoroughly examine the athlete who exhibits apparent inappropriate pain, sensory symptoms, or motor weakness. These symptoms will persist and/or progress on frequent re-examinations. The passive stretch test (gentle stretching of the ischemic muscle causing dramatic increase in pain) and the palpation test (pressure on the involved compartment, which is noted to be markedly tense and tender) are specific signs of the compartment syndrome process and are helpful in establishing the diagnosis. Compartment pressure measurements[21, 25] with possible decompressive fasciotomy type surgery[26] should be performed immediately. Failure to do so can result in irreversible muscle necrosis and joint contractures. Preventive measures to avoid this condition include the routine use of flexibility and stretching exercises prior to weight lifting and other activities.

Reflex Sympathetic Dystrophy

Crushing injuries to the upper extremity during sporting activities may result in a participant's complaining of chronic pain described as burning and persistent in nature. This intensity of the pain will appear to be out of proportion to the severity of the primary injury and will often be associated with tenderness and markedly increased sensitivity of the entire upper extremity. Such a clinical picture is quite suggestive of reflex sympathetic dystrophy. This syndrome is manifested by four more or less constant characteristics: (1) intense or unduly prolonged pain, (2) vasomotor disturbance, (3) delayed functional recovery, and (4) various associated trophic changes.[16] While the etiology is unknown, the most tenable hypothesis is of a widespread disturbance of centrally mediated autonomic regulation.[8, 20] Awareness of this entity of pain of apparently unwarranted magnitude is critical to appropriate early treatment and avoidance of progression to more chronic dystrophy. Vigorous and judicious physical therapy with hand usage and dynamic splinting, mild analgesic and anti-inflammatory medication, and the occasional course of tapering corticosteroids[5, 16] appear to be the best early treatment measures. Pain management techniques such as stellate ganglion blocks, transcutaneous electrical nerve stimulation, biofeedback, or electroacupuncture[41] are appropriate for more chronic cases but are much less predictable in their efficacy. Early recognition is the key to successful treatment.

Conclusion

While complaints of arm pain, cramping, numbness, and impaired dexterity are common in the athlete, compression neuropathy in the forearm, wrist, and hand are surprisingly rare. When one considers the intensity of the athlete's training program as well as the tremendous forces to which these areas are subjected, it is amazing that more problems in this regard do not occur. When compressive neuropathy is diagnosed, however, appropriate changes in the technique and frequency of the individual activity as well as appropriate adjustment in the equipment used for the particular sport can often allow participation in athletic endeavors without permanent adverse problems.

REFERENCES

1. Baird, D. B., Friendenberg, Z. B.: Delayed ulnar-nerve palsy following a fracture of the hamate. J. Bone Joint Surg. 50A:570, 1968.
2. Carr, D., Davis, P.: Distal posterior interosseous nerve syndrome. J. Hand Surg. 10A:873, 1985.
3. Casten, D. F., Betches, A. M.: Reflex sympathetic dystrophy, Surg. Gynecol. Obstet. 100:97, 1955.
4. Chan, C. S., Chow, S. P.: Electroacupuncture in the treatment of post-traumatic sympathetic dystrophy (Sudeck's atrophy). Br. J. Anaesth. 53:899, 1981.
5. Christensen, K., Jenson, E. M., Noer, I.: The reflex dystrophy syndrome response to treatment with systemic corticosteroids. Acta Chir. Scand. 148:653, 1982.
6. Dellon, A. L., Mackinnon, S. E.: Radial sensory nerve entrapment in the forearm. J. Hand Surg. 11A:199, 1986.
7. Dobyns, J. H., Obrian, E. T., Linscheid, R. L., et al.: Bowler's thumb: diagnosis and treatment. A review of seventeen cases. J. Bone Joint Surg. 54A:751, 1972.
8. Drucker, W. R., Hubay, C. A., Holden, W. D., et al.: Pathogenesis of post traumatic sympathetic dystrophy. Am. J. Surg. 97:454, 1959.
9. Eversman, W. W.: Compression and entrapment neuropathies of the upper extremity. J. Hand Surg. 8:759, 1983.
10. Frontera, W. R.: Case Report—Cyclist's palsy: clinical and electrodiagnostic findings. Br. J. Sports Med. 17:91, 1983.
11. Fulkerson, J. P.: Transient ulnar neuropathy from Nordic skiing. Clin. Orthop. 153:230, 1980.
12. Green, D. P.: Operative Hand Surgery, Vol. 2. New York, Churchill Livingstone, 1982.
13. Green, D. P.: Diagnostic and therapeutic value of carpal tunnel injection. J. Hand Surg. 9A:850, 1984.
14. Hang, Y.-S.: Tardy ulnar neuritis in a Little League baseball player. Am. J. Sports Med. 9:244, 1981.
15. Kopell, H. P., Thompson, W.A.L.: Pronator syndrome. N. Engl. J. Med. 259:713, 1958.
16. Kozin, F., Ryan, L. M., Carerra, G. F., et al.: The reflex sympathetic dystrophy syndrome (ASDS). III. Scintigraphic studies, further evidence of the therapeutic efficacy of systemic cortico-steroids and proposed diagnostic criteria. Am. J. Med. 70:23, 1981.
17. Linscheid, R. L.: Personal communication.
18. Linscheid, R. L., Dobyns, J. H.: Athletic injuries of the wrist. Clin. Orthop. 198:141, 1985.
19. Lister, G. D., Besole, R. B., Kleinert, H. E.: The radial tunnel syndrome. J. Hand Surg. 4:52, 1979.
20. Lorente, de No, R.: Analysis of the activity of the chains of internuncial neurons, J. Neurophysiol. 1:207, 1938.
21. Matsen, F. A., III, Clawson, D. K.: Compartmental syndromes. Clin. Orthop. 113:2, 1975.
22. Minkow, F. V., Bassett, F. H., III: Bowler's thumb. Clin. Orthop. 83:112, 1972.
23. Morrey, B. F.: The Elbow and Its Disorders. Philadelphia, W. B. Saunders, 1985, p. 692.
24. Morris, H. H., Peters, B. H.: Pronator syndrome: clinical and electrophysiologic features in seven cases. J. Neurol. Neurosurg. Psychiatry 39:461, 1976.
25. Murbarak, S. J., Hagens, A. R.: Acute compartment syndromes: diagnosis and treatment with the aid of the wick catheter. J. Bone Joint Surg. 60A: 1091, 1978.

26. Murbarak, S. J., Hagens, A. R.: Acute compartment syndromes. Surg. Clin. North Am. 63:539, 1983.
27. Nisenfield, F. G., Neviaser, R. J.: Fracture of the hook of the hamate: a diagnosis easily missed. J. Trauma 14:612, 1974.
28. North, J., Dietz, V., Mauritz, K. H.: Cyclist's palsy. J. Neurol. Sci. 47:111, 1980.
29. Parkes, A. R.: Traumatic ischemia of peripheral nerves. Br. J. Surg. 32:403, 1944.
30. Pickering, T. G.: Runner's radial palsy. N. Engl. J. Med. 305:768, 1981.
31. Roles, N. C., Maudsley, R. H.: Radial tunnel syndrome—resistant tennis elbow as a nerve entrapment. J. Bone Joint Surg. 54B:499, 1972.
32. Schreiber, S. N., Leibowitz, M. R., Burnstein, L. H.: Limb compression and renal impairment (crush syndrome) following narcotic overdose. J. Bone Joint Surg. 54A:168, 1972.
33. Seddon, H. J: Three types of nerve injury. Brain 66:237, 1943.
34. Shea, J. D., McClain, E. J.: Ulnar-nerve compression syndromes at and below the wrist. J. Bone Joint Surg. 51A:1095, 1969.
35. Sprofkin, B. E.: Cheiralgia paresthetica—Wartenberg's disease. Neurology 4:857, 1954.
36. Stellbrink, G.: Compression of the palmar branch of the median nerve by atypical palmaris longus muscle. Hand Chir. 4:155, 1972.
37. Stern, P. J., Kutz, J. E.: An unusual variant of anterior interosseous nerve syndrome. J. Hand Surg. 5:32, 1983.
38. Struthers, J.: Anatomical and Physiological Observations, Part I. Edinburgh, Sutherland and Knox, 1854.
39. Struthers, J. : On a peculiarity of the humerus and humeral artery. Month. Med. Sci. 8:264, 1948.
40. Sunderland, S: Nerves and Nerve Injuries. Baltimore, Williams & Wilkins, 1968, p. 749.
41. Talesnick, J.: The palmar cutaneous branch of the median nerve and the approach to the carpal tunnel. J. Bone Joint Surg. 55A:1212, 1973.

CHAPTER

11

Vascular Injuries to the Athletic Hand

E. F. Shaw Wilgis, M.D.

While vascular injuries in the athlete's hand are rare, they are seen occasionally. An understanding of their etiology underlies their treatment and hopefully their prevention.

While most vascular injuries that involve repeated minor blunt trauma and such serious late consequences as thrombosis and aneurysm, open injuries involving lacerations and direct vascular trauma are occasionally encountered. Both the arterial and the venous systems can be injured, although the major complications come from acute arterial injury.

One such complication is hemorrhage. With this in mind, Halstead once wrote, "True it is as I have so often said, that the surgeon's method of dealing with the blood vessels is a criterion of his proficiency in his art—one of the chief fascinations of surgery is the management of wounded vessels, the avoidance of hemorrhage." He continued, "The only weapon with which the unconscious patient can immediately retaliate upon the incompetent surgeon is hemorrhage. If he bleeds to death, it may be presumed that the surgeon is to blame; whereas, if he dies of pneumonia, peritonitis or other infection or from an unphysiological operative performance, the surgeon's incompetence may not be so evident."

Because unrecognized or untreated vascular injuries can lead to gangrene or contracture, it is incumbent upon the treating physician to identify and properly manage them. Most open vascular injuries encountered in the athlete are associated with fractures. Any compound fracture of a long bone in the upper extremity or hand must be inspected with the thought that the bone could have lacerated an adjacent vessel. The most obvious sign of such an injury, of course, is excessive bleeding from a wound.

Appropriate pressure dressing at the scene will, in most cases, provide adequate control of hemorrhage. At the hospital and prior to operation, an extensive evaluation of the vascular system should be made, including visualization of the arterial tree by various angiographic techniques. During the operative exposure of the fracture, the vessels should be visualized and repaired if necessary. An injury with sufficient damage to cause a laceration in all likelihood will need resection of the involved zone of injury and direct repair and/or bridging of the defect with venous interposition graft.

Direct blunt trauma sometimes associated with fractures can also cause disruption of the vascular tree. The most common site of this kind of vascular injury is at the joint level where, to allow for motion, there is a looser anatomic arrangement of vessels than there is proximal and distal to it. Injuries to the clavicle and shoulder region can damage the underlying subclavian and axillary arteries. As the vessels course over the first rib they can be caught between the clavicle and first rib and severed. Venous injury in this region is also common and can present with a large hematoma that must be evacuated before the vessel is repaired. If a hematoma is allowed to resolve, there will be scarring in the surrounding brachial plexus region with resultant damage. Damage to the axillary artery following shoulder dislocation has been reported and should be suspected if the involved arm shows signs of vascular insufficiency or if an expanding hematoma is detected in the supraclavicular and axillary space. Surgical exploration is required and should not be unduly delayed for arteriographic studies. Contrast angiography or digital subtraction angiography through the venous route should be done for localization of the injury, but if massive bleeding is present, as evidenced by shock, surgery should be undertaken immediately. Axillary artery injury associated with shoulder dislocation is a serious complication and mortality has been reported. The sports doctor faced with a patient with acute shoulder dislocation must be aware of this complication.

Injury to the brachial artery in the region of the elbow is a common complication of fracture-dislocation of the elbow and supracondylar fracture of the humerus. The physician should study the distal pulses, and if they are diminished or absent, should institute further diagnostic testing including Doppler evaluation, pulse volume recording, and/or contrast visualization of the arterial tree to demonstrate whether acute occlusion or rupture of the brachial artery has occurred. When direct surgical repair of the brachial artery is required, all damaged vessels must be excised before anastomosis is attempted because damaged intima will cause thrombosis if left in place. If there is a gap remaining after the area of damage is excised, then interpositional vein grafting using a vein of the same size from another limb, preferably the leg, should be done. Once arterial repair has been accomplished the distal muscle group should be evaluated for compartmental swelling and a fasciotomy done if necessary.

The most common vascular injury in the forearm is compartmental pressure elevation associated with acute trauma or chronic repetitive trauma, which can lead to muscle ischemia and eventual contraction is left untreated. If this complication is suspected, intercompartmental tissue pressure measurement by either Whiteside's technique or the Wick-Catheter method should indicate whether fasciotomy is necessary.

At the hand and wrist level, direct injuries are less common, but dislocation of the wrist can rupture the radial ulnar artery and produce ischemic changes in the hand. With injuries at this level, a surgeon must be aware of the anatomic variations in the hand. In approximately 20 percent of the population, either the radial or the ulnar artery does not contribute to the superficial palmar arch, thereby making the contralateral artery the most important in the hand. The presence of capillary filling is *not* adequate evidence that circulation is sufficient. Under these circumstances, digital pressure recordings of each individual digit should be taken to see if the blood supply to the remainder of the hand is within normal limits with the occlusion of one or more of the major arteries.

Acute angulated fractures in the region of the proximal phalanges of the digits can cause arterial embarrassment to the distal part of the finger. In this situation, the surgeon's primary concern is to reduce the fracture adequately. When this is done, the circulation of the digit distally often improves dramatically and essentially returns to normal. However, if circulation is not improved, then revascularization of the digit should be performed.

Of far more importance, in terms of both numbers of cases and potential complications, is vascular injury from blunt trauma, which can be found in any sport involving repetitive impact of the hand. Such injuries have been reported in baseball, handball, and volleyball and can include thrombosis and aneurysm formation in the wrist and digital vessels.

Mechanism of Injury

The arterial wall is composed of the intima, media, and adventitia, and depending on the level of damage within the arterial wall, either thrombosis or aneurysm formation can occur. Damage to the intima alone usually results in thrombosis within the lumen. When the intima is damaged, subendothelial connective tissue is exposed; circulating platelets attach to the connective tissue and undergo a secretory process known as the release action. During this reaction, the contents of certain intracellular granules are expelled from within the platelet into the surrounding plasma. The release reaction is not simply a disruption of the platelet; rather, it is a specific secretory process similar to the release of chemical amines from the adrenal medulla. The platelet components that enter the plasma have important biologic activity, i.e., they induce the release reaction in additional platelets, causing the process to be self-perpetuating. When the platelets aggregate, a platelet thrombus forms. The two most common causes of surface-induced thrombosis are injury to the normal endothelium, such as repetitive trauma, and an ulcerated atherosclerotic plaque that attracts platelets to the exposed subendothelial connective tissue. The combination of trauma and atherosclerotic plaquing within one region predisposes it to thrombus formation, which of course, makes the athlete in the older age range much more prone to thrombosis of the small vessels of the wrist and hand.

The arterial tree of the hand is subject to blunt trauma where it is not protected by fascial structures. The ulnar artery is vulnerable from the distal border of the continuation of the transverse carpal ligament until it enters the protection of the palmar fascia. A force applied to the ulnar aspect of the palm will crush the ulnar artery against the unyielding hook of the hamate. The term "hypothenar hammer syndrome" has been applied to the spectrum of injuries to which the ulnar artery is susceptible in this region.

There are several reports in the literature of blunt injury to the radial and ulnar arteries in sports enthusiasts. Kostianen and Orava[3] have reported three cases of this syndrome in volleyball players. In all of these cases, young volleyball players experienced symptoms of impaired circulation in the hands and on examination showed poor flow through the radial and/or ulnar arteries of the right wrist due to repeated ball and floor impact during volleyball training and playing. The most interesting aspect of this report is that all three of these patients were treated conservatively with cessation of smoking and vasodilating agents. The vascular lesions were reversible and all three players continued to play after a period of rest and treatment. Seen at 4 months and 1 year postincident, the pulses were essentially normal. This, then, represents the first stage of the problem, i.e., traumatic vasospasm essentially produced by chronic repetitive trauma. In two of the cases, the apparently thrombosed arteries were spontaneously opened during 8 weeks of treatment with rest and vasodilatation, indicating that these were probably vasospastic conditions. What is important is that these conditions were diagnosed early when rest and pharmacologic treatment could eliminate the need for surgery. Further, they prevented additional damage by the use of protective padding or covers on the palm and forearm area.

Similarly, the digital vessels are vulnerable to trauma as they exit from the protection of the palmar fascia. In an interesting report Lowrey, Chadwick, and Waltman[4] described digital vessel trauma resulting from repetitive impact in baseball catchers. In order to secure better control and to permit the one-handed catch, catchers now have less padding and a thinner preformed pocket in their mitts, and the incidence of digital vessel trauma has increased. They studied 22 professional catchers with the Allen's test, the Doppler flow test, and radioactive angiography. Only 9 of the 22 athletes had evidence of normal circulation in the left index finger—the digit that receives the repetitive impact. Twenty-one of the 22 had normal circulation in the right hand. Of the 13 athletes with decreased circulation in the index finger, two had a positive Allen's test and all had impaired flow. Interestingly enough, of the nine athletes who had normal circulation, all used a thick golf glove or handball glove beneath the catcher's mitt, and three also used some type of sponge. In four of the catchers with impaired flow to the index finger, there was also evidence of impairment of flow to the radial digital vessel of the middle finger. This report indicates that repetitive trauma does in fact alter the circulation and in a certain percentage of cases does cause thrombosis of the digital vessels. They also indicate that more padding in the catcher's mitt can prevent this digital vessel injury. Certainly any catchers who have had cold intolerance and evidence of vascular change should use extra padding to prevent additional trauma and further thrombosis.

Further corroboration was provided in another report by Buckhout and Warner[1] who reviewed the digital perfusion of handball players and

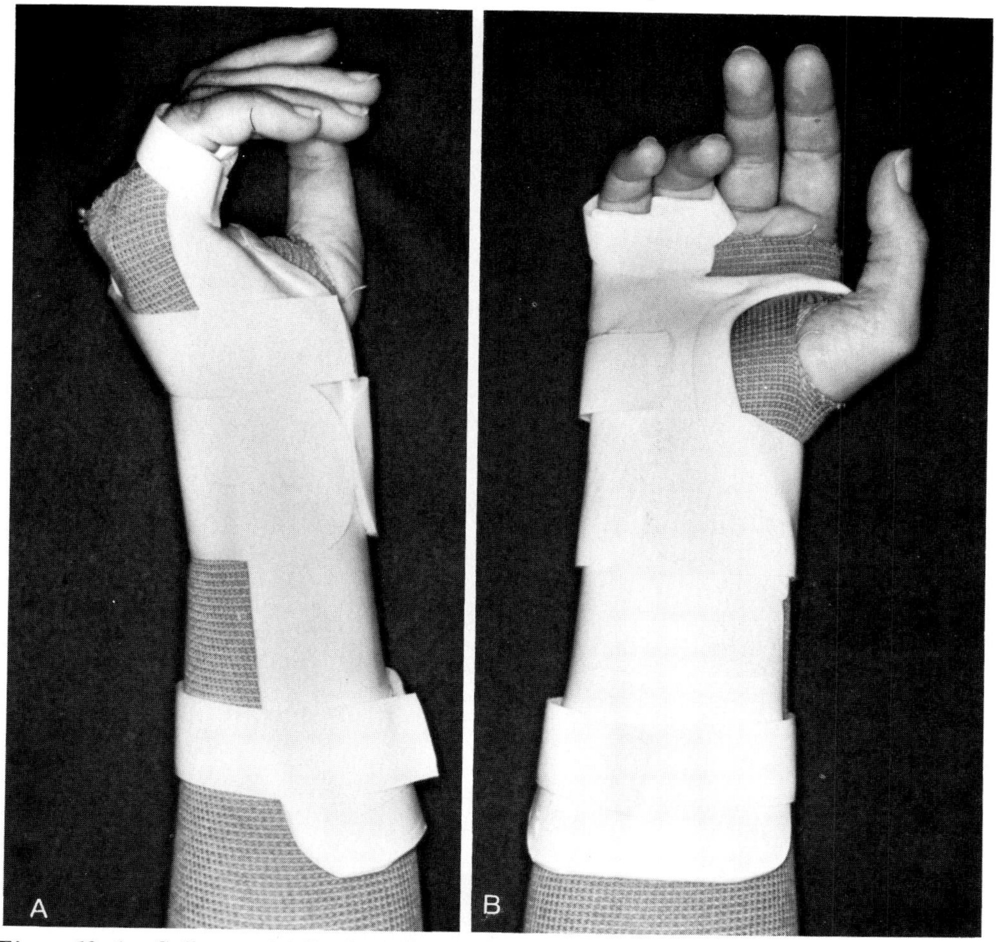

Figure 12–1. Splint used following metacarpal fractures. The MCP joints are positioned in flexicn with the IP joints excluded.

and limited joint flexion. This position also relaxes the deforming forces from the intrinsic muscles. The proximal interphalangeal (PIP) and distal interphalangeal (DIP) joints are usually excluded to prevent inadvertent stiffness due to overimmobilization. If there is concern about digital rotation, the physician may request buddy taping of the fractured digit to an adjacent digit. If maximum control of rotation is essential, the interphalangeal joints are included at neutral position in the splint (Fig. 12–2). With stable base and proximal shaft fractures, a well-molded wrist splint may provide sufficient support while allowing full digital range of motion (Fig. 12–3). All casts and splints should be well-molded to maintain architectural integrity, keeping in mind both the longitudinal and the transverse arches important to hand function.

The initiation of active range of motion is dependent on fracture stability. With closed reduction, active motion is usually begun 3 weeks postinjury. Passive motion is begun when the fracture is clinically healed —approximately 6 weeks postinjury. In cases in which rigid types of

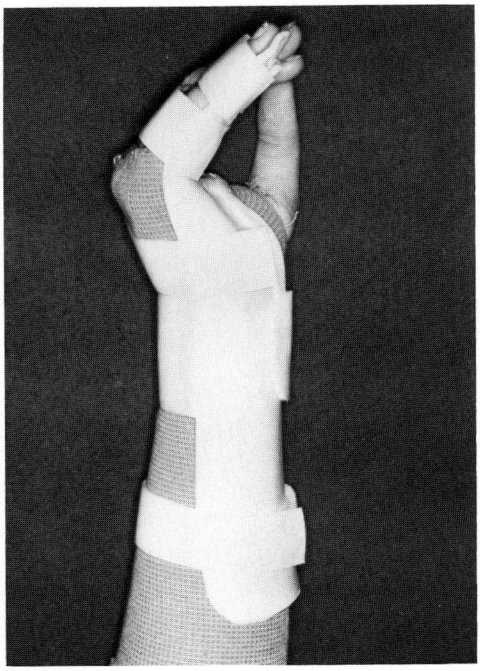

Figure 12–2. "Safe" position resting pan splint.

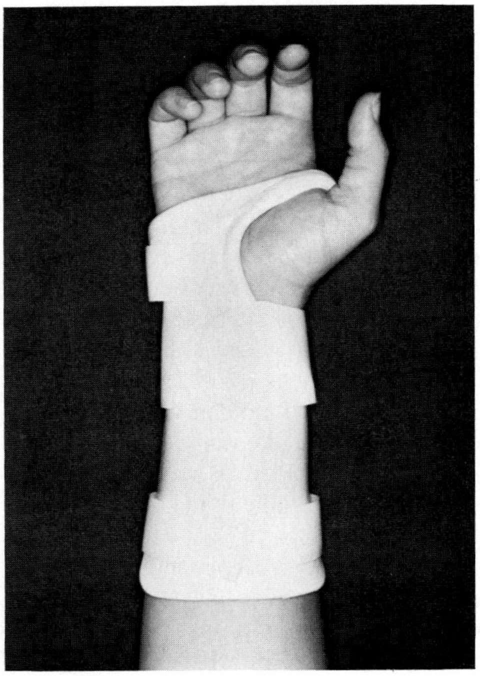

Figure 12–3. Custom-fitted wrist immobilization splint.

internal fixation are used (e.g., screws, AO plates), fracture stability may be sufficient to allow active and passive range of motion within the first postoperative week. Interval splint wear between exercise sessions is necessary until the fracture is clinically healed.

Problems associated with metacarpal fracture management must be recognized and addressed by the therapist. These may include (1) excessive edema, (2) tendon adherence, (3) joint contracture, and (4) intrinsic muscle contracture.

Edema is a common problem with blows to the hand that result in soft tissue damage as well as metacarpal fracture. Methods of controlling dorsal hand edema include elevation, light compressive dressings, Isotoner gloves, elastic wraps, and Jobst stockinettes.

Extensor tendon adherence is more common than flexor tendon adherence at the metacarpal level. Due to the amount of soft tissue between the metacarpals and flexors, adherence of the flexor tendons is rarely a problem. On the dorsum of the hand, the extensor tendons immediately overlie the periosteum and significant trauma may produce scar adhesions that result in MCP joint extensor lags and extrinsic extensor tendon tightness. Open reduction and internal fixation techniques may contribute further to extensor tendon adherence. Beneficial treatment techniques for minimizing extensor tendon adhesions include (1) isolated extensor digitorum communis (EDC) exercises, (2) scar massage and retraction, (3) Silastic pressure molds, and (4) functional electrical muscle stimulation (FES). Isolated EDC exercises are done by extending the MCP joints while maintaining the IP joints in flexion (Fig. 12–4). Scar massage and retraction are performed to soften and elongate adhesions. Scar retraction consists of passive manipulation of adhesions in the opposite direction of active tendon pull. For example, a scar over the dorsum of the hand is

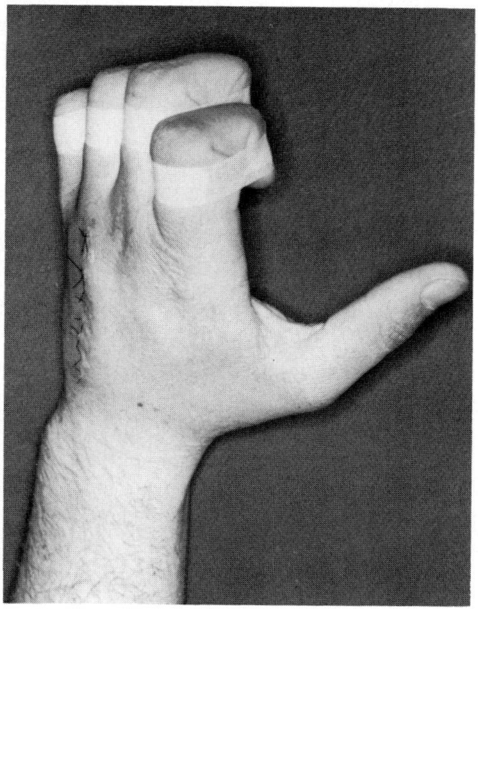

Figure 12–4. Isolated active MCP joint extension facilitates excursion of the extensor digitorum communis.

mobilized in a distal direction during active extension and a proximal direction during active flexion. Silastic pressure molds (e.g., Otoform-K, Silastic Elastomer) apply firm positive pressure over scar tissue, which induces stretching and realignment of collagen bundles and reduces vascularity. This pressure may also produce ischemia, which retards synthesis of collagen fibers.[12] FES is beneficial in enhancing tendon excursion and muscle strength. The "active" electrode is placed on the EDC muscle belly. This modality is excellent for home use and may be employed in conjunction with scar retraction techniques. The reader is referred to *Functional Electrical Stimulation–A Practical Clinical Guide*[2] for further instruction on the use of this modality.

To decrease extrinsic extensor tendon tightness, composite digital flexion with simultaneous wrist flexion is performed. If the fracture is clinically healed, the digits may be taped in flexion and a light weight placed on the dorsum of the hand for a more aggressive stretch (Fig. 12–5).

MCP joint extension contractures often develop if close attention is not directed toward proper positioning and exercise, especially with head and neck fractures. As mentioned earlier, the MCP joints are placed in flexion to maintain maximum collateral ligament length. Once range of motion exercises are initiated, isolated MCP joint exercises are emphasized. Motion may be encouraged through use of Velcro finger trappers (Fig. 12–6). If sufficient bone healing has occurred, digital flexion taping (Fig. 12–7) or periodic dynamic flexion splints (Fig. 12–8) may prove beneficial in increasing flexion. Sufficient bone healing should be determined by the physician before advancing to these more aggressive measures.

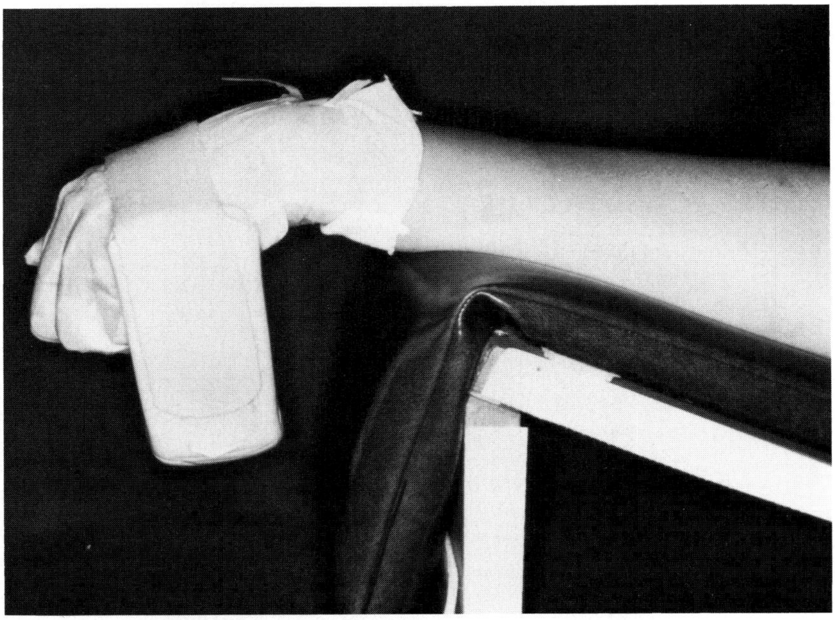

Figure 12–5. Composite flexion taping in combination with a dorsal wrist weight places stretch on the extrinsic extensor tendons.

Figure 12–6. Velcro trappers help isolate MCP joint motion during exercise.

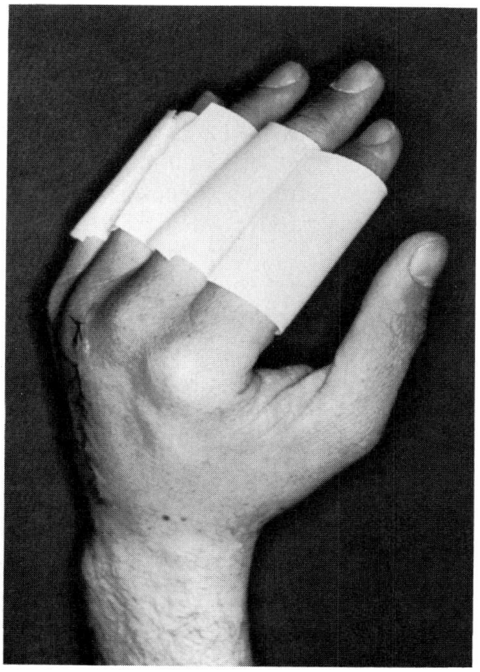

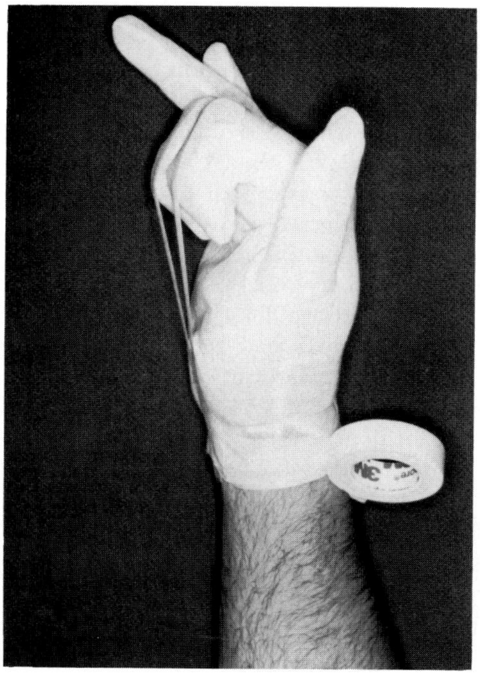

Figure 12–7. Finger flexion taping is performed to increase passive joint mobility. Additional layers of tape are used to serially increase joint flexion.

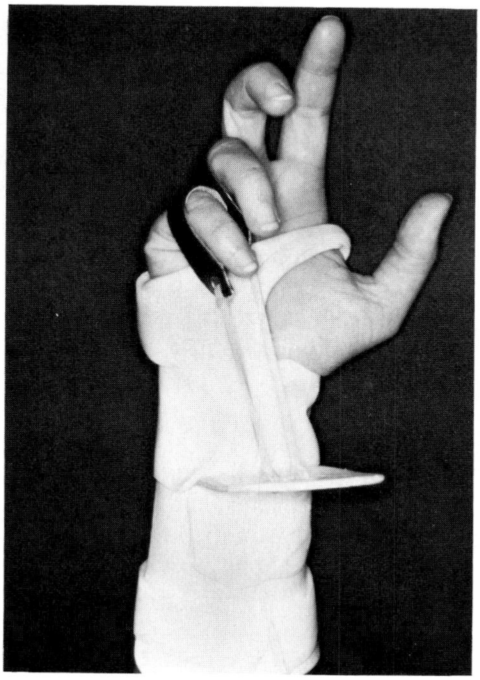

Figure 12–8. Dynamic MCP joint flexion splint.

While intrinsic tightness is a less common problem, it may result from the direct trauma and edema of severe crushing injuries. While it is necessary to immobilize metacarpal fractures in the intrinsic plus position, this further promotes intrinsic tightness. Patients are instructed in intrinsic stretches once it is safe to begin motion. The interphalangeal joints are passively held in flexion while the MCP joint is passively extended.

Strength-building programs, permissible as early as 6 weeks postinjury, should be initiated at the discretion of the physician based on fracture consolidation. The patient should be placed on a gradual progressive strength-building program for the entire upper extremity, not just the hand.

Continued protection is often necessary once the athlete is allowed to return to practice or competition, especially with contact sports. Splints must provide sufficient protection for the specific injury, be compatible with participation in the given sport, and comply with athletic regulations pertaining to splints on the hand. The therapist must acquire information regarding "illegal equipment," since different sports and leagues have varying rules. Integrating these factors, the therapist must use ingenuity in designing and fabricating an appropriate splint. The ideal splint protects the fracture site itself, as well as the areas proximal and distal to it. Protective splinting of any type following metacarpal fractures should include rigid dorsal support, as well as some type of shock-absorbing material to protect against blows to the dorsum of the hand. Some type of wrist support is required for metacarpal base fractures, whereas a well-molded palmar bar (Fig. 12–9) may provide sufficient support for shaft fractures. A protective splint for metacarpal head and neck fractures should extend beyond the MCP joints; however, the interphalangeal joints may be excluded to allow increased function (Fig. 12–10). This latter splint may be hand based or forearm based depending on the degree of bone healing and protection needed. Most athletic associations permit playing casts composed of GE RTV-11 silicone rubber compound* with the addition of external padding (Fig. 12–11). This material is strong and provides moderate protection yet is semiflexible and does not pose any danger to other players participating in contact sports. However, it is somewhat bulky and athletes needing fine hand coordination may not find it suitable.

Although normal range of motion and strength are usually restored following metacarpal fractures, a few potential problems do exist as mentioned previously, and it is important that these be anticipated and addressed early in the therapeutic process. Appropriate early intervention will greatly reduce or avoid the development of limited MCP joint motion and extrinsic extensor tendon tightness.

Proximal Phalanx Fractures

Phalangeal fractures are among the most frequently seen fractures in athletes, and of these, fractures of the proximal phalanx are probably the most common. The complex anatomic structures surrounding the proximal phalanx make injury to this area particularly difficult to manage. The

---

* General Electric Co., Silicone Products Division, Waterford, NY 12188.

Figure 12–9. A well-molded palmar bar moderately supports the metacarpals.

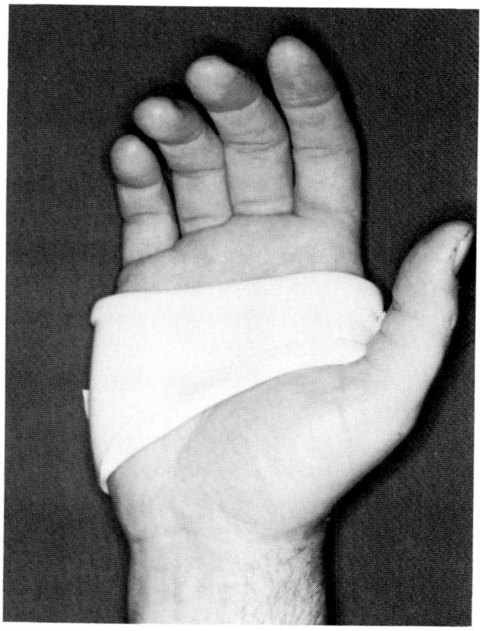

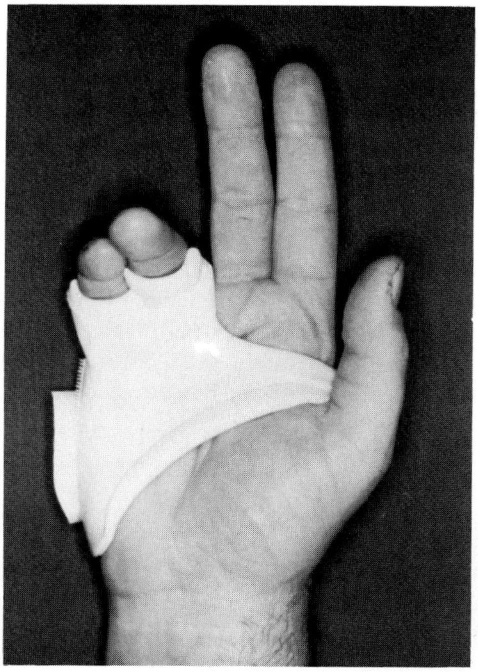

Figure 12–10 A hand-based splint with the MCP joints in flexion may be used to support metacarpal head and neck fractures.

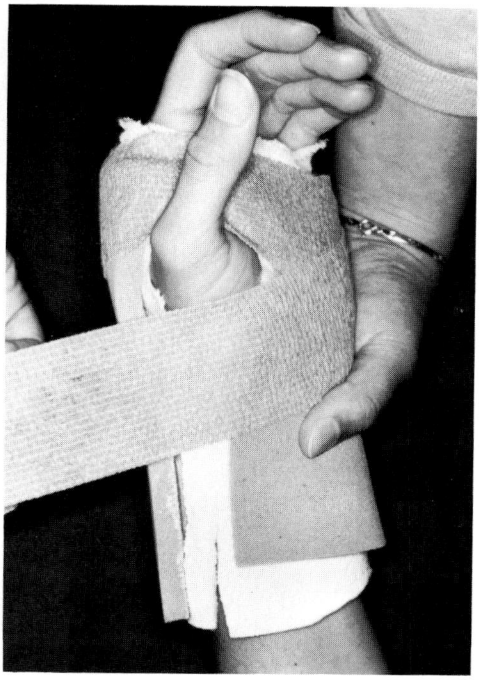

Figure 12–11. Application of a playing cast composed of GE RTV-11 silicone rubber compound.

close proximity of the digital flexor tendons lying volar to the phalanx and the central extensor mechanism and lateral bands lying dorsal often make maintenance of tendon glide after injury difficult. This problem is certainly compounded when either of the important articulations of the MCP or PIP joints are involved, in which case limited joint mobility also occurs.

The position of immobilization is dependent upon the location of the fracture. Base and shaft fractures are immobilized in the intrinsic plus position, also referred to as the "safe" position. This position includes the wrist in approximately 25° of dorsiflexion, the MCP joints in 70° of flexion, and the interphalangeal joints in full extension (see Fig. 12–2). Unlike the MCP collateral ligaments, the PIP collateral ligaments are tight throughout the entire range of motion. Therefore, the PIP joints are placed in extension to minimize the risk of developing flexion contractures. Slight PIP joint flexion may be indicated in transverse fractures of the proximal phalanx to prevent recurvatum type angulation. Stable head and neck fractures are placed in a digital splint maintaining the interphalangeal joints in full extension (Fig. 12–12). If they are unstable, the physician may request the aforementioned safe position splint.

The course of rehabilitation following a proximal phalanx fracture can be quite variable depending on the exact type and location of the fracture and on the chosen method of reduction. As a general rule, there is adequate fracture consolidation to allow active range of motion exercises at 3 weeks postinjury and passive range of motion between 5 and 6 weeks. As with metacarpal fractures, rigid internal fixation can permit active and passive range of motion within the first postoperative week. Interval splint wear between exercise sessions is necessary until the fracture is clinically healed.

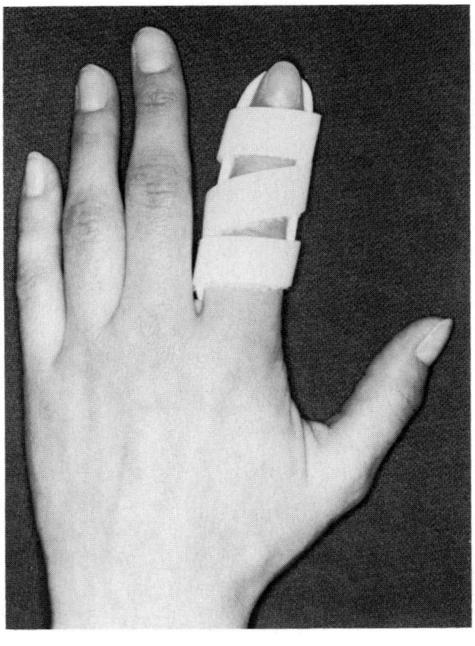

Figure 12–12. A digital extension splint may be used for stable head and neck fractures of the proximal phalanx.

Therapy programs following proximal phalanx fractures must be closely monitored and tailored to fit the needs of the individual injury to avoid potential problems, which may include (1) limited excursion of the flexor digitorum superficialis (FDS) and flexor digitorum profundus (FDP), (2) limited active extension of the PIP joint, and (3) capsular tightness.

Limited FDS and FDP excursion is addressed with isolated tendon gliding exercises and the use of functional electrical muscle stimulation (FES). Various cadaver and intraoperative studies have been performed to determine the excursion needed by the FDS and FDP to produce flexion at their joints of action.* The differential tendon gliding exercise has been shown to produce 11 mm of excursion between the FDS and FDP at the wrist level.[31] This exercise is performed by first making a fist, then taking the intrinsic minus position, and ending with full digital extension (Fig. 12–13). Composite digital and wrist flexion followed by composite digital and wrist extension (Fig. 12–14) maximizes glide of the FDS, approximately 49 mm at the wrist level.[30] Blocking exercises are performed by holding the MCP joint in extension to isolate active PIP joint flexion and

* See refs. 5, 13, 17, 24, 26, 29, 30, 31.

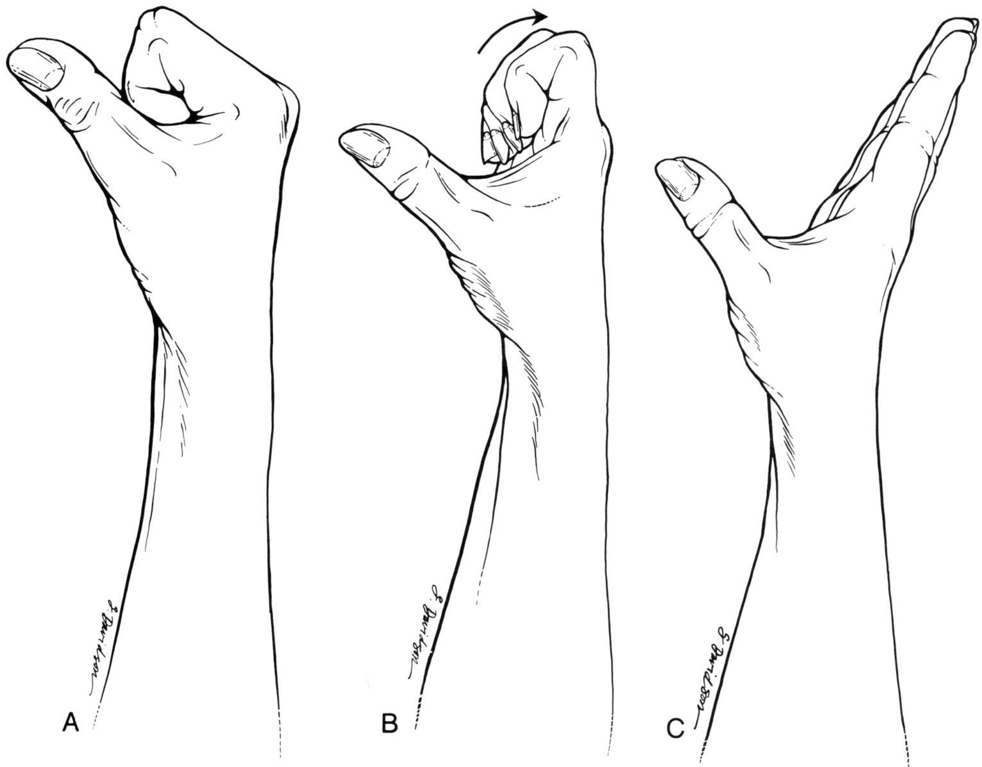

Figure 12–13. Differential tendon gliding exercise. Active finger flexion (*A*) followed by (*B*) positioning of the digits in the intrinsic minus position and concluding with (*C*) full extension of the digits. (From Cannon, N.M.: Enhancing flexor tendon glide through tenolysis . . . and hand therapy. J. Hand Ther. 2:122, 1989.)

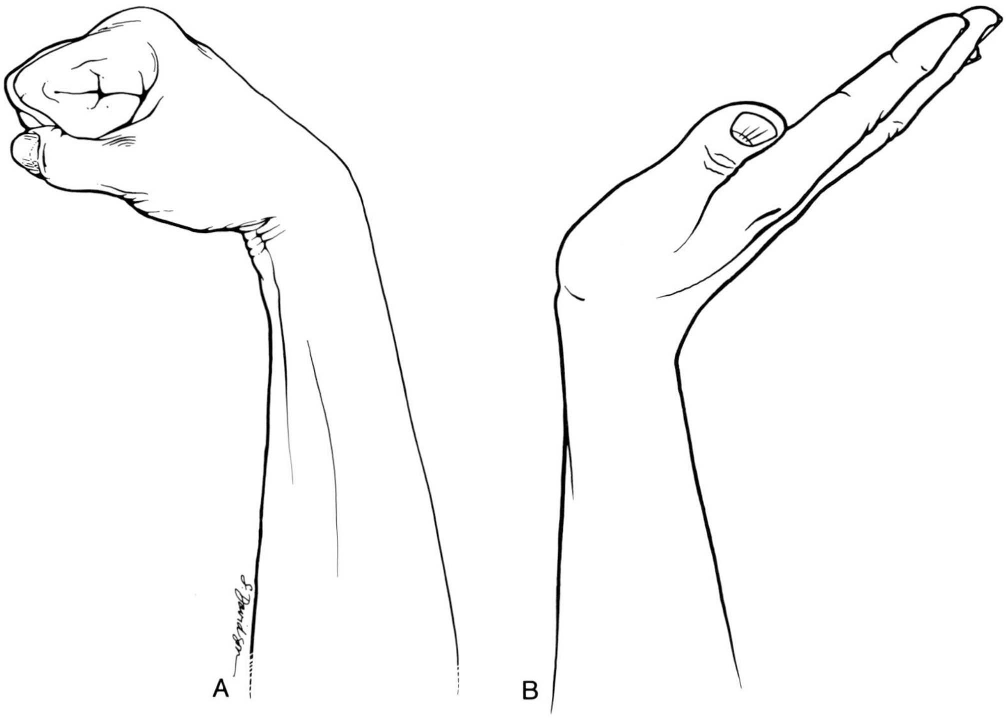

Figure 12–14. Active wrist and finger flexion (*A*) followed by active wrist and finger extension (*B*) maximizes excursion of the FDS. (From Cannon, N.M.: Enhancing flexor tendon glide through tenolysis . . . and hand therapy. J. Hand Ther. 2:122, 1989.)

holding the PIP joint in extension to isolate DIP joint flexion (Fig. 12–15). Flexion of a single digit while the others are held in full extension isolates excursion of the FDS (Fig. 12–16). All of these exercises are beneficial and should be included in the athlete's exercise program. FES to the extrinsic flexor tendons can also enhance tendon excursion and strength of these muscles.[2]

PIP joint extensor lags are also addressed through specific exercise. With the MCP joints blocked in flexion, the patient performs active PIP and DIP joint extension (Fig. 12–17), which isolates the intrinsic and extrinsic tendon contributions to PIP joint extension.

Capsular tightness at the PIP joint is often seen with intra-articular head and neck fractures. Any trauma to an articular surface predisposes it to post-traumatic arthritic changes. Volar capsular tightness, resulting in a PIP joint flexion contracture, can often be curtailed by assuring that the PIP joint is held at neutral during the initial splint fabrication. If a PIP joint flexion contracture develops, it can usually be resolved early through the appropriate use of static or dynamic extension splints. The prefabricated Safety Pin Splint (Fig. 12–18) is useful for contractures of 25° or less, while a custom-fitted short dorsal outrigger splint is indicated for contractures greater than 25° (Fig. 12–19). Dorsal capsular tightness, resulting in a PIP joint extension contracture, is addressed with prolonged passive stretches

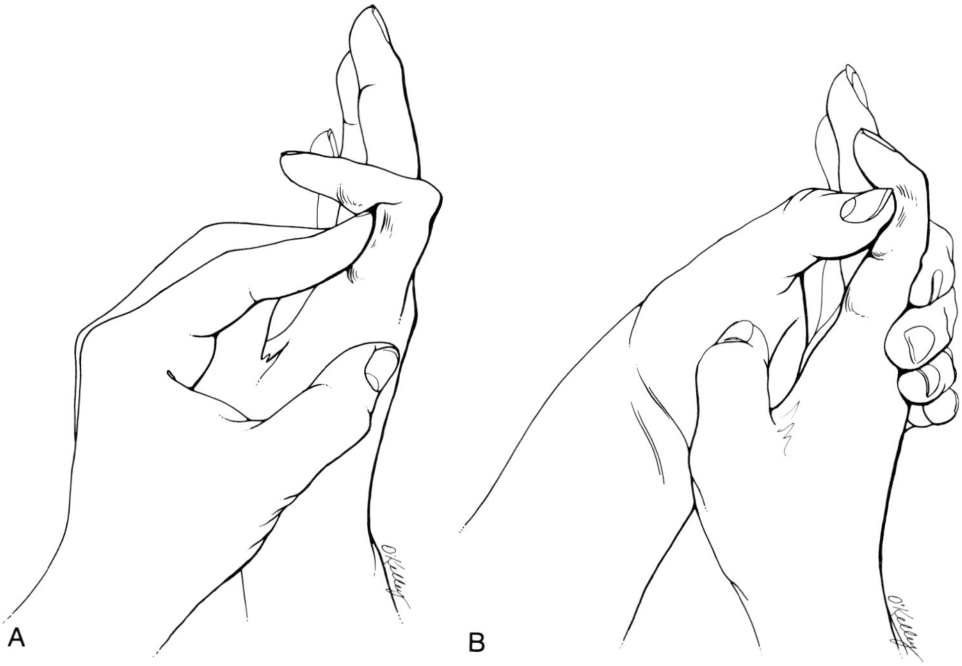

Figure 12–15. *A,* Blocking exercise to the PIP joint. *B,* Blocking exercise to the DIP joint. (From Cannon, N.M.: Enhancing flexor tendon glide through tenolysis . . . and hand therapy. J. Hand Ther. 2:122, 1989.)

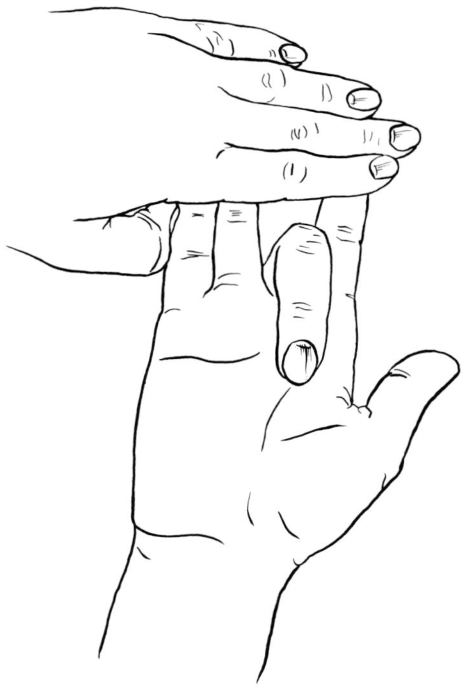

Figure 12–16. Isolated FDS exercises allow for independent glide of the flexor digitorum superficialis. (From Cannon, N.M.: Enhancing flexor tendon glide through tenolysis . . . and hand therapy. J. Hand Ther. 2:122, 1989.)

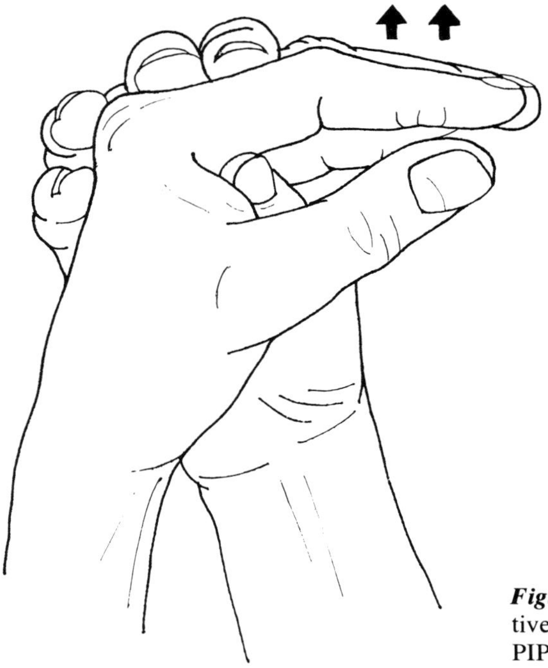

Figure 12–17. Isolated active extension exercise to the PIP joints.

into flexion. This can be performed manually, with the use of digital flexion taping, or through dynamic flexion splinting (Fig. 12–20).

When the fracture is clinically stable, the athlete may often return to practice with protective splinting. Rigid internal fixation in combination with a protective external splint may allow return as early as 3 weeks postoperatively. With the exception of base fractures, rigid digital splints

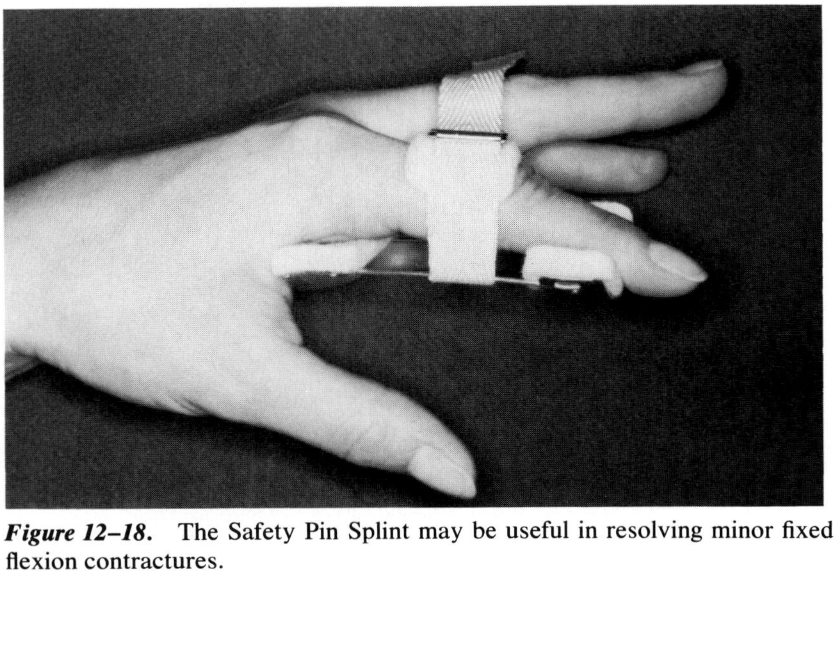

Figure 12–18. The Safety Pin Splint may be useful in resolving minor fixed flexion contractures.

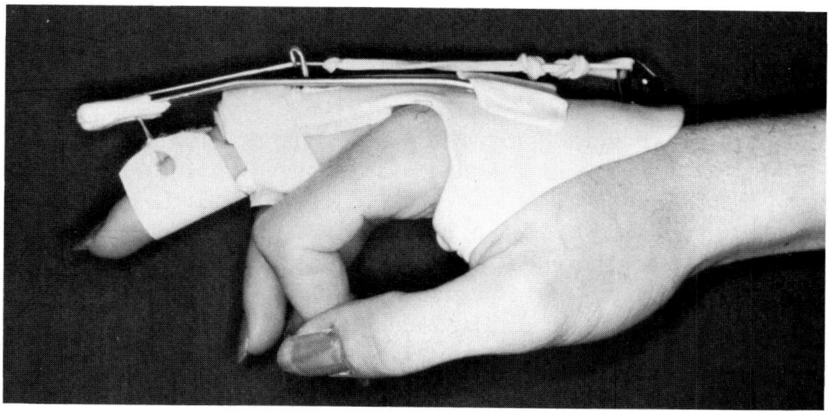

Figure 12–19. A low profile short dorsal outrigger splint may be indicated for severe fixed flexion contractures of the PIP joint.

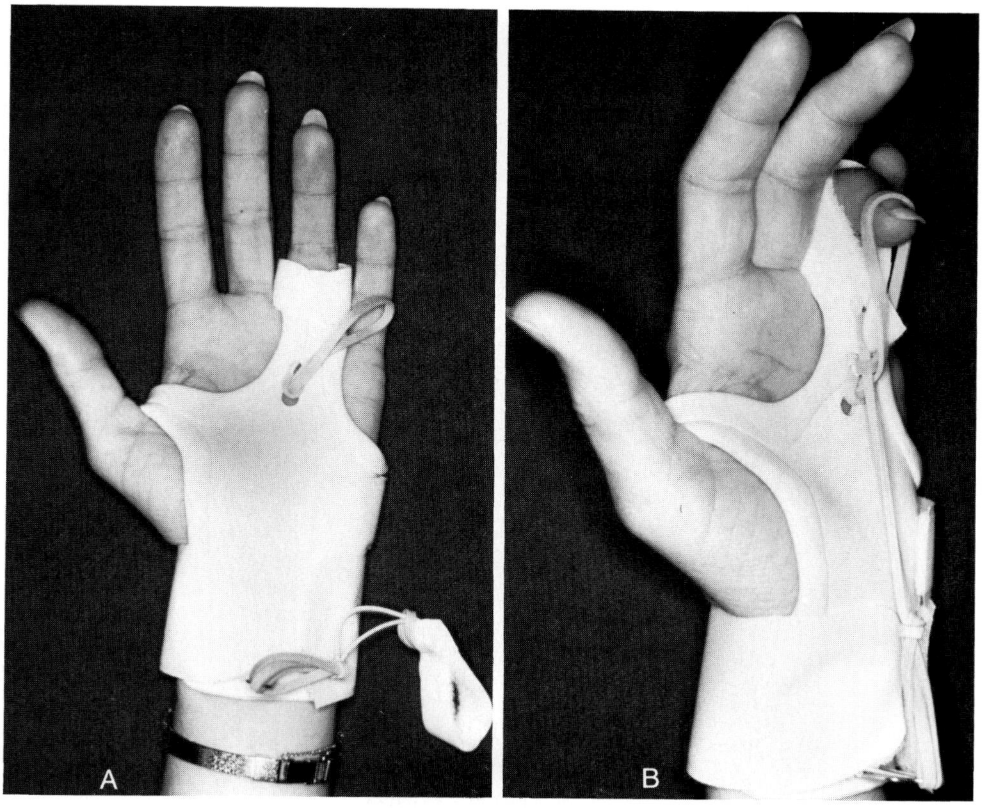

Figure 12–20. A dynamic PIP joint flexion splint.

such as cylinder casts (Fig. 12–21) or digital extension gutter splints provide the best protection for a healing fracture. With base fractures, it is often necessary to include the MCP joint in the splint. Unfortunately, these splints do not allow good mobility of the hand. A flexible alternative is buddy taping with athletic tape or custom-made Velcro straps (Fig. 12–22). This technique helps protect against torque and rotational forces, but one must realize that it offers only minimal protection. It is difficult to provide maximum protection to such a small and vulnerable area while allowing good mobility of the hand. Grip strengthening programs are initiated at the discretion of the physician based on achievement of fracture consolidation, usually by 6 to 8 weeks postinjury. Athletes who participate in contact or ball-handling sports should not be allowed to return to competition until 6 weeks postinjury due to the high risk of reinjury.

Without proper management, proximal phalanx fractures can be quite debilitating and require further surgery. Common complications, such as tendon adhesions and capsular tightness, must be resolved with appropriate intervention. As internal fixation techniques continue to be refined and popularized, these problems may be minimized with the onset of earlier and more aggressive treatment.

TENDON INJURIES

Avulsion of the Flexor Digitorum Profundus

Avulsion of the flexor digitorum profundus from its bony insertion on the distal phalanx occurs primarily during contact sports, in particular football and wrestling when a moving opponent's jersey is suddenly

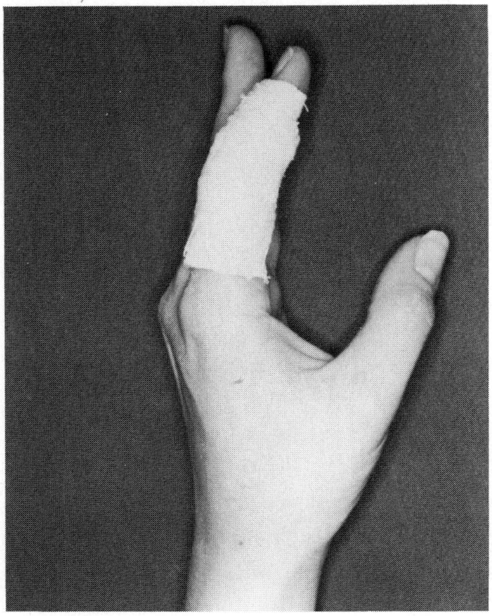

Figure 12–21. Plaster cylinder cast.

Athletes may continue to participate in play provided the splint is secure and worn continuously. There is usually no appreciable hindrance in athletic performance, except in those sports requiring fine dexterity.

Boutonnière Deformity

Boutonnière deformity is caused by disruption of the central slip and dorsal transverse retinacular fibers over the PIP joint. Left untreated, the lateral bands will sublux volar to the PIP joint axis and progressively thicken and shorten, the oblique retinacular ligament will also tighten, and secondary joint changes may occur.[6] The final clinical picture is one of PIP joint flexion and DIP joint hyperextension.

With a closed injury, optimal results are obtained with early diagnosis and prompt initiation of an appropriate splinting and exercise program. Factors that positively influence the final result include (1) early initiation of a conservative program, (2) continuous immobilization of the PIP joint in full extension, and (3) DIP joint flexion exercises with the PIP joint at neutral position. Without prompt attention, this injury can progress to a PIP joint fixed flexion contracture with secondary joint changes making conservative management more difficult and often less effective. If a fixed flexion contracture has developed, this must first be resolved though appropriate extension splinting. Beneficial splints include a short dorsal outrigger with lumbrical bar for contractures greater than 25° and a Safety Pin Splint for less severe contractures. Once full passive extension has been obtained, the PIP joint is immobilized continously in neutral position. Acute injuries are splinted for 6 weeks, whereas chronic injuries of more than 3 weeks duration are splinted for 8 weeks. The authors recommend a digital cylinder cast holding the PIP joint at neutral with the MCP and DIP joints excluded. A lateral radiograph assists in verifying full PIP joint extension within the cast (Fig. 12–26). The patient is seen every 2 weeks

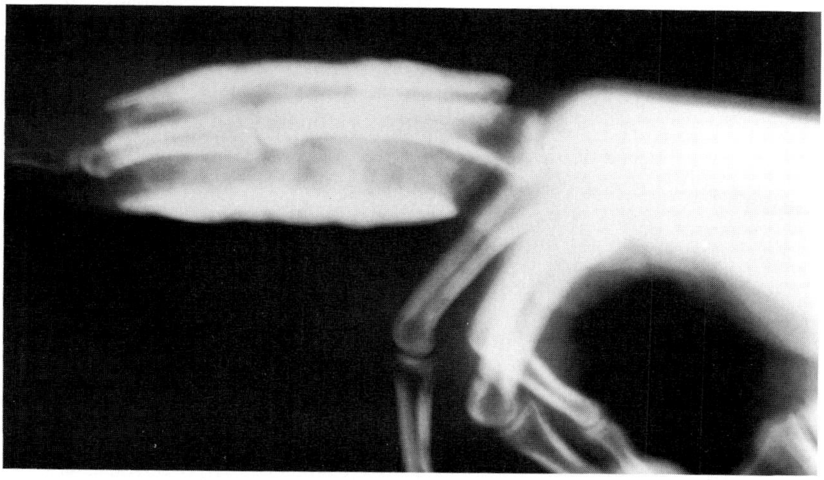

Figure 12–26. A radiograph verifies the position of the PIP joint within the cylinder cast.

for cast changes and to insure compliance with cast wear. The athlete may participate in sports during this time if the cast is secure and worn continuously.

Although holding the PIP joint at neutral assists in repositioning the lateral bands dorsal to the PIP joint axis, it also places tension on the lateral bands and oblique retinacular ligament, resulting in increased tenodesis of the DIP joint into hyperextension.[6] To help stretch the lateral bands and oblique retinacular ligament back to their physiologic length, active and passive DIP joint flexion exercises should be performed.

Following 6 to 8 weeks of PIP joint immobilization, active exercises are initiated with interval extension splinting. The aggressiveness of the program is dependent upon PIP joint motion. The primary goal is to regain flexion while maintaining PIP joint extension. Passive flexion exercises, dynamic flexion splinting, and splint wear are influenced by this goal.

Conservative management should always be attempted before surgical intervention. Results following acute injuries managed conservatively are usually excellent; results following chronic injuries are not as favorable but usually include a functional arc of motion. If the digit does not respond well to conservative measures, there are a variety of surgical procedures to rebalance the extensor mechanism. These techniques require preoperative as well as specific postoperative therapy and splinting.

DISLOCATIONS AND LIGAMENTOUS INJURIES

General Considerations

Dislocations and ligamentous injuries are common among athletes. These injuries are often minor but can result in chronic pain, stiffness, and joint instability and are vulnerable to further injury if not given adequate medical treatment. Management following dislocations, stable fracture-dislocations, and partial tears and many complete tears of the collateral ligaments is conservative. The initial goals of treatment include decreasing edema, stabilizing the affected joint(s) to allow healing of the soft tissue structures, and encouraging protected range of motion when appropriate, all of which will subsequently reduce pain associated with movement. Although only conservative management is discussed here, the therapist must be aware that surgical intervention is often necessary following unstable dislocations with associated fracture[7] and that controversy exists as to whether complete ligamentous tears should be surgically repaired.

Injuries at the digital PIP joint level are more common than at the MCP joint due to the vulnerable location of the PIP joint and differing anatomy. The MCP joint is less susceptible to injury due to its protected position at the base of the fingers, its ligamentous and supporting structures, and its condyloid joint, which allows motion in both flexion and extension and abduction and adduction. The PIP joint is a hinge joint with a bicondylar configuration that allows only flexion and extension; therefore, it is more resistive to stresses. Its stability is derived mainly from the strong attachment of the collateral ligaments and volar plate into the base of the middle phalanx.

Dorsal Proximal Interphalangeal Joint Dislocations

Three types of dislocations may occur at the PIP joint: dorsal, volar, and lateral. Of these, dorsal dislocation is by far the most common. The mechanism of injury is usually hyperextension of the PIP joint, frequently sustained in ball-handling sports. With dorsal dislocation, the volar plate is torn, either directly from bone or with a chip of bone from the volar base of the middle phalanx.

Conservative management is recommended for pure dislocations and most stable fracture-dislocations. Following closed reduction, the digit is placed in a dorsal extension block splint with the PIP joint positioned in flexion (Fig. 12–27). Approximately 30° of PIP joint flexion is usually adequate, but greater amounts are sometimes required to maintain a satisfactory reduction. Once the initial acute edema and pain have subsided, approximately 1 week postinjury, the patient is encouraged to begin active and passive flexion exercises within the splint. Buddy taping the injured digit to an adjacent digit to prevent PIP joint hyperextension may replace splinting at approximately 2 to 3 weeks in dislocations without associated fracture. Buddy taping at all times for

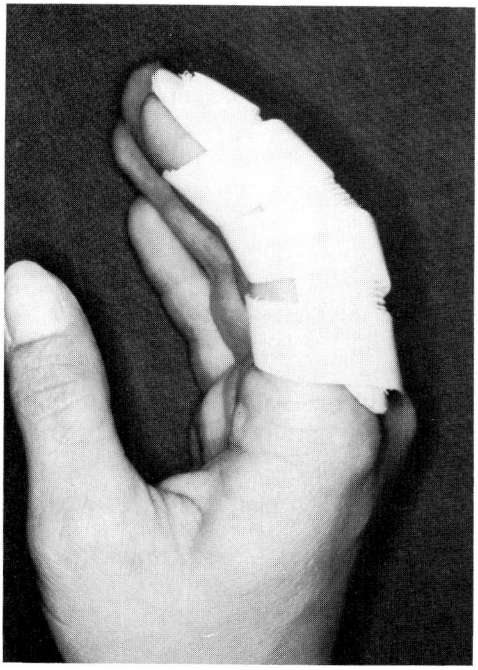

Figure 12–27. Dorsal blocking splint to the PIP joint.

an additional 3 weeks and up to 3 months postinjury during sports is encouraged.

Following dislocation with associated fracture, the dorsal extension block splint is continued until 6 weeks with active and passive flexion exercises performed within the splint. From the third to sixth week, the splint is adjusted weekly to increase PIP joint extension in 10° increments. At 6 weeks, buddy taping is used for light protection during activity and sports to discourage hyperextension of the PIP joint. Joint swelling may persist for months. One-inch Coban wrap is helpful in controlling edema and patients tend to appreciate the light support it offers.

Normally, full range of motion is easily restored with an aggressive exercise program. Occasionally, there may be a slight residual fixed flexion contracture due to scarring at the volar plate, and some type of intermittent extension splint may be needed to resolve the contracture.

Collateral Ligament Injuries at the PIP Joint

An incomplete tear (sprain) of a collateral ligament at the PIP joint is managed with buddy taping and controlled range of motion exercises. The injured finger is taped to an adjacent digit, preferably the digit on the side of the injured ligament to avoid any additional deviation forces. Velcro tapes or sturdy athletic tape is placed around the proximal and middle phalanges to secure the digits together but allow unrestricted PIP joint motion. The tape is worn continuously for 3 to 5 weeks or until there is no pain on a lateral stress test or palpation over the involved ligament. Buddy taping is continued for up to 3 months during participation in sports. The exact length of time in buddy tapes may be quite variable depending upon the individual sport and the specific stresses the joint is subject to during competition. Generally, pain should be of key importance in determining the need for prolonged protection during sports participation. Active range of motion should be encouraged from the outset. As with most injuries to a small joint, edema is usually prevalent. Coban wrapping is helpful in reducing joint swelling.

The authors also treat most complete collateral ligament tears at the PIP joint with buddy taping. Complete ruptures are often extremely painful, swollen, and unstable. A digital extension splint with sides that provide adequate lateral support and good joint alignment may be necessary for the first 1 to 2 weeks to promote healing and decrease pain and edema. However, splint wear should not be prolonged for fear of joint stiffness. After approximately 3 days of immobilization, the splint should be removed a few times each day for gentle exercise within buddy tapes. The athlete can usually return to play almost immediately with the use of buddy tapes.

Collateral Ligament Injuries at the Digital Metacarpophalangeal Joints

Conservative management of incomplete and complete tears consists of 3 weeks of immobilization with the MCP joints in 60° to 70° of flexion. An adjacent digit is often included in the splint for increased stability and comfort. At 3 weeks, active and gentle passive range of motion exercises are initiated. Splinting may be continued intermittently if joint pain persists.

During the first 3 weeks, the patient can participate in sports only if able to comply with splint wear. At 3 weeks, buddy taping is used, but this provides only minimal protection due to the laxity of the MCP joint collateral ligaments when the digits are in extension.

Ulnar Collateral Ligament Strain at the Thumb Metacarpophalangeal Joint

The ulnar collateral ligament of the thumb MCP joint is subject to injury when sudden stress into abduction is applied to the thumb or when repeated microtrauma to the area causes stretching and weakening of the ligament. Although traditionally referred to as "gamekeeper's thumb," this injury is more aptly termed "skier's thumb" due to its frequent occurrence during a fall on an outstretched hand when the skier's thumb is caught in the ski pole. This condition is not unique to skiers: it also occurs in other sports such as hockey, polo, baseball, and wrestling to name a few.

Treatment of this type of strain consists of a cast or splint immobilizing the thumb in approximately 40° to 45° of abduction and the MCP joint in slight flexion. Immobilization is continued for 4 to 6 weeks depending on the severity of the injury. Pain upon stress or palpation is a good indicator of the length of immobilization needed. Preferably, a short opponens splint (Fig. 12–28) is used since it allows good hand function. If it is possible to immobilize the wrist without jeopardizing athletic participation, a wrist and thumb static splint (Fig. 12–29) provides greater protection and more adequate immobilization of the

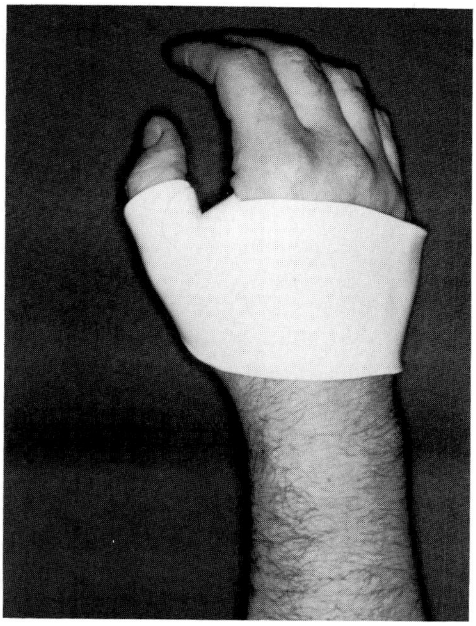

Figure 12–28. Short opponens splint.

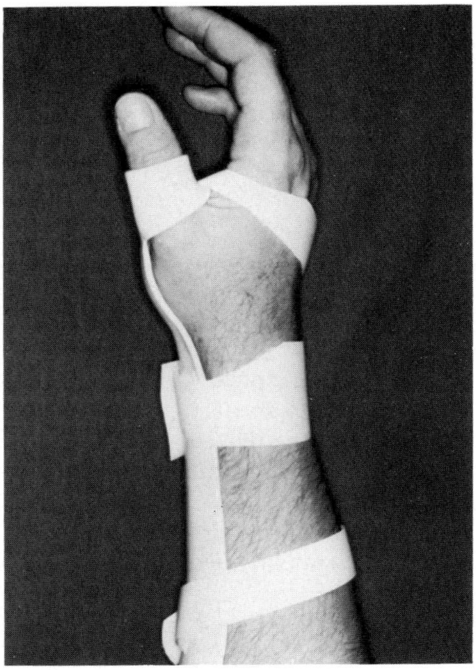

Figure 12–29. Wrist and thumb immobilization splint with the IP joint excluded.

thumb carpometacarpal (CMC) and MCP joints. Both splints serve as a protective device in the early healing stages and also as a preventive measure once healing has occurred. The short opponens splint may be especially beneficial for long-term use during activities that stress the thumb or in athletes with chronic weakened and stretched ulnar collateral ligaments.

All athletes should be evaluated for the appropriate playing splint to avoid injury to a noninvolved joint. For example, a short opponens splint can sometimes be a fulcrum for injury to the thumb IP joint if excessive force is applied to the tip of the thumb. In sports where this is likely to occur, it might be best to include the thumb IP joint in the splint.

If the league will not allow a rigid thermoplastic short opponens splint, a playing cast made of RTV 11 silicone rubber compound or athletic taping may be used. Taping provides only minimal protection and should be considered only if the former two devices are unacceptable.

An ulnar collateral ligament strain of the thumb MCP joint is a common athletic injury. If managed early and properly, it can be resolved with minimal loss of competitive time and full restoration of strength and function.

TENDINITIS/TENOSYNOVITIS

General Management

Athletes who participate in sports that require repetitive motions such as cross-country skiing, golf, rowing, and tennis may be susceptible to tendinitis. Load, resistance, and impact of the objects used in many of these sports are contributory factors.

Conservative management of tendinitis consists of three basic phases: (1) rest, (2) reconditioning, and (3) ongoing rehabilitation during return to competition. Rest encompasses rigid splints, gentle exercises, anti-inflammatory measures, and avoidance of painful activities. The ideal splint places the inflamed tendon in a shortened or relaxed position. The splint is removed for gentle exercise to prevent additional fibroblastic scar formation and loss of tensile strength due to immobilization. It has been shown that immobilization causes a loss of glycosaminoglycans (GAGs)[1], which are important in scar architecture. Tendon tensile strength has also been shown to decrease with immobilization and stress deprivation.[9, 11] Useful modalities may include ice massage, contrast baths, iontophoresis, ultrasound phonophoresis, and high voltage pulsating direct current.[4, 10, 15, 21, 27] These therapeutic techniques should not be attempted before obtaining a thorough knowledge of their indications and contraindications and receiving instruction in their proper administration. Frequently, oral anti-inflammatory medication is prescribed or a local corticosteroid injection is administered by the physician at the onset of this phase.

Reconditioning is initiated once pain and inflammation have subsided, following approximately 2 to 6 weeks of rest. During this phase, flexible counterbalance supports replace rigid splints; these limit extremes of motion while allowing functional activity. These supports are integrated into a structured reconditioning program that begins with warm-up and stretching, followed by progressive resistive exercises to strengthen specific muscles. General warm-up exercises, such as calisthenics or jogging, increase cardiovascular output and muscle temperature. An increase in muscle temperature helps facilitate metabolic processes and a drop in muscle viscosity produces more rapid, forceful, and smooth contractions.[22] Nirschl recommends warming-up to a light sweat.[20] Stretching exercises are performed to enhance flexibility, which may decrease the incidence of musculotendinous injuries. The strengthening program, performed within the patient's comfort limits, consists of a gradual progression from eccentric isotonic to concentric isotonic and finally isokinetic exercises. Eccentric exercises may be beneficial in the rehabilitation of tendinitis conditions since resistance is used as the muscle fibers lengthen. This places the musculotendinous unit under stress but usually does not recreate the stresses which caused the problem. If pain or swelling occur after exercise, icing of the affected area for approximately 10 minutes may be beneficial. During the final stages of the reconditioning phase, the athlete completes a "functional progression" in which he simulates the actions necessary to perform his sport. The intensity and duration of sport activity are gradually increased over a given period of time until the athlete has adequate strength to return to competition. Athletic participation may be allowed earlier if the activity can be modified to avoid aggravating movements.

During return to competition, stretching and flexibility exercises are continued to minimize muscle injury. Flexible supports should also be continued if compatible with the sport.

Management of Tendinitis at Specific Locations

Three common sites of tendinitis are the first dorsal compartment, the flexor carpi radialis (FCR) tunnel, and the lateral epicondyle. Stenosing tenosynovitis at the first dorsal compartment is referred to as DeQuervain's disease. It stems from a constriction of the extensor pollicis brevis (EPB) and abductor pollicis longus (APL) within their fiberosseous tunnel over the radial styloid. FCR tendinitis may occur from constriction, compression, or inflammation as the tendon passes through the tunnel at the wrist created by the split insertion of the transverse carpal ligament into the tubercle of the scaphoid and the crest of the trapezium.[25] Epicondylitis may appear laterally, medially, or posteriorly; however, lateral epicondylitis is by far the most common. Lateral epicondylitis is related to activities that increase tension and stress to the wrist extensor and supinator muscles, such as in the backhand stroke in tennis. Repeated overloading and stress to these areas may cause vascular compromise as well as microscopic tendinous tears, commonly in the extensor carpi radialis brevis (ECRB). Specific management of these three inflammatory conditions will be addressed using the previously mentioned phases as guidelines.

In the initial phase, all three of these problems are often treated with an anesthetic-steroid injection by the physician, after which the appropriate rigid splint is fitted. In the management of DeQuervain's disease, a wrist and thumb immobilization splint is fitted to relax the EPB and APL. Appropriate positioning includes the wrist in approximately 15° of dorsiflexion, the thumb CMC joint in 40° of abduction, and the MCP joint in 10° of flexion, and the IP joint is excluded. The appropriate splint for FCR tendinitis holds the wrist in 10° of volar flexion and slight radial deviation to place the FCR in a shortened position. A wrist splint is also indicated for lateral epicondylitis; however, the wrist is positioned in 30° of dorsiflexion to minimize tension on the ECRB. Splints are worn at all times except during bathing and two daily exercise sessions. Gentle isolated exercises, including stretches, are performed to the appropriate muscles. Modalities that may prove beneficial include contrast baths for DeQuervain's disease and iontophoresis for lateral epicondylitis. Iontophoresis uses an electrical current to allow ions to pass through a semipermeable membrane.[4] This permits the noninvasive administration of medications into the body tissue. The strength and duration of the current determines the quantity and distribution of the drug. It is the authors' experience that four treatments of 2 ml of 4% lidocaine and 1 ml of 4% dexamethasone sodium phosphate administered every other day just distal to the lateral epicondyle provides relief in approximately 50 percent of the cases.

As mentioned previously, the focus of the reconditioning phase is maximizing strength while integrating flexible counterbalance supports when possible. Progressive resistance exercises are preceded by active warm-up and stretching to minimize muscle injury. With DeQuervain's disease, Walker recommends resistive exercises that increase forearm, grip, and pinch strength.[27] With FCR tendinitis, attention is directed toward strengthening of the wrist flexor muscles. In the authors' experience with lateral epicondylitis, the upper extremity strengthening program designed by Nirschl for isotonic exercise[19] and the Baltimore Therapeutic Equipment (BTE) Work Simulator for isokinetic exercise have proven beneficial in managing this population. The exercises proposed by Nirschl are excellent in increasing strength, endurance, and flexibility in the wrist, elbow, forearm, and shoulder.[19]

There are a variety of flexible supports on the market. For DeQuervain's disease, a soft thumb spica support may be helpful (Fig. 12–30). For tendinitis at the wrist, the Lion's Paw may be used; however, it is somewhat bulky (Fig. 12–31). At the present time, it is difficult to find comfortable anatomically designed supports that adequately control motion. Arm bands are helpful in the treatment of lateral epicondylitis. They function by compressing the involved extensor muscle-tendon complex, thereby constraining normal expansion that occurs with contraction. Nirschl refers to this compression as a counterforce against the contracting extensor musculotendinous unit, which either disseminates or reduces the muscular contractile force.[18] The byproduct of this counterforce limits overload at the origin of the ECRB. The authors recommend the Aircast Pneumatic Armband (Fig. 12–32), which contains an aircell that concentrates pressure on the involved muscle. It is worn during activity and exercise.

Treatment during the return to competition phase includes precompetition stretching of the involved muscles and wearing of flexible supports when possible. Movements that aggravate previous tendinitis

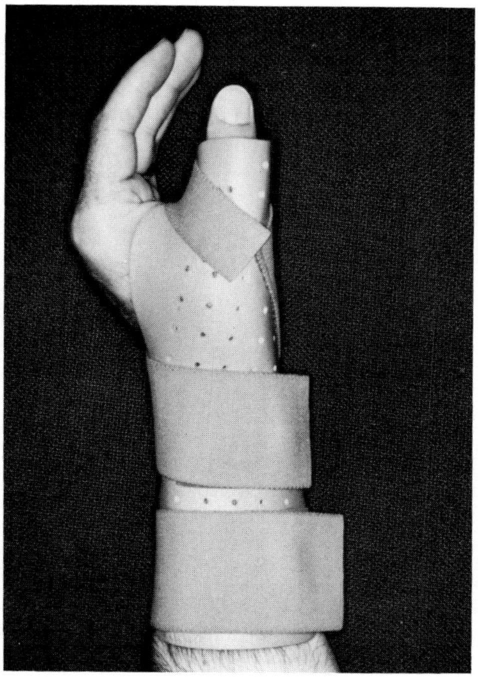

Figure 12–30. Soft thumb spica support (Alimed, Inc., Dedham, MA; North Coast Medical, Inc., San Jose, CA).

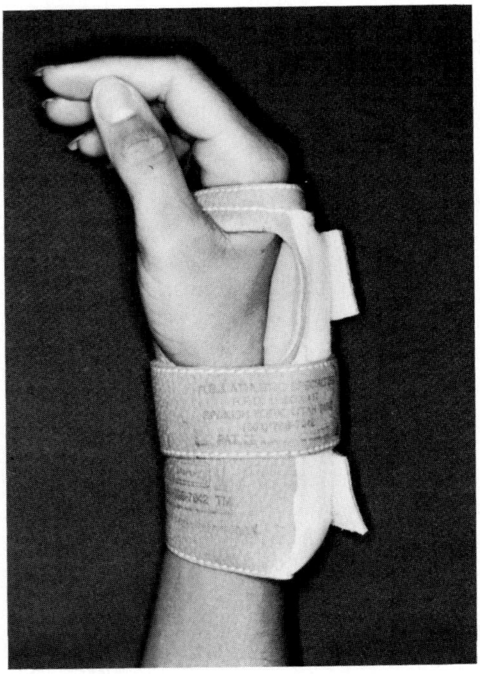

Figure 12–31. The Lion's Paw (R.B.J. Athletic Specialties, Spanish Fork, UT).

conditions should also be modified to alleviate excessive stress to these areas.

Conservative management of tendinitis often alleviates the pain, thereby avoiding surgical intervention. In some chronic cases, surgical intervention may be mandated.

NERVE COMPRESSION SYNDROMES

Upper extremity compression neuropathies are somewhat uncommon in athletes. They may occur from direct contusion of the tissues

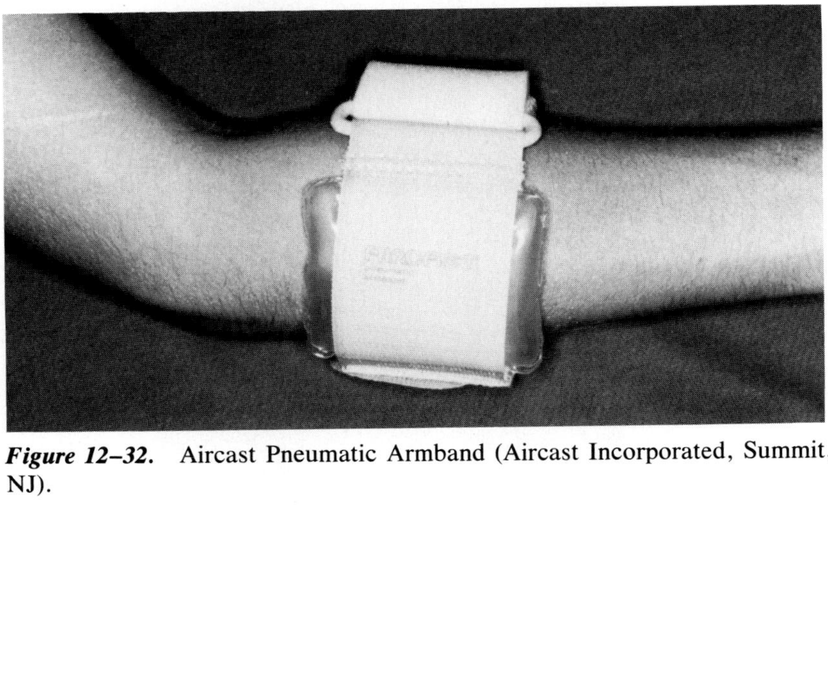

Figure 12–32. Aircast Pneumatic Armband (Aircast Incorporated, Summit, NJ).

overlying peripheral nerves or from vigorous repetitive athletic activity that produces inflammation and tissue swelling leading to nerve compression, usually in closed passages such as the carpal, cubital, or ulnar tunnels. Nerve compression syndromes are treated similarly to tendinitis conditions, beginning with rest and progressing to reconditioning and finally return to competition.

Carpal Tunnel Syndrome

Carpal tunnel syndrome (CTS) is one of the most common of all the nerve compression syndromes. It results from increased pressure within the carpal tunnel that compresses the median nerve. The mechanism of compression may be acute wrist trauma as with a carpal fracture, cumulative trauma as in hitting a ball repetitively with the wrist (e.g., volleyball), prolonged positions in the extremes of wrist motion, or highly repetitive finger or wrist motion inherent in some sports. The onset is usually gradual and symptoms are often ignored until there is an actual sensory deficit or notable weakness that affects athletic performance. When managed acutely, CTS can be resolved through conservative means, but if ignored, surgical intervention may become necessary.

The initial phase of conservative treatment consists of splinting, gentle exercises, and contrast baths. The physician may also inject the carpal canal with a steroid and/or prescribe an oral anti-inflammatory medication. The splint immobilizes the wrist in 0° to 15° of dorsiflexion while allowing full digital and thumb range of motion. By inhibiting wrist motion, potential compression to the median nerve is minimized. We prefer a custom-fitted wrist immobilization splint made of a low temperature thermoplastic. An array of prefabricated wrist supports is available if one lacks the skills and materials to fabricate a custom-fitted splint. When choosing a prefabricated splint, one must take into consideration basic splinting principles to insure patient comfort and avoid potential trauma to soft tissues. The 10½ inch wrist support with Velcro closure by Ezy Wrap is comfortable and allows good hand function (Fig. 12–33). The splint is worn at all times except during bathing and exercise sessions.

Chronic tenosynovial inflammation is frequently associated with CTS and can result in tendon adhesions in the carpal tunnel. If the tendons become adherent to one another they move through the carpal tunnel as a unit or "plug" instead of individually, thus causing pressure on the median nerve.[28] A simple method to evaluate limited tendon excursion is to compare flexor digitorum superficialis (FDS) tendon glide of the involved hand with that of the noninvolved hand. Isolated tendon gliding exercises (such as those described for proximal phalanx fractures) can facilitate tendon glide and promote healing while avoiding adherence of the tendon system due to possible fibroblastic scar formation from immobilization. The patient is encouraged to perform these exercises three times daily.

To complement the exercises, contrast baths are performed once daily to help promote increased blood exchange, metabolism, and

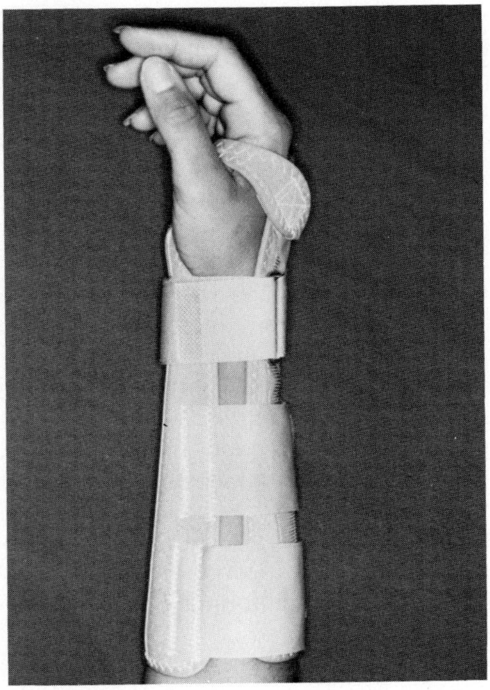

Figure 12–33. Ezy Wrap wrist support (Ezy Wrap, De Funiak Springs, FL).

phagocyte activity, which is thought to reduce inflammatory byproducts in the area. This initial stage of treatment should be continued for 4 to 6 weeks.

The next phase of treatment is initiated when carpal tunnel symptoms become quiescent. At this time, gentle progressive resistance exercises may be necessary to return the patient to normal strength. The patient is also educated regarding avoidance or modification of aggravating movements.

Continued protection may be indicated in instances in which the athlete is prone to stress the median nerve in the carpal tunnel. Flexible wrist supports that limit the extremes of wrist motion and splints or gloves with shock-absorbing qualities are beneficial. Shock-absorbing materials such as Viscolis, Neoprene, and Sorbothane can be used as splint inserts or liners. Many types of prefabricated antivibration gloves or pads are currently available (Fig. 12–34) (see Table 12–1).

Many patients have benefitted from a therapeutic management program, thereby avoiding surgical intervention. For this reason, a nonoperative approach to management of CTS should be considered.

Hand Splinting

Splints play an integral part in the rehabilitation process, from the acute phase through return to competition. Traditionally, splints consist of a low temperature thermoplastic, conform to standard positions of protection, and conform to specific splinting principles. Protective

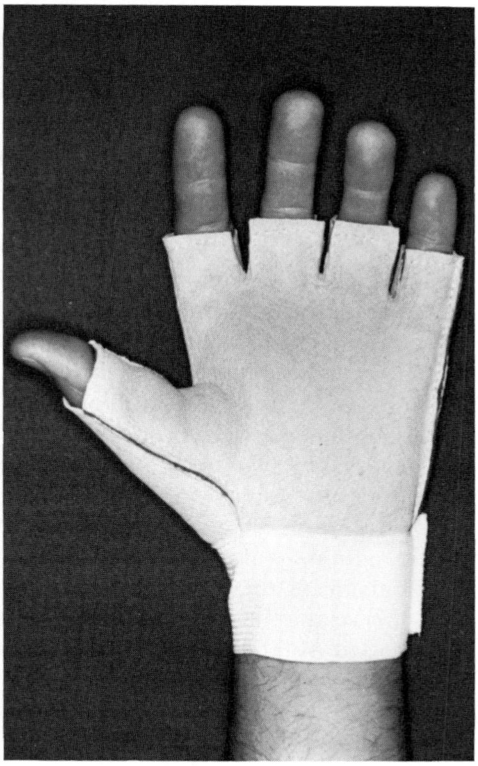

Figure 12–34. Anti-vibration glove (Steel Grip, Inc., Danville, IL).

splints for athletes may vary from the traditional materials and positions but splinting principles are constant. Two splints are often necessary: a protective splint for sports is positioned to facilitate athletic performance and often consists of a flexible material, while a traditional splint is worn when the athlete is not involved in play.

Splints serve a variety of purposes: they provide protection, restrict undesired motion, prevent deformity, and resolve tendon tightness or joint contracture. To effectively achieve its goal, a splint must meet specific criteria. An understanding of the basic principles of hand splinting and a familiarity with the array of current thermoplastics and materials allow the therapist to design and fabricate the optimal splint. Creativity is often needed to appropriately adapt the splint to the special needs of the sport and patient while safely protecting the injury.

SPLINTING PRINCIPLES

The principles basic to traditional splint fabrication are founded upon a knowledge of hand anatomy, kinesiology, and biomechanics. Each area in itself merits elaborate study, which the reader is encouraged to pursue. Key points will briefly be mentioned.

Anatomy

Several important anatomic considerations pertain to hand arches, skin creases, bony prominences, superficial nerves, and ligamentous structures. The three structural arches of the hand, two transverse and one longitudinal, contribute to object manipulation and function. Splints must be carefully contoured to the hand to support and preserve these arches.

Skin creases are used as external landmarks for underlying anatomic structures. A splint designed to allow motion at a particular joint should not interfere with its corresponding skin crease. For example, a splint fabricated to immobilize the wrist but allow full digital motion should not extend beyond the distal palmar flexion crease as this corresponds to the fourth and fifth metacarpal heads.

Excessive pressure produced by improper splint fit can traumatize the cutaneous surface and underlying soft tissues. Especially prone to these pressure forces are bony prominences and superficial nerves. These structures are accommodated through contouring of the thermoplastic, allotment of additional space, the use of foam inserts, or simply by exclusion of that area in the splint. The superficial branch of the radial nerve and the ulnar nerve at the cubital tunnel are two sites often compressed by poorly fitting forearm-based hand splints or posterior elbow splints.

Ligamentous structures must be honored in both static and dynamic splints. Prolonged lateral stress to a joint can lead to overstretching of a collateral ligament with resultant joint instability and pain (Fig. 12–35).

Kinesiology

Kinesiologic considerations relate to basic external anatomic configurations and the changes that occur as the thumb and digits move through an arc of motion. A splint designed to allow motion must be fitted to accommodate anticipated changes in the arches and bony prominences.

Biomechanics

Biomechanical principles deal with pressure, forces, and mechanical advantage. Advantageous use of these principles enhances patient comfort and maximizes splint effectiveness. The principle that pressure is directly proportional to the area of force application implies that as the surface area of a splint increases pressure diminishes. Achieving contiguous splint fit also minimizes pressure through a uniform application of force. When applying the concept of a lever system to a splint, mechanical advantage indicates the relationship between the lengths of the force arm and resistance arm.[8] Simply stated, as the length of the forearm trough increases, the force or pressure transferred to the hand decreases. All of these principles imply that longer, wider splints that are well-contoured result in optimal comfort. Two thirds the length and

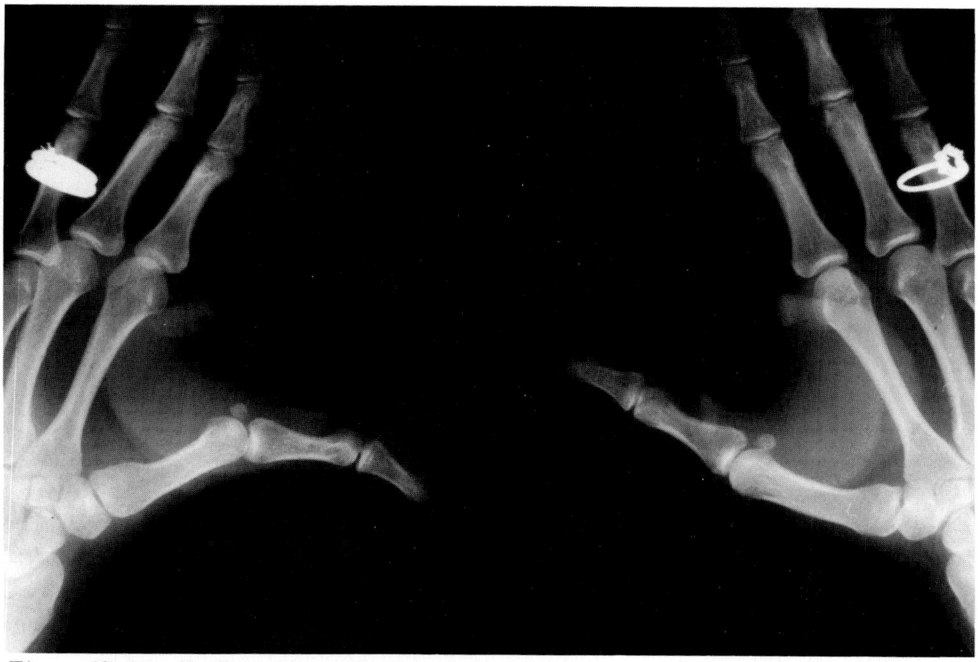

Figure 12–35. Radiograph on the left demonstrates excessive stress being applied to the thumb MCP joint ulnar collateral ligament during the construction of a web spacer splint. Radiograph on the right demonstrates minimal stress being applied to the collateral ligament with proper splint fabrication (From Cannon, N.M., et al.: Manual of Hand Splinting, New York, Churchill Livingstone, 1985.)

one half the width of the forearm are the recommended measurements for a forearm-based splint.

Rotational forces are pertinent to dynamic splints. A 90° angle of traction to the bone being mobilized maximizes the available rotational force. An angle significantly greater or lesser than 90° could result in joint distraction or damage to the articular surfaces.[8]

TYPES OF SPLINTS

The term "splint" encompasses numerous devices and supports with varying characteristics. Unfortunately, no standardized classification system presently exists. Traditionally, splints have been classified into one of two categories: static or dynamic. Static splints have no moveable parts and are typically used to support or immobilize a joint. Dynamic splints mobilize joints through means of traction devices. Protective splints for sports fall under the static category. Other characteristics may include rigid versus flexible and custom-fitted versus prefabricated.

Rigid splints are desirable following a fracture to provide protection and support while awaiting bony healing. Although rigid support is necessary, hard plastics may not be acceptable in contact sports due to the risk of injury to other players. To avoid reinjury or injury to another player, athletes who have sustained hand fractures should be restricted from competition. Flexible splints may replace rigid splints when there is radiographic evidence of adequate bony healing. Although flexible splints provide less protection than rigid ones, they generally help decrease pain and prevent excessive undesired motion. Of course, the degree of movement is dependent upon the flexibility of the material.

Soft splints are a good alternative, when rigid support is no longer necessary.[3] Playing casts made of GE RTV-11 silicone rubber compound are accepted by most leagues. These supports provide moderate protection yet do not pose any danger to opponents. This cast consists of three layers of RTV-11 compound impregnated with rolled gauze. The layers are applied over a surgical glove with a shock absorbent foam placed over the last layer. An elastic wrap is used to secure the foam, and the cast is allowed to cure for 3 to 4 hours. Once cured, the elastic wrap is removed and the cast is cut along one side of the hand for easy removal and reapplication. The cast is secured with an elastic wrap, Coban, or athletic tape for wear during practice or competition (Fig. 12–36). Due to the bulkiness and closed cell nature of the cast, a traditional thermoplastic splint is worn at all other times. The authors have found this cast especially beneficial following metacarpal, carpal, and distal radial or ulnar fractures when rigid support is no longer required due to sufficient bony healing.

There are a variety of prefabricated flexible supports on the market. Design and materials vary according to the purpose of the support. Some supports provide warmth while others are designed to limit extremes of motion. Neoprene supports aid in retaining the body's natural warmth while providing gentle uniform compression. Warmth helps keep soft tissues more pliable and hopefully less susceptible to injury. Support is only minimal and range of motion is not restricted. Flexible splints that limit extremes of motion may be beneficial in the treatment of carpal tunnel syndrome and tendinitis conditions. Some supports limit motion in only one plane and others in more than one. When choosing a prefabricated splint, keep in mind basic splinting principles to maximize patient comfort and minimize any potential trauma to soft tissues.

MATERIALS

The full armamentarium of splinting materials must be available to the therapist when fabricating splints. An appreciation of the unique characteristics and properties of each material allows the splintmaker to determine the optimum type to be used for the support and protection of a particular injured part (Table 12–1).

Most splints utilize low temperature thermoplastic materials, the majority of which are plastic combined with varying amounts of rubber. A high plastic content will generally give the material good drapeability and contour, whereas the amount of rubber will determine the elasticity

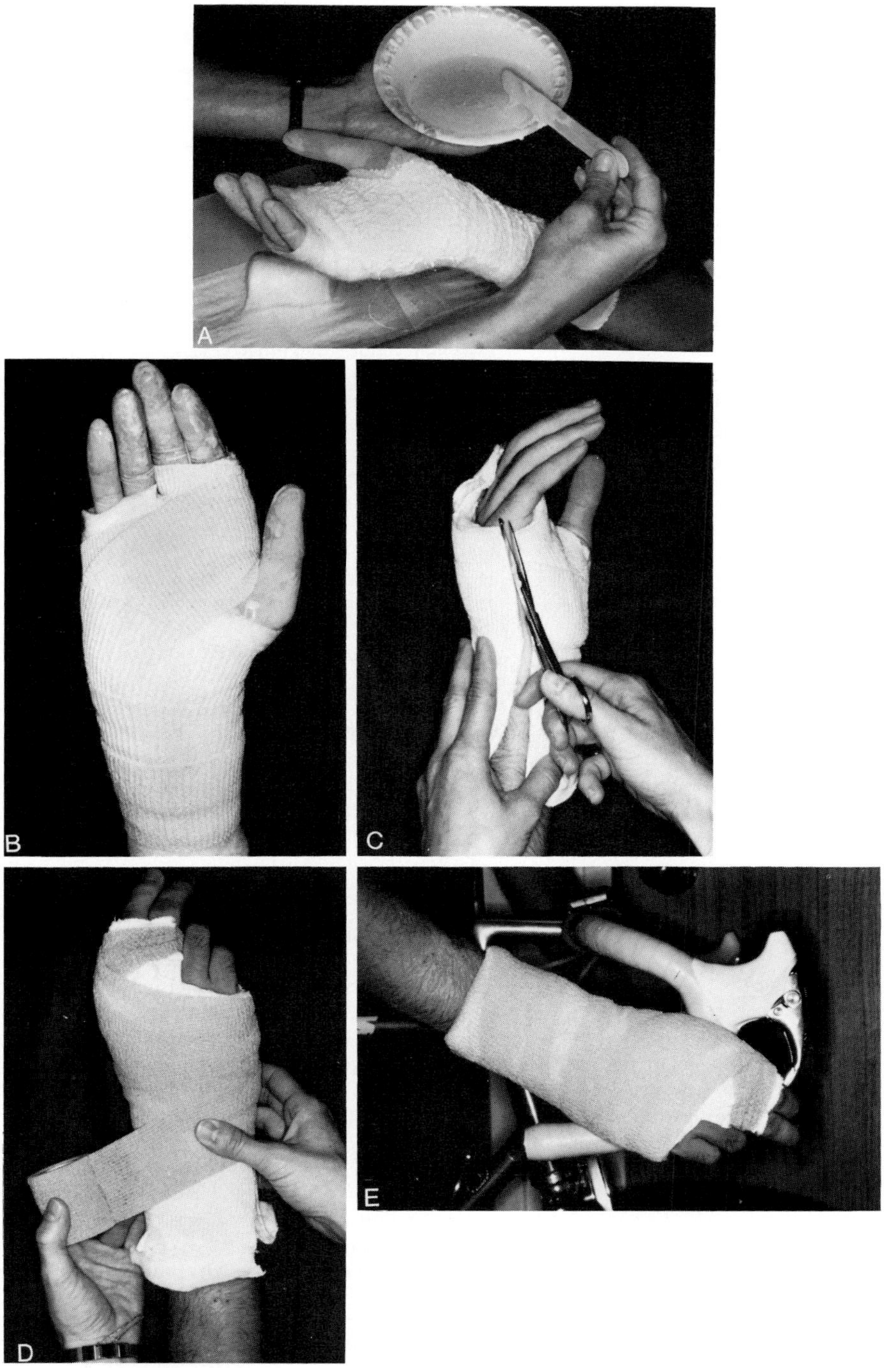

Figure 12–36. Fabrication of a soft cast for a cyclist with index and long metacarpal fractures. *A,* A surgical glove was applied to the hand and covered with three layers of gauze impregnated with GE RTV-11 silicone rubber compound. *B,* A strong elastic tape was applied over the final layer of RTV-11. The cast was allowed to cure for approximately 4 hours during which time the patient periodically grasped his handlebars for good conformity. *C,* The cast was removed by cutting it along the uninjured side of the hand. D, During cycling, the cast was reapplied and secured with Coban wrap. *E,* The cast allowed excellent functional use of the hand during cycling while supporting the metacarpal fractures.

Table 12–1 Splint and Related Materials for Hand Injuries

Splint Materials

LOW TEMPERATURE THERMOPLASTICS		
Polyform (Plastic polymer)	Good drapability with excellent stretch No memory Excellent contourability Excellent rigidity and impact strength	Smith and Nephew Rolyan, Inc. N93 W14475 Whitaker Way Menomonee Falls, WI 53051
Polyflex II (Plastic polymer and rubber)	Good draping and contourability Good resilient stretch with slight memory Excellent rigidity-resists fatigue Ideal for larger splints	Smith and Nephew Rolyan, Inc. N93 W14475 Whitaker Way Menomonee Falls, WI 53051
Orthoplast (Transpolyisoprene)	High rubber content Offers some stretch with good memory Good rigidity, yet lightweight Ideal for circumferential splinting due to flexibility	Johnson & Johnson Products New Brunswick, NJ 08903
Aquaplast-T (Non-sticky polycaprolactone with surface coating)	Clear when heated enabling control of pressure points over small areas Good conforming qualities Excellent elasticity when heated Good memory with repeated heating Excellent rigidity with small splints	WFR Aquaplast Corporation Post Office Box 327 Ramsey, NJ 07446

Others—Ezeform (plastic polymer), Orthoform (transpolyisoprene), Hexcelite (polymers, filler, and pigment impregnated onto cotton netting), Aquaplast (original sticky) (polyepsilon caprolactone), Monorthos (polycaprolactone other polymers and pigment), Green Stripe Aquaplast (polycaprolactone with or without surface coating), Burns Quality Aquaplast (Blue Stripe), Kay-Splint Series 3 (plastic polymer), K-Splint Isoprene (plastic polymer), Kay Splint (plastic polymer), JU 1000 Splinting Compound (plastic polymer), MR 2000 Splinting Compound (plastic polymer), RS 3000 Splinting Compound (plastic polymer).

HIGH TEMPERATURE THERMOPLASTICS
Vinyl (polyvinyl chloride), Kydex (copolymer of polyvinyl chloride and acrylic), W-Clear (transparent polyester-based orthotic material) (copolyester of polyethylene terephthalate).

Playing Cast Materials

RTV-11	Liquid based silicone rubber compound, cured with a catalyst Impregnated with gauze during application Usually padded externally (often with Slo-Foam) Requires 3–4 hours to completely cure	General Electric Company Silicone Rubber Products Div. Waterford, NY 12188 (518) 237–3330

Table 12–1 Splint and Related Materials for Hand Injuries *Continued*

3-M Scotchrap	Semi-rigid support wrap External padding can be used pending specific regulations for competition	3-M Orthopaedic Products Div. 6850 South Harlem Avenue Bedford Park, IL 60501
	Shock Absorbent Materials	
Neoprene	Closed cell rubber available in variety of thicknesses Retains maximum body heat Provides uniform compression	Local distributor of divers' supplies
Sorbothane	Visco-elastic polymer Elasticity and flowability Can absorb 94% of energy in dynamic load displacement tests High compression resistance	IEM Orthopaedics 251 West Garfield Road Aurora, Ohio 44202
Viscolis	Visco-elastic polymer Has elasticity and flowability Excellent fine-vibration shock absorber High resistance to compression	Chattanooga Corporation Visco-Elastic Products 101 Memorial Drive Post Office Box 4287 Chattanooga, TN 37405
	Foam Materials	
Polycushion	Soft, closed cell foam with adhesive backing Resists compression well Available in ¼ and ⅛ inch thickness	Smith and Nephew Rolyan, Inc. N93 W14475 Whitaker Way Menomonee Falls, WI 53051
Slo-Foam	Soft, visco-elastic foam product with adhesive back Fluid-like support conforms to hand Resists impact, shock and vibration	North Coast Medical, Inc. 450 Salmar Avenue Campbell, CA 95008
	Splint Inserts	
Otoform-K (Transpolyisoprene)	Paste form of silicone elastomer cured catalyst Amount of catalyst used will affect firmness of finished rubber mold Good contourability for interfacing splints Good shock absorbing quality	WFR Aquaplast Corporation Post Office Box 327 Ramsey, NJ 07446
Elastomer (Silastic 382, Medical Grade)	Liquid based silicone elastomer cured with a catalyst Produces firm, closed cell rubber mold Excellent contouring for interfacing with splints Good shock-absorbing quality	WFR Aquaplast Corporation Post Office Box 327 Ramsey, NJ 07446

Table 12–1 Splint and Related Materials for Hand Injuries *Continued*

	Padded Gloves	
Anti-vibration gloves	Leather or jersey glove with Viscolis insert Available in a variety of sizes and styles	Steel Grip, Inc. 700 Garfield Street Danville, IL 61832

and memory. Most low temperature thermoplastics may be softened at 160° F by the use of wet or dry heat. Working times vary according to manufacturer, but generally fall between 3 and 6 minutes. The authors have found the two materials, Polyform and Orthoplast, to be versatile enough for most hand splinting needs. Polyform, with its high plastic content, has excellent stretching and molding capabilities, producing an exact fit with good contour. When cured, Polyform is quite rigid. Orthoplast, in contrast, has a higher rubber component, which provides better flexibility and elasticity. These characteristics make Orthoplast the preferred material for larger, more circumferential types of splints where exact contour is not so important. There are numerous thermoplastics available with similar characteristics and also with other features. The splint material should be chosen on the basis of its ability to meet the requirements of the injury for which the splint is being fabricated and the experience and preferences of the therapist.

Early protective splinting for return to competition usually requires some type of padding or lining for comfort and shock absorption. Again, a wide variety of materials are available for customizing the splint to the athlete's injury and the needs of the sport. Several types of foam are available in various densities, and most have peel-off adhesive backing for easy application. Polycushion is an excellent all-purpose, closed cell foam used primarily as a splint interface for patient comfort. Slo-Foam is a viscoelastic foam that provides fluidlike support and can be contoured to the hand through warmth and body heat, making it quite comfortable. Although it is soft to the touch, Slo-Foam is firm on impact, making it a good shock absorber.

Medical grade silicone compounds, such as Otoform-K, Silastic Elastomer, and GE RTV-11 silicone rubber compound also have excellent shock-absorbing capabilities and may be useful in the preparation of athletic splints. Otoform-K and Elastomer are excellent splint interfaces as they will contour to a specific area and cure in less than 5 minutes. Elastomer and RTV-11 can also be used in combination with gauze for soft splints.

Conclusion

The primary goal of this chapter is to familiarize the professional treating hand injuries with the basic principles and precautions in managing the more common hand problems. Treatment of athletic hand injuries should be undertaken only by highly qualified medical professionals who are cognizant of the unique anatomic structures and healing requirements of the hand. These are the individuals who can facilitate early return to competition without risk of further injury or complications. It is the unquestionable desire of the athlete, coach, trainer, therapist, and physician to allow return to competition as early as possible. This process requires a team effort with open communication among all involved.

REFERENCES

1. Akeson, W.H., Amiel, D., Mechanic, G.L., et al.: Collagen cross-linking alterations in joint contractures: changes in the reducible cross-links in periarticular connective tissue collagen after nine weeks of immobilization. Connect. Tissue Res. 5:15, 1977.
2. Benton, C.A., Baker, L.L., Bowman, B.R., et al.: Functional Electrical Stimulation—A Practical Clinical Guide. Downey, CA, Rancho Los Amigos Rehabilitation Engineering Center, 1981.
3. Bergfeld, J.A., Weiker, G.G., Andrish, J.T., et al.: Soft playing splint for protection of significant hand and wrist injuries in sports. Am. J. Sports Med. 10:293, 1982.
4. Boone, D.C.: Applications of iontophoresis. Clin. Phys. Ther., 2:99, 1981.
5. Boyes, J.H.: Bunnell's Surgery of the Hand, 4th ed. Philadelphia, J.B. Lippincott, 1964.
6. Burton, R.: Extensor tendons—late reconstruction. In Green, D.P., (ed.): Operative Hand Surgery, 2nd ed. New York, Churchill Livingstone, 1988.
7. Dray, G., Eaton, R.: Dislocations and ligament injuries in the digits. In Green, D.P., (ed.): Operative Hand Surgery, 2nd ed. New York, Churchill Livingstone, 1988.
8. Fess, E.W., Philips, C.A.: Hand Splinting. Principles and Methods. St Louis, C.V. Mosby, 1987.
9. Gelberman, R.H., Woo, S.L., Lothringer, K., et al.: Effects of early intermittent passive mobilization on healing canine flexor tendons. J. Hand Surg. 7:170, 1982.
10. Harris P.R.: Iontophoresis: clinical research in musculoskeletal inflammatory conditions. J. Orthop. Sports Phys. Ther. 4:109, 1982.
11. Hitchcock, T.F., Light, T.R., Bunch, W.H., et al.: The effect of immediate constrained digital motion on the strength of flexor tendon repairs in chickens. J. Hand Surg. 12A:590, 1987.
12. Johnson C.L.: Physical therapists as scar modifiers. Phys. Ther. 64:1381, 1984.
13. Kaplan, E.B.: Anatomy and kinesiology of the hand. In Flynn, J.E., (ed.): Hand Surgery, 2nd ed. Baltimore, Williams & Wilkins, 1975.
14. Leddy, J.P., Packer, J.W.: Avulsion of the profundus tendon insertion in athletes. J. Hand Surg. 2:66, 1977.
15. Lehmann, J.F., Warren, C.G., Scham, S.M.: Therapeutic heat and cold. Clin. Orthop. 99:207, 1974.
16. Mason, M.L., Allen, H.S.: The role of healing of tendons: an experimental study of tensile strength. Ann. Surg. 113:424, 1941.
17. McGrouther, D.A., Ahmed, M.R.: Flexor tendon excursions in "no-man's land." Hand 13:129, 1981.
18. Nirschl, R.P.: The etiology and treatment of tennis elbow. J. Sports Med. 2:308, 1974.
19. Nirschl, R.P.: Tennis elbow. Primary Care 4:367, 1977.
20. Nirschl, R.P., Sobel, J.: Conservative treatment of tennis elbow. Physician Sports Med. 9(6):43, 1981.
21. Roy, S., Irvin, R.: Sports Medicine. Prevention, Evaluation, Management and Rehabilitation. Englewood Cliffs, NJ, Prentice Hall, 1983.
22. Safran, M.R., Seaber A.V., Garrett, W.E.: Warm-up and muscular injury prevention. An update. Sports Med. 8:239, 1989.
23. Savage, R.: The influence of wrist position on the minimum force required for active movement of the interphalangeal joints. J. Hand Surg. 13B:262, 1988.

24. Simmons, B.P., DeLa Caffiniere, J.Y.: Physiology of flexion of the fingers. In Tubiana, R. (ed.): The Hand, Vol. I. Philadelphia, W.B. Saunders, 1981.
25. Steichen, J.B., Call, W.H., Kleinman, W.B.: Flexor carpi radialis tunnel syndrome. Orthop. Trans. 5:108, 1981.
26. Verdan, C.: Tendon Surgery of the Hand. New York, Churchill Livingstone, 1979.
27. Walker, S.E.: Treatment of soft tissue inflammatory problems of the forearm and hand. Presented at the American Society of Hand Therapists Annual Meeting, March 5, 1983.
28. Walker, S.E.: Hand therapy management for cumulative trauma disorder: acute phase through work capacity testing. Presented at the Cumulative Trauma Disorders and Ergonomics Meeting of the National Safety Council, May 16, 1984.
29. Wehbe, M.A.: Differential tendon gliding in the hand. J. Hand Surg. 9:596, 1984.
30. Wehbe, M.A., Hunter, J.M.: Flexor tendon gliding in the hand. I. In vivo excursions. J. Hand Surg. 10A:570, 1985.
31. Wehbe, M.A., Hunter, J.M.: Flexor tendon gliding in the hand. II. Differential gliding. J. Hand Surg. 10A:575, 1985.

INDEX

Note: Page numbers in *italics* refer to illustrations; page numbers followed by t refer to tables.

Aircast Pneumatic Arm Band, for epicondylitis, 263, *264*
Anesthetic agents, local, use of, for injured athletes, 6
Aneurysms, of ulnar artery, 233
Angiography, after fractures, 230
Annular pulley(s), finger, *178,* 178–179
Anterior interosseous nerve syndrome, *217,* 217–218
Anti-inflammatory drugs, for muscle injury, 25
Artery(ies). See entries under specific arteries.
Arthrodesis, at scaphoid bone, *119*
  for scapholunate dissociation, 115, *119*
  for ulnar translocation, 121, *122*
Arthrography, of carpal ganglion, 109
  of lunotriquetral ligament, 119, *120*
  of metacarpophalangeal joint, thumb, 99
  of midcarpal region, 119, *120*
  of radiocarpal space, 119
  of scapholunate dissociation, 115, *117*
Arthroplasty, for intra-articular metacarpophalangeal joint fracture, 54
Articular cartilage, 12–15
Avascular necrosis, of capitate bone, 170
  of scaphoid bone, 160
Axillary artery, injury of, 230
Axonotmesis, 26, 210t

Baseball catchers, index finger injury in, 232
Baseball finger. See *Mallet finger.*
Bennett's fracture-dislocation, of metacarpophalangeal joint, thumb, 83–85, *84*
Bicycling, and palsy, 222
  and ulnar nerve injury, 222
Biomechanics, of splints, 268–269
Blood supply, of hand, 231, 232
  vincular, 179, *179*
Bone(s), 9–12
  cancellous, 9, 10
  cell types in, 9
  composition of, 9
  electric potentials of, 27
  electric stimulation of. See *Electrical stimulation.*
  fractures of. See *Fracture(s).*
  grafts of, for fracture gaps, 12
    for scaphoid nonunion, 159–160, 162, *163, 164*
  healing of, 10–12, 27–28
  remodeling of, 9
    after fractures, 10
    and electric fields, 27–28
Bone morphogenic protein (BMP), and fracture healing, 12
Boutonniere deformity, 62, *65,* 65–68, *186–190,* 186–192
  after volar dislocation of proximal interphalangeal joint, 62, 69–70, 176, 186–192
  pseudo-, 62, 69–70, 191–192, *193*
  treatment of, 66–68, *67,* 189–191, 255–256
    cylinder cast, *255*
    safety pin splint, 189–191, *190,* 255
    surgical reconstruction, 68, *190,* 191, *192*
Bowler's thumb, 218, *219*
Boxer's fracture, metacarpal bones, 136
Boxer's knuckle, 193–194, *194*
Brachial artery, elbow-fracture dislocation and, 230
Brewerton view, of hand fractures, 133, *134*
Bunnell safety pin splint, *67*

Calcium hydroxyapatite, in bone, 9
Callus formation, in bone fracture, 10
Cancellous bone, 9
Capitate bone, fractures of, 167–170
Carpal bone(s). See also names of specific carpal bones.
  fracture-dislocations of, 171
  fractures of, 156–171
  instability of, 111–112, *113*
Carpal ganglion, 109–111, *110*
Carpal tunnel, axial view of, *212*
Carpal tunnel syndrome, 218
  and tendinitis/tenosynovitis, 265–266
Carpometacarpal joint, anatomy of, 76–82, *77*
  dislocations of, 77–82, *78, 79*
    treatment of, 80–82, *81*
Cartilage, articular, 12–15
  composition of, 13
  drying of, 13
  healing of, 14–15
  immobilization effects on, 15
  injury of, 14
  zones of, 13–14
Cheiralgia paresthetica, 224
Child, mallet finger deformities in, 74, 180–181, *181,* 185
  Salter-Harris fracture in, proximal phalanx, small digit, 146–147
Chondrocytes, cartilage injury and, 14
Clawing deformity, 138–139, *139*
Cleland's ligament, 55
Collagen, in bone, 9
  in cartilage, 13
  in ligaments, 15
    after immobilization, 18
  in muscles, 22
  in tendons, after injury, 20
    at insertion, 19
  in wound healing, 8
Compartment syndrome, 224–225
Compressive neuropathies. See *Neuropathy(ies), compressive.*
Computed tomography, of hook of hamate fracture, *169*
  of scaphoid fracture, 159
Connective tissue, of muscles, 22
    after injury, 23
  of nerves, 25
Continuous passive motion (CPM), and articular cartilage, 15
  for immobilized tendon, 21
Contrast baths, for carpal tunnel syndrome, 265–266
Corticosteroids, effects of, on bones, 29
    on joint surfaces, 28–29
    on ligaments, 28–29
    on tendons, 28–29
CPM. See *Continuous passive motion (CPM).*
Cruciform pulley(s), *178,* 178–179
Cubital tunnel, *213*
Cyclist's palsy, 222
Darrach operation, in triangular fibrocartilage excision, 126
Deformity(ies). See names of specific types, e.g. *Boutonniere deformity.*
DeQuervain's disease, 262–264
Dexamethasone sodium phosphate, for tendinitis of first dorsal compartment, 262
DIP joint(s). See *Interphalangeal joint(s), distal (DIP).*
Doppler test, for vascular injury, 230
Dorsal impaction syndrome, 111
Dorsal intercalated segment instability (DISI) deformity, and scaphoid fracture, 158
Drop finger. See *Mallet finger.*
Drugs, anti-inflammatory, for tendinitis, 25
  corticosteroid, 28–29, 124
  dexamethasone sodium phosphate, for tendinitis, 262
  lidocaine, for tendinitis, 262
  local anesthetic, 6
DRUJ. See *Radioulnar joint(s), distal (DRUJ).*
Dystrophy, sympathetic, 225

Eaton-Littler tenodesis, for thumb dislocation, 80–81, *81*
Elbow(s), anatomy of, 214, *214*
  dislocation of, brachial artery injury and, 230
  "tennis," 223
Electrical stimulation, 239–240, 245
  and healing, of fractures, 27–28, 159
    of soft tissue, 28
    of tendons, 239–240, 245, 253
  failure of, 28
  methods for, 29
Endomysium, 22
Endoneurium, 25
Endotenon, 19
  in healing tendons, 20
Epicondylitis, 262
Epimysium, 22
Epineurium, 25
Epitenon, 19
  in healing tendons, 20, 21
Epithelial regeneration, in wound healing, 8
Exercise(s). See also *Rehabilitation.*
  and ligament healing, 18
  and muscle development, 22–23
Extensor digiti quinti proprius muscle, 175, 176
Extensor digitorum communis muscle, 176, *176*
  exercises for, 239, *239*
  extensor hood injury and, 53–54
Extensor hood(s), 176
  injury to, 53–54
Extensor indicis proprius muscle, 175, 176
Extensor pollicis brevis muscle, 175

Extensor pollicis longus muscle, 175
Extensor tendon(s), anatomy of, 175–176, *177*
function of, 176
injuries of, at metacarpophalangeal joint, 192–196
boxer's knuckle, 193–194, *194*
dislocation-subluxation and, 194–196, *196*

Fascicles, of tendons, 19
Fasciotomy, for compartment syndrome, 225
of forearm, 230
Fibroblasts, in ligaments, 15
Fibroplasia, in wound healing, 8, 16–17
Finger(s), extensor mechanism of, 176–178, *177*
flexor mechanism of, 178–179
pulley mechanism in, *178*
injuries of. See also specific sites of injury.
digital joint, 49–76
extra-articular fractures as, 129–153
vincular blood supply of, 179, *179*
Finklestein sign, in superficial radial nerve compression, 224
Flexor carpi radialis tunnel, tendinitis at, 262–264
Flexor digitorum profundus muscle, 178–179, *179*
exercises for, *245,* 245–246
tendon insertion avulsions of, 74–76, *75, 197–202,* 197–203, 250–253, *252, 253*
Flexor digitorum superficialis muscle, 178–179, *179*
exercises for, 245–246, *245–247*
Flexor tendon(s), of finger, *178,* 178–179
of hand, blood supply of, 179, *179*
Fracture(s). See also specific sites or names of fractures.
healing of, 10–12, 27–28
bone morphologic protein and, 12
callus formation in, 10
hematoma formation in, 10
medullary union in, 10, 11
primary union in, 10, 11
immobilization period following, 12
management of, 2–3, 12
rehabilitation in, 239–250
nonunion/delayed union of, 11–12
bone graft for, 12
causes of, 11
electrical stimulation for, 27–28
radiography of, 133–135
terms for, 135
sports participation and, 2–4
"worst case scenario," 3
stabilization of, 11
Freer elevator, for volar plate dislocation, 69

Gamekeeper's thumb, 88
Ganglion, dorsal carpal, 109–111, *110*
Gloves, padded, 269, *269*
Golfers, hook of hamate fracture in, 165–166
Graft, bone, for fracture gaps, 12
for scaphoid nonunion, 159–160, 162, *163, 164*
Grayson's ligament, 55
Growth factors, for wound healing, 8
Guyon's canal, *213, 221*
ulnar neuropathy and, 220
Gymnastics, and distal posterior interosseous nerve syndrome, 223
and wrist pain, 111, 119
diagnosis of, 119

Hamate bone, fractures of, 164–166, 221, *221,* 232
computed tomography of, *169*
radiography of, *165,* 166, *167–169*
Hand(s), bones of, 9. See also names of specific bones.
healing of, 7–30
injuries of, compressive neuropathies as, 216–226
digital joint, 49–92
extra-articular fractures as, 129–153
sports-related, 37–48
literature review of, 37–39
Methodist Sports Medicine Center survey of, 39–43, 42t
Olympic Training Center survey of, 44–46, 44t–46t
thumb, 77–85, 91–92, 95–105
ligaments of, 15–16. See also names of specific ligaments.
muscles of, 21–25, 176–179, *177*. See also names of specific muscles.
nerves of, 25–27, 210–216. See also names of specific nerves.
tendons of, 18–19, 175–179, *177–179*. See also names of specific tendons.
vincular blood supply of, 179, *179*
Hematoma(s), 10, 230
Hook of hamate bone fracture(s), 164–166
computed tomography of, *169*
hypothenar hammer syndrome and, 232
radiography of, *165,* 166, *167–168*
ulnar artery injury and, 232
ulnar nerve injury and, 221, *221*
Hypothenar hammer syndrome, 232

Inflammation, cell reaction in, 7–8
in bone fractures, 10
hematoma formation and, 10
in ligament injury, 16
in soft tissue wounds, 7
use of corticosteroids and, 28–29

Injury(ies), sports-related. See *Sports-related injuries* and specific anatomic sites.
Intercalated segment instability deformity, and scaphoid fracture, 158
Interosseous muscle(s), of hand, 176–178, *177*
Interosseous nerve syndrome, *217*, 217–218, 223–224
Interphalangeal joint(s), distal (DIP), anatomy of, 55–56, *56*
deformity of, hyperextension as, 70
mallet finger as. See *Mallet finger*.
exercises for, 246, *247*
extensor tendons of, 176–178, *177*
flexor tendons of, *178*, 178–179, *179*
injury(ies) of, dislocations as, 71
flexor digitorum profundus avulsion as, 74–76, *75*, *197–202*, 197–203
fracture-dislocations as, 71–72
intra-articular fractures as, 71–72
volar plate, 68–70
splinting for, 245–255, *254*
proximal (PIP), 55–71
anatomy of, 55–56, *56*
deformity of, boutonniere. See *Boutonniere deformity*.
swan neck as, 69–70, 180
exercises for, 246–248, *247*, *248*
extensor tendons of, 176–178, *177*
flexor tendons of, 178–179, *178–179*
injury(ies) of, articular fractures as, 56–59, *57*
collateral ligament, 55, 60, 63–65, *64*, 258
dislocations as, 60–63, *61*, *63*, 69–70, 176, 186–190, *186–190*, *192*, 257–258
flexure contracture as, 246–249, *248*, *249*
fracture-dislocations as, 59–60
volar plate, 68–70

Jahss reduction maneuver, for fraction of metacarpal neck, 139, *140*
"Jammed finger," 60–63. See also *Interphalangeal joint(s), proximal*.
"Jersey finger," 74–76, *75*, *197–202*, 197–203, 250–253, *252*, *253*
Joint(s). See also names of specific joints.
articular cartilage, 12–15
Juncturae tendinum, 176

Kapandji procedure, for triangular fibrocartilage degeneration, 124, *125*
Karate, and metacarpophalangeal joint injuries, 193–194
Kienböck's disease, 170
Kinesiology, of splints, 268
Kirschner wires, for fixation of scaphoid fracture, 158, *159*, *163*
for interphalangeal joint dislocation, 60, 62
for interphalangeal joint fracture, 71
for metacarpal neck fractures, 139–141, *140–142*
for metacarpal shaft fractures, 143, 144, *144*
for metacarpophalangeal joint fracture, 54
for proximal phalanx base fracture, 148
for proximal phalanx diaphyseal fracture, *149*, 150
for thumb injuries, carpometacarpal joint dislocations and, 80–81
fractures and, 91–92
mallet finger and, 182, 185
ulnar collateral ligament dislocations and, 89
for volar plate dislocation, 70

Lidocaine, for tendinitis of first dorsal compartment, 262
Ligament(s). See also names of specific ligaments.
adaptation of, to stress, 16
bone insertion of, 16–18
composition of, 15–16
function of, 15
healing of, 16–18
immobilization and, 18
laxity of, 108
physical conditioning and, 17–18
remodeling of, after injury, 17
repair of, 17
rupture of, 16–18
viscoelastic properties of, 16
Lion's Paw, for wrist tendinitis, 263, *264*
Local anesthetic agents, use of, for injured athletes, 6
Lumbrical muscle(s), 176–178, *177*
Lunate bone, fractures of, 170
Lunotriquetral ballottement test, 118–119
Lunotriquetral ligament, 118–120, *120*, 123, *125*, 126

Mallet finger, 72–74, *73*, *180*, 180–185, *181*, *184*
in children, 74, 180–181, *181*, 185
treatment of, 72–74, *73*, 181–185, *182*, *183*, *254*, 254–255
Mallet thumb, 182, 185, *185*
Median nerve, *210–212*, 211–212
compression of, *216*, 216–219, *217*, *219*, 265–266
"Meniscoid," of wrist, 111
Mesotenon, 19
Metacarpal bone fracture(s), 129–145, 166, *169*

Metacarpal bone fracture(s) (*continued*)
  anesthesia for, 136
  athletic field evaluation of, 132
  hamate bone fractures and, 166, *169*
  management of, 236–242, *237–241, 243, 271*
  mechanism of, *130,* 130–132
  oblique, *137,* 137–138
  of metacarpal neck, 138–141
    angulation of, 138, *139–141*
    reduction of, 133–141, *140–141*
  of metacarpal shaft, *142–144,* 142–145
  of thumb, 145
  physical evaluation of, 132–133
  radiography of, 133, *134, 135*
    terms for, 135
  spiral, 136–137, *137,* 144–145
Metacarpophalangeal (MCP) joint(s), of finger, 50–54
    anatomy of, 50
      tendon relationships in, 176
    collateral ligament injuries of, 52–53
    contractures after fracture of, 240–242, *241*
    dislocations of, 50–52
      complex, 50–51, *51*
      irreducible, 50–51, *51*
      treatment of, 52, *52*
    extensor tendon injuries of, 192–196, *196*
      boxer's knuckle, 193–194, *194*
      dislocation-subluxation and, 194–196, *196*
      extensor hood, 53–54
    intra-articular fracture of, 54
    rehabilitation of, 240–242, *241, 243*
  of thumb, anatomy of, 82, 95
    collateral ligament injuries of, 85–91, 95–105
      arthrography of, 99
      diagnosis of, 86–87, *87,* 96–100, *97–99*
      radiography of, 98–99, *99, 100*
      rehabilitation of, 103–104, 258–260, *259–260*
      treatment of, 88–90, *90,* 101–104, *102–104*
    dislocations of, 82–85
    fractures of, interphalangeal, 91–92
      intra-articular, 83–85, *84*
    function of, 95–96
Methodist Sports Medicine Center, survey of hand/wrist sports-related injuries by, 39–43, 40t–42t
Muscle(s). See also names of specific muscles.
  composition of, 22
  connective tissue of, 22, 23
  healing of, 23–25
    in elderly, 24
  immobilization of, 24
  injuries of, 23–25
  of hand, 21–25
  of wrist, *210*
  repair of, 23–25
Myofiber, 22

Naviculo-capitate fracture, 168
Necrosis, avascular, of capitate bone, 170
  of scaphoid bone, 160
Nerve(s). See also names of specific nerves.
  disruption of, 25–27, 210t, 216–223
    axonotmesis in, 26
    neuropraxia in, 25–26
    neurotmesis in, 26
  macro-anatomy of, 25–26, 209–216
    carpal tunnel, axial view, *212*
    cubital tunnel, *213*
    elbow and forearm, volar surface, *210*
    Guyon's canal, *213*
    wrist, volar surface, *211, 215*
  micro-anatomy of, 25–27
  repair of, 26–27
Neuropathy(ies), compressive, 209–226
    compartment syndrome as, 224–225
    of median nerve, 216–219
      anterior interosseous nerve syndrome as, *217,* 217–218
      bowler's thumb and, 218, *219*
      carpal tunnel syndrome as, 218, 265–266
      palmar cutaneous nerve compression as, 218
      pronator syndrome as, *216,* 216–217
    of radial nerve, 222–224
      cheiralgia paresthetica as, 224
      distal posterior interosseous nerve syndrome as, 224–225
      radial tunnel syndrome as, 223
      resistant tennis elbow as, 223
      syndrome of, 223–224
    of ulnar nerve, cyclist's palsy as, 222
    reflex sympathetic dystrophy as, 225
    treatment of, 264–266
    types of, 209–210, 210t
Neuropraxia, 25–26, 210t
Neurotmesis, 26, 210t
Node of Ranvier, 25

Olympic Training Center, survey of hand/wrist sports-related injuries by, 44t–46t, 44–46
Opponens splint, for metacarpophalangeal collateral ligament strain, *259,* 259–260
Osteoblasts, 9
Osteoclasts, 9
Osteocytes, 9

Palmar bar, for metacarpal fracture, 242, 243
Palmar cutaneous nerve compression, 218
Palsy, "cyclist's," 222
  runner's radial nerve, 223

Pencil, used in reduction of small digit fracture, 146, *147*
Perimysium, 22
Perineurium, 23
Periosteum, in callus formation, 10
Peritenon, 19
Phalanx bone fracture(s), 129, 146–153, 180–185, *184*
  anesthesia for, 136
  athletic field evaluation of, 132
  finger circulation and, 231
  management of, 242, 244–250, *244–251*
  mechanism of, *130,* 130–132
  pencil reduction of, 146, *147*
  physical examination of, 132–133
  radiography of, 133, *134, 135*
    terms for, 135
  site of, distal phalanx as, 151
    middle phalanx as, 151
    proximal phalanx as, *146,* 146–150, *149, 150,* 231
Phalen's sign, in carpal tunnel syndrome, 218
PIP joint(s). See *Interphalangeal joint(s), proximal (PIP).*
Pisiform bone fracture(s), 170
  and ulnar nerve injury, 221, *221*
Posterior interosseous nerve syndrome, 221–224
Pronator syndrome, *216,* 216–217
Proteoglycans, in bone, 9
  in cartilage, 13
Pseudo-boutonniere deformity, 62, 69–70, 191–192, *193*
Pulley system, finger, *178,* 178–179

Racquet sports, and hook of hamate fracture, *165,* 165–166
Radial artery, injury to, in volleyball players, 232
Radial collateral ligament, of thumb, injury of, 91, 101–104, *104*
    chronic, 90–91, 102–103, *103*
    diagnosis of, 86–87, *87,* 96–100, *97–99*
    historical review of, 87–88
    mechanism of, 86, 96
    treatment of, 88–90, *90,* 101–104, *102–104*
  rehabilitation of, 258–260
Radial nerve, 214, *214, 215*
  compression of, 222–224
Radial tunnel syndrome, 223
Radiography, of collateral ligament injuries, 99, *99, 100*
  of fractures, general principles of, 133–135
    in hand, 133, *134*
    in hook of hamate, *165,* 166, *167–169*
    in metacarpals, 133, *134, 135*
    in phalanges, 133, *134, 135*
    in scaphoid, 156, *157, 158, 162*
Radioulnar joint(s), distal (DRUJ), injuries of, 123–126
Radioulnar joint(s) (*continued*)
  subluxation of, *124, 125*
  ulnar shortening of, *125,* 126
Ranvier, node of, 25
Reflex sympathetic dystrophy, 225
Rehabilitation, 235–275
  after metacarpophalangeal fractures, *239–241,* 239–242, *243*
  after proximal phalangeal fractures, 244–250
    exercises for, 245–248, *245–248*
  for boutonniere deformity, 256
  for carpal tunnel syndrome, 265–266
  for flexor digitorum profundus avulsion, 252–253
  for mallet finger, 254–255, *255*
  for metacarpophalangeal joint injuries, 258–260
    of collateral ligaments, 258–259
  for tendinitis/tenosynovitis, 261–264
  general principles of, 235–236, 256–257
    phases in, 236
Retinacular ligament(s), of hand, 178, *178*
Rolando's fracture-dislocation, of metacarpophalangeal joint, 85
Runner's radial nerve palsy, 223

Safety pin splint, for boutonniere deformity, *67*
  for palmar dislocation of proximal interphalangeal joint, 189–191, *190*
  for phalangeal fracture, 246, *248*
Sagittal band(s), of hand, 176
  function of, 176, *177*
Salter-Harris fracture, proximal phalanx, *146,* 146–148, *147*
  in child, 146–147
Satellite cells, in myofibers, 22, 23
  in nerves, 25
Sauve-Kapandji procedure, *125*
Scaphoid bone, dorsal intercalated segment instability deformity of, 158
  fracture of, 11, 156, 168
    bone grafting for, 160, 161, *163*
    distal third, 162, *164*
    mechanism of injury in, 156
    middle third, 157–160, *158, 159*
    nonunion of, 159–160, *161–164,* 163–164
    proximal third, 160–162
    radiography of, 156, *157, 162*
  scapholunate disability of, 112–118
    diagnosis of, 112–115, *113–117*
    treatment of, 115–118, *118, 119*
Schwann cells, 25
  and reponse to electrical stimulation, 28
Sesamoid bone(s), in metacarpophalangeal joint, 82
Shoulder dislocation, axillary artery injury and, 230
  venous injury and, 230
Silastic pressure molds, for splinting, 239–240

Ski pole injury(ies), 96
 to thumb metacarpophalangeal joint, 96, 132
Snuffbox, anatomic, and wrist fracture, 156
Soft tissue injury(ies), healing of, 7–8. See also specific sites.
 of fingers, 4
 of wrist, 107–126
 sports participation and, 4–6
Splints, for boutonniere deformity, *255*, 255–256
 for carpal tunnel syndrome, 265–266, *266*
 for flexor digitorum profundus avulsion, *252*, 252–253
 for injured hand, 235–275
 for mallet finger, 182, *182, 183, 254*, 254–255
 for metacarpal bone fractures, 236–239, *237, 238*, 242, *243*
 for metacarpophalangeal joint collateral ligament injuries, 258–260, *259, 260*
 for proximal interphalangeal collateral ligament injuries, 258
 for proximal interphalangeal joint dorsal dislocations, *257*, 257–258
 for proximal phalangeal fractures, *238*, 243, *244*, 246–250, *246–251*
 for tendinitis/tenosynovitis, 262–264, *263, 264*
 materials for, 270, 272–274t, 274
 principles of, 267–269
  anatomy and, 268
  biomechanics and, 268–269
  kinesiology and, 268
 types of, 269–270
Sports participation. See also specific injuries.
 after fractures, 2–4, 129–130, 250
 after soft tissue injuries, 4–6
 after tendinitis/tenosynovitis, 261
 age and nature of injury and, 5
 anesthetic agents and, 6
 general principles of, 1–6, 235–236
 playing cast for, *243*
Sports-related injuries, management of. See also *Rehabilitation; Splints*.
 guidelines for, 2, 235–236
 immobilization of fractures in, 12
 philosophy of, 1–6
 sports participation and, 1–6
Steinmann pin, for fixation of metacarpal shaft fracture, *142*
Stener lesion, 89, 90
Steroids. See also *Corticosteroids*.
 for triangular fibrocartilage injury, 124
Swan neck deformity, after interphalangeal joint injury, 180
 after volar plate injury, 69–70
 of thumb, 92
"Sweater finger." See *"Jersey finger."*
Sympathetic dystrophy, 225
Synovitis. See also *Tendinitis*.
 of wrist, 111
 rehabilitation for, 261–264

Tendinitis, at first dorsal compartment, 262
 at flexor carpi radialis tunnel, 262–264
 drugs for, 25, 262
 rehabilitation for, 261–264
 splinting for, 262–264, *263, 264*
  Lion's Paw in, 263, *264*
 sports participation and, 261
Tendon(s). See also names of specific tendons.
 anatomy of, 18–19, 175–179, *177–179*
 function of, 18–19
 healing of, 19–21, 253
  adhesion formation in, 21
 immobilization effects of, 21
 inflammation of. See *Synovitis; Tendinitis*.
 injuries of, 19–21
 repair of, 21
 vascular supply of, 19
Tennis elbow, 223
Tenocytes, 19
Tensile strength, of wound, 8
Terminal extensor tendon. See also *Mallet finger*.
 avulsion of, 245–249, *254*, 254–255
TFC. See *Triangular fibrocartilage (TFC)*.
Thumb, 76–92
 carpometacarpal joint of, anatomy of, 76–82, *77*
  dislocation of, 77–82, *78, 79, 81*
 collateral ligament injuries to, 85–91, 95–105, *259*, 259–260, *260*
 dislocation of, 77–83, *78, 79, 81*
  tenodesis for, 80–81, *81*
 fractures of, 83–85, *84*, 91–92, 145
 gamekeeper's, 88
 mallet deformity of, 182, 185
 metacarpal joint of. See *Metacarpophalangeal joint (MCP), of thumb*.
 Rolando's fracture-dislocation of, 85
 sesamoid bones of, 82
 Stener lesion in, 89, 90
 volar plate and, 69–70, 82–83
Thumb spica support, for deQuervain's disease, 263, *263*
Tinel's sign, in carpal tunnel syndrome, 218
 in nerve injury, 25
 in pronator syndrome of median nerve, 217
 in radial nerve compression, 224
Tomography, computed, of hook of hamate fracture, *169*
  of scaphoid fracture, 159, *160*
 of scaphoid fracture, 159
Trapezium bone, anatomy of, 76–77, *77*
 fractures of, 170

Triangular fibrocartilage (TFC), avulsions
of, *124, 124, 124–126, 125*
degeneration of, 123–126, *125*
injuries of, 123–126, *124, 125*
Triquetrum bone, fractures of, 171
Triquetrolunate instability, 118–120

Ulnar artery, aneurysm of, 233
blunt injury and, 232
hypothenar hammer syndrome and, 232
wrist dislocation and, 231
Ulnar collateral ligament, of thumb, injury of, 85–91, 101–104
chronic, 90–91, 102–103, *103*
diagnosis of, 86–87, *87,* 96–100, *97–99*
historical review of, 87–88
mechanism of, 86, 96
treatment of, 88–90, *90,* 101–104, *102–104*
Ulnar nerve, *211–213, 212, 215*
compression of, 219–222
Ulnar shortening, in triangular fibrocartilage injury, *125,* 126
Ulnar translocation, 120–122, *121, 122*

Vascular injury(ies), aneurysms as, 233
etiology of, 229–233
blunt trauma and, 230–233
clavicle injury and, 230
dislocation of wrist and, 231
elbow fracture-dislocation and, 230
forearm trauma and, 230–231
fractures and, 229–230, 231
repeated trauma and, in ball players, 232–233
shoulder dislocation and, 230
mechanism of, 231
Vincular blood supply, 179, *179*
Volar intercalated segment instability (VISI) deformity, 118, 119
Volar ligament, 76–77, *77*
injury of, 78–82
Volar plate, anatomy of, 55
in dislocation of metacarpophalangeal thumb joint, 69–70, 82–83
Volar plate (*continued*)
in fracture-dislocation of proximal interphalangeal joint, 60
injuries of, 68–70
Volleyball, and radial artery injury, 232

Wallerian degeneration, after nerve injury, 25, 26
Wartenberg's disease, 234
Watson's maneuver, for scapholunate dissociation, 112, *114*
Web spacer splint, *269*
Wolfe's law, of bone remodeling, 9, 27
Wounds, healing of, 7–8
epithelial regeneration and, 8
fibroplasia in, 8
growth factors and, 8
tensile strength of, 8
inflammation of, 7
Wrist(s), anatomy of, 156, *210–212, 215*
fractures of, 156–171. See also names of specific bones.
nerves of, 209–216, *211–213, 215*
soft tissue injuries of, 107–126
carpal instability and, 111–112, *113*
dorsal impaction syndrome and, 111
mechanism of, 108–109
meniscoid, 111
occult dorsal carpal ganglion and, 109–111, *110*
scapholunate disability and, 112–117, *113–119*
synovitis and, 111
triangular fibrocartilage, 123–126, *124, 125*
triquetrolunate instability and, 118–120, *120*
ulnar translocation and, 120–122, *121, 122*
sports-related injuries of, literature review of, 37–39
Methodist Sports Medicine Center survey of, 40t, 41t, 42t
Olympic Training Center survey of, 44–46, 44t–46t
sprained, 107–108